Geriatric Education FOR Emergency Medical Services

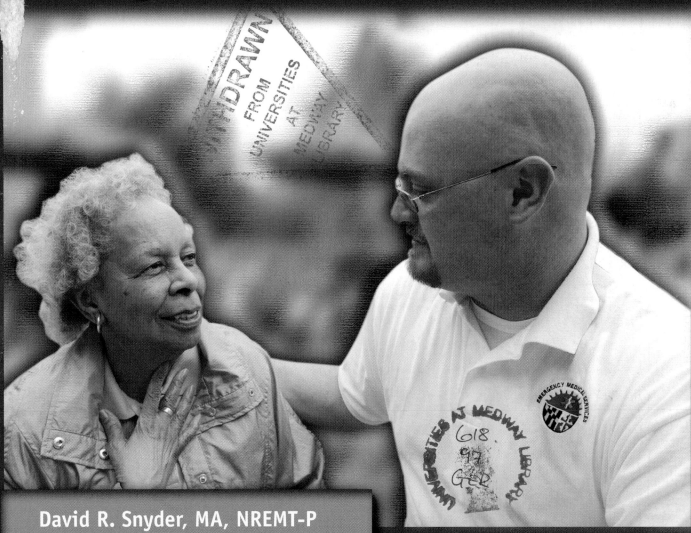

David R. Snyder, MA, NREMT-P
Editor

Colleen Christmas, MD
Editor

Jones and Bartlett Publishers
Sudbury, Massachusetts
Boston   Toronto   London   Singapore

American Geriatrics Society

Executive Vice President: Linda Hiddemen Barondess
Associate Vice President, Professional Education and Special
  Projects: Nancy Lundebjerg, MPA
Senior Consultant, AGS Foundation for Health in Aging:
  Patricia Connelly
Manager, Professional Education and Special Projects:
  Linda Saunders
Manager, Professional Education and Special Projects: Dennise McAlpin

American Geriatrics Society
The Empire State Building
350 Fifth Avenue, Suite 801
New York, NY 10118
(212) 308-1414
www.americangeriatrics.org

Jones and Bartlett Publishers

World Headquarters
40 Tall Pine Drive
Sudbury, MA 01776
978-443-5000
info@jbpub.com
www.jbpub.com

Jones and Bartlett Publishers Canada
6339 Ormindale Way
Mississauga, ON L5V 1J2
CANADA

Jones and Bartlett Publishers International
Barb House, Barb Mews
London W6 7PA
UK

Production Credits

Chief Executive Officer: Clayton Jones
Chief Operating Officer: Donald W. Jones, Jr.
Executive V.P. & Publisher: Robert W. Holland, Jr.
V.P., Design and Production: Anne Spencer
V.P., Manufacturing and Inventory Control: Therese Bräuer
Director, Sales and Marketing: William Kane
Publisher: Kimberly Brophy
Associate Editor: Carol Brewer
Senior Production Editor: Linda S. DeBruyn
Production Editor: Julie C. Bolduc

Senior Marketing Manager: Alisha Weisman
Director, Interactive Technology: Adam Alboyadjian
Interactive Technology Assistant: Dawn Mahon Priest
Design Manager: Kristin E. Ohlin
Cover Design: Shawn Girsberger
Interior Design and Composition: Nesbitt Graphics, Inc.
GEMS Diamond Logo Concept: Amy M. Snyder
Printing and Binding: Courier Kendallville
Cover Printing: Lehigh Press

This textbook is intended as a guide to the appropriate procedures to be employed when rendering emergency care to the geriatric population. It is not intended as a statement of the standards of care required in any particular situation, because circumstances and the patient's physical condition can vary widely from one emergency to another. Nor is it intended that this textbook shall in any way advise emergency personnel concerning legal authority to perform activities or procedures discussed. Such local determination should be made only with the aid of legal counsel.

Notice: The patients described in the case studies throughout this text are fictitious.

Additional credits appear on page 381, which constitutes a continuation of the copyright page.

Copyright © 2003 by American Geriatrics Society and Jones and Bartlett Publishers, Inc.

ISBN-13: 978-0-7637-2086-5
ISBN-10: 0-7637-2086-0

Library of Congress Cataloging-in-Publication Data
Geriatric education for emergency medical services / David R. Snyder,
Colleen Christmas, editor[s] ; American Geriatrics Society [and]
National Council of State Emergency Medical Services Training
Coordinators, Inc.
    p. ; cm.
  Includes bibliographical references and index.
  ISBN 0-7637-2086-0 (alk. paper)
    1. Aged--Diseases. 2. Falls (Accidents) in old age 3. Medical
emergencies. 4. Emergency medical services.
    [DNLM: 1. Emergencies--Aged--Programmed Instruction. 2. Emergency
Medical Technicians--education. 3. Geriatrics--education. WB 18.2 G369
2003] I. Snyder, David R. II. Christmas, Colleen. III. American
Geriatrics Society. IV. National Council of State Emergency Medical
Services Training Coordinators.
  RC952.5 .G433 2003
    618.97--dc21   2002151383
6048

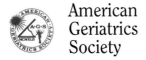

American Geriatrics Society

National Council of State EMS Training Coordinators

Dear EMS Provider:

The American Geriatrics Society (AGS) and the National Council of State EMS Training Coordinators (NCSEMSTC) have partnered to bring you *Geriatric Education for Emergency Medical Services (GEMS)*, the first and only national continuing education curriculum for prehospital professionals focusing specifically on the care of geriatric patients.

The demographics underlying our support of this curriculum are compelling. The U.S. population aged 65 and older has risen dramatically in the 20th century, increasing from 3 million in 1990 to 34.3 million today. Approximately 34% of calls (3.4 million responses) for emergency medical services involve patients over the age of 60. Older adults have unique, and oftentimes multiple, medical needs. This text thoroughly covers all the special needs of the older population and will help ensure that older adults receive the specialized treatment they require from prehospital professionals in the moments when geriatric training skills are most needed.

The AGS and NCSEMSTC invited representatives from eleven national organizations concerned with emergency medical services for geriatric patients and formed the GEMS Steering Committee. Together we created a comprehensive, indispensable tool for the prehospital provider.

On behalf of the American Geriatrics Society and the National Council of State EMS Training Coordinators, we thank you for taking the time to learn how to improve the emergency care you provide to older adults.

Sincerely,

Jerry C. Johnson, MD
President
American Geriatrics Society

Dwight W. Corning
Chairman
National Council of State EMS
Training Coordinators

Brief Contents

Contents

8   Respiratory Emergencies   144

9   Cardiovascular Emergencies   162

10   Neurological Emergencies   174

14 Elder Abuse and Neglect 282

15 Improving Quality of Life 304

P Procedures and Home Health Devices 318

A Appendix A: Organizations and Services for Older People 346

B Appendix B: Medication Guide 347

C Appendix C: Home Safety Checklist 349

Glossary 358

Index 366

Additional Credits 381

Geriatric Education for Emergency Medical Services

The American Geriatrics Society (AGS) and the National Council of State EMS Training Coordinators (NCSEMSTC) are pleased to bring you *Geriatric Education for Emergency Medical Services* (GEMS), a new national continuing education curriculum.

This exciting new program is the first of its kind—designed specifically for First Responders, EMTs, Paramedics, and any other emergency care provider. GEMS represents the most credible and complete source of prehospital medical information on older adults. It addresses all of the special needs of the older population, including the geriatric objectives as identified in the EMT-Basic, Intermediate, and Paramedic National Highway Traffic Safety Administration (NHTSA) National Standard Curricula.

Chapter Resources

The GEMS course is designed to give EMS providers the education and confidence they need to effectively treat older patients. This textbook is the core of the GEMS course with features that will reinforce and expand on the essential information. These features include:

GEMS Diamond

The GEMS diamond was created to help providers remember what is different about the older patient. These issues should be considered when assessing every older patient:

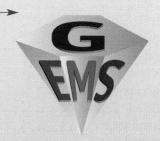

G—Geriatric: older patients are different and may present atypically

E—Environmental assessment: the environment may contain clues to the cause of the emergency

M—Medical assessment: older patients tend to have a variety of medical problems

S—Social assessment: older patients may have less of a social network

Case Study

Each chapter contains multiple case studies. Case studies prompt providers to think about what they might do if they encountered a similar situation in the field. A summary of each case study appears at the end of the chapter.

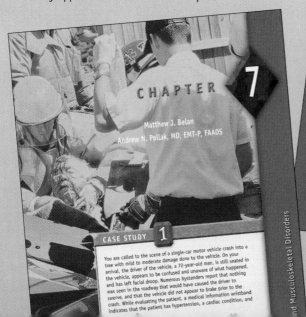

CHAPTER 7

Matthew J. Belan
Andrew N. Pollak, MD, EMT-P, FAAOS

CASE STUDY 1

You are called to the scene of a single-car motor vehicle crash into a tree with mild to moderate damage done to the vehicle. On your arrival, the driver of the vehicle, a 72-year-old man, is still seated in the vehicle, appears to be confused and unaware of what happened, and has left facial droop. Numerous bystanders report that nothing was seen in the roadway that would have caused the driver to swerve, and that the vehicle did not appear to brake prior to the crash. While evaluating the patient, a medical information wristband indicates that the patient has hypertension, a cardiac condition, and

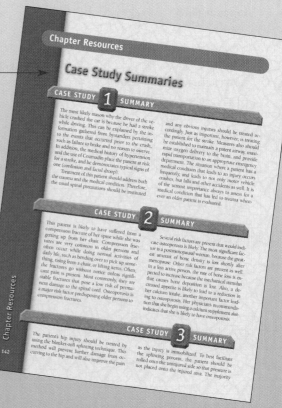

Chapter Resources

Case Study Summaries

CASE STUDY 1 SUMMARY

The most likely reason why the driver of the vehicle crashed the car is because he had a stroke while driving. This can be explained by the information gathered from bystanders pertaining to the events that occurred prior to the crash, such as failure to brake and no reason to swerve. In addition, the medical history of hypertension and the use of Coumadin place the patient at risk for a stroke, and he demonstrates typical signs of one (confusion and facial droop).

Treatment of this patient should address both the trauma and the medical condition. Therefore, the usual spinal precautions should be instituted and any obvious injuries should be treated accordingly. Just as important, however, is treating the patient for the stroke. Measures also should be established to maintain a patent airway, maximize oxygen delivery to the brain, and provide rapid transportation to an appropriate emergency department. The situation where a patient has a medical condition that leads to an injury occurs frequently, and leads to not only motor vehicle crashes, but falls and other accidents as well. It is of the utmost importance always to assess for a medical condition that has led to trauma whenever an older patient is evaluated.

CASE STUDY 2 SUMMARY

This patient is likely to have suffered from a compression fracture of her spine while she was getting up from her chair. Compression fractures are very common in older persons and often occur while doing normal activities of daily life, such as bending over to pick up something, rising from a chair, or lifting items. Often, the fractures go without notice unless significant pain is present. Most commonly, they are stable fractures that pose a low risk of permanent damage to the spinal cord. Osteoporosis is a major risk factor predisposing older persons to compression fractures.

Several risk factors are present that would indicate osteoporosis is likely. The most significant factor is a postmenopausal woman, because the greatest amount of bone density is lost shortly after menopause. Other risk factors are present as well. In a less active person, the rate of bone loss is expected to increase because the mechanical stimulus that causes bone deposition is lost. Also, a decreased appetite is likely to lead to a reduction in her calcium intake, another important factor leading to osteoporosis. Her physician's recommendation that she begin using a calcium supplement also indicates that she is likely to have osteoporosis.

CASE STUDY 3 SUMMARY

The patient's hip injury should be treated by using the blanket-roll splinting technique. This method will prevent further damage from occurring to the hip and will also improve the pain as the injury is immobilized. To best facilitate the splinting process, the patient should be rolled onto the uninjured side so that pressure is not placed onto the injured area. The majority

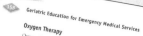

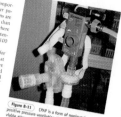

ALS Icon

Alerts providers that the information is for advanced life support (ALS) personnel.

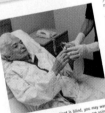

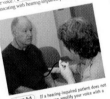

Communication Tip

Tips to remind providers of communication issues, and how to communicate properly.

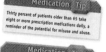

Medication Tip

Tips to remind providers of the importance of documenting medications, medication reactions, incorrect dosing, and other medication issues to keep in mind when working with an older patient.

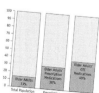

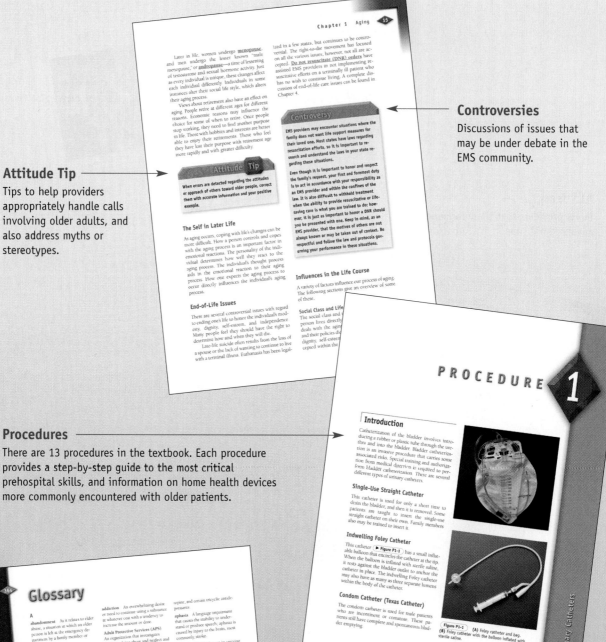

Attitude Tip

Tips to help providers appropriately handle calls involving older adults, and also address myths or stereotypes.

Controversies

Discussions of issues that may be under debate in the EMS community.

Procedures

There are 13 procedures in the textbook. Each procedure provides a step-by-step guide to the most critical prehospital skills, and information on home health devices more commonly encountered with older patients.

Glossary Terms

Comprehensively defined in the glossary at the end of the textbook, and an online glossary is available at www.GEMSsite.com.

GEMS Course Resources

The GEMS course is supported by a complete teaching and learning system. This system includes the textbook plus the following resources:

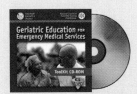

ToolKit CD-ROM

ISBN: 0-7637-2271-5

Preparing for a GEMS course is easy with the resources found on this CD-ROM including:

- Lecture Outlines that outline the topics covered in the text
- PowerPoint presentations that correspond to the lecture outlines
- Image Bank providing you with the most important images found in the text

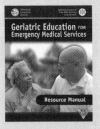

Resource Manual

ISBN: 0-7637-2270-7

An invaluable source of information, the Resource Manual contains:

- Helpful tips and guidelines for teaching a GEMS course
- Lecture outlines that offer a script for the PowerPoint presentations
- Skill station strategies and activities
- Scenarios that will keep providers engaged in group discussions
- Administrative forms for the Course Coordinator's convenience

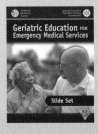

Slide Set

ISBN: 0-7637-2272-3

These 35mm slides are keyed to the PowerPoint presentations and lecture outlines for the Course Coordinator's convenience. Both ALS and BLS slides are included.

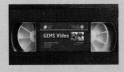

Video

ISBN: 0-7637-2273-1

Containing real-life footage from the field, this video will captivate students and show them how to perform important skills and procedures.

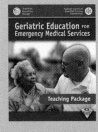

Teaching Package

With ToolKit CD-ROM
ISBN: 0-7637-2269-3

The Teaching Package combines the GEMS textbook, ToolKit CD-ROM or Slide Set, Resource Manual, and Video in one convenient box.

With Slide Set
ISBN: 0-7637-2268-5

Technology Resources

www.GEMSsite.com

Make full use of today's teaching and learning technology with www.GEMSsite.com, a community of GEMS faculty and providers.

Find a GEMS Course

Locate an upcoming GEMS course in your area.

Find a GEMS Course Coordinator

Locate a GEMS Course Coordinator in your area.

About GEMS

Course preview, ALS and BLS course schedules, and information on how to start a GEMS course of your own.

GEMS Community

News and resources for faculty and providers, plus GEMS bulletin board and e-mail list serve.

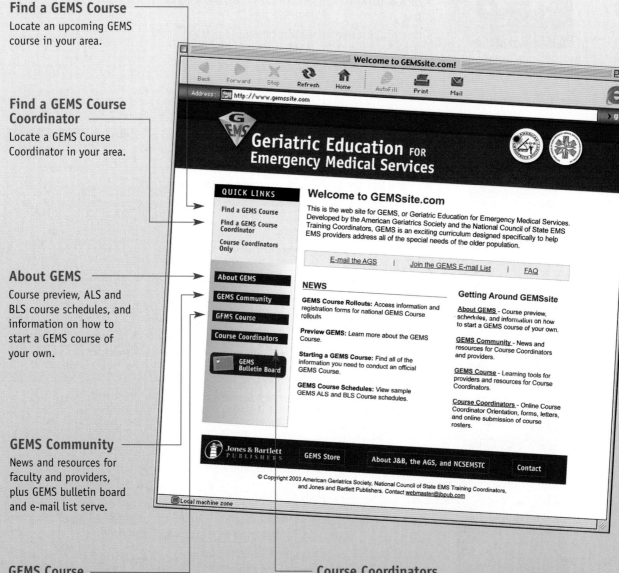

GEMS Course

Learning tools for providers and resources for faculty. Providers can continue their education outside of class with:

♦ Online Pretests to prepare for class with instant results and feedback

♦ Web Links to present current information and to expand on important information

♦ Online Glossary to expand medical vocabulary

♦ GEMS Scenarios to encourage critical thinking and aid comprehension of course material

Course Coordinators

Online Course Coordinator Orientation, forms, letters, GEMS course publicity, and online submission of course rosters, an easy alternative to paperwork.

Acknowledgments

Editors

David R. Snyder, MA, NREMT-P
Colleen Christmas, MD

Contributors

Luis F. Amador, MD
University of Texas Medical Branch
Galveston, Texas

Vicki Bacidore, RN, MS
Loyola University Medical Center
Maywood, Illinois

Roxy Barnes, RN
Vancouver Fire Department
Vancouver, Washington

Matthew J. Belan
University of Maryland School of
Medicine
Baltimore, Maryland

Susan K. Bowles, PharmD
Dalhousie University
Halifax, Nova Scotia

Russ Calhoun, BS, REMT-P
Oklahoma State University
Oklahoma City, Oklahoma

Chris Coughlin, MEd, CEP
Glendale Community College
Glendale, Arizona

Heather Davis, MS, NREMT-P
UCLA Center for Prehospital Care
Los Angeles, California

Barbara Dodge, BA, NREMT
Nebraska Department of Health
and Human Service
Lincoln, Nebraska

Teresita M. Hogan, MD, FACEP
Resurrection Medical Center
Chicago, Illinois

Jennifer Kapo, MD
University of Pennsylvania
Philadelphia, Pennsylvania

Marian P. LaMonte, MD, MSN
University of Maryland School of
Medicine
Baltimore, Maryland

Jeffrey T. Lindsey, MEd, MS, EMT-P
Estero Fire Rescue
Fort Myers, Florida

Robert L. Maher, Jr, PharmD
Duquesne University School of
Pharmacy
Pittsburgh, Pennsylvania

David E. Milkes, MD
Stanford University School of
Medicine
Stanford, California

Eric C. Nager, MD, FAAEM
Franklin Square Hospital
Baltimore County Fire Department
Baltimore, Maryland

Michael O'Keefe, MS, NREMT-P
Vermont Department of Health
Burlington, Vermont

Michael D. Panté, NREMT-P
Robert Wood Johnson University
Hospital
New Brunswick, New Jersey

James R. Pierce, LCDR, NC, USN
Naval Medical Center
Portsmouth, Virginia

Andrew N. Pollak, MD, EMT-P,
FAAOS
University of Maryland School of
Medicine
Baltimore, Maryland

Robert C. Salinas, MD, CAQ(G)
University of Oklahoma Health
Sciences Center
Oklahoma City, Oklahoma

LCDR Christopher Schmidt, NC, USN
Naval Hospital
Jacksonville, Florida

Jack Schwartz, JD
Maryland Assistant Attorney
General
Baltimore, Maryland

David L. Seabrook, MPA, EMT-P
Vancouver Fire Department
Vancouver, Washington

William H. Seifarth, MS, NREMT-P
Maryland Institute for Emergency
Medical Services Systems
Baltimore, Maryland

Ann Marie Spellbring, PhD, RN
University of Maryland School of
Nursing
Baltimore, Maryland

Kevin Spelman, AHG
Tai Sophia Institute
Laurel, Maryland

George Triadafilopoulos, MD
Stanford University School of
Medicine
Stanford, California

Andy Trohanis, MA, EMT-B
Maryland Institute for Emergency
Medical Services Systems
Baltimore, Maryland

James D. Upchurch, MD, NREMT-P
PHS Indian Hospital
Crow Agency, Montana

Sue Fryer Ward, MSW, LCSW, BCD
Maryland Department of Aging
Baltimore, Maryland

James R. Webster, MD, MS
Northwestern University Medical
School
Chicago, Illinois

Reviewers

Marie Bernard, MD
University of Oklahoma College of
Medicine
Oklahoma City, Oklahoma

Nicole Brandt, PharmD, CGP, BCPP
University of Maryland School of
Pharmacy
Baltimore, Maryland

Reviewers, continued

Loree Cook-Daniels, MS
Adult Abuse Review
Glendale, Wisconsin

Steven R. Counsell, MD, AGSF
Indiana University School of
Medicine
Indianapolis, Indiana

Sam R. Cunningham, BA, EMT-P
Georgia Department of Human
Resources
Columbus, Georgia

Rodger Green, EMT-P
Lincoln, Nebraska

Linda K. Honeycutt
Milford, Michigan

Thomas W. Jackson, MD
MCG Center for Senior Health
Augusta, Georgia

David Kuchta, RN, NREMT-P, BSAS
Mississippi State Department of Health
Jackson, Mississippi

Kathleen A. McLeron, PA-C, MICP
Department of Health and Social
Services
Juneau, Alaska

Robert G. Nixon, BA, EMT-P
LifeCare Medical Training
Walnut Creek, California

Judith Ruple, PhD, RN, NREMT-P
University of Toledo
Toledo, Ohio

David L. Seabrook, MPA, EMT-P
Vancouver Fire Department
Vancouver, Washington

Antonio Suarez, MSA, NREMT-P
Robert Wood Johnson University
Hospital
New Brunswick, New Jersey

The GEMS course was piloted in Maryland in August 2002, Utah in September 2002, and New Jersey in December 2002. Many thanks to the pilot participants for their review and critique of the course components which resulted in further improvement and refinement of the GEMS course materials.

Maryland Pilot Participants

Augustus W. Bowlings III, Dana Nicole Brooks, Terrell Buckson, Stacy Bussing, Larry Cohen, Jon S. Cooper, Steve Cox, Nicola J. Dattilio, Mark Demski, Earle Mark Dubel, Michael Fold, Steven K. Frye, Robert E. Gambel III, Erica Haberman, Ethel Hall, Darren Howell, Jennifer Hughes, Gerald L. Kyle, Kevin L. Lewis, Glenn H. Luedtke, Tracey L. Marvel, Frederick D. Monday, George Morgan, Jay M. Myers, Ralph Neil, Michelle M. New, John Newman, James G. Pirtle, Robert Powell, Patty Reger, Houston Reynolds, Marie A. Rosich-Sisk, Matthew Rzegocki, Michael Shapiro, Jennifer K. Simmons, Charles J. Simpson, Jr., John B. Smith, Ian St. John, Russ Strickland, Judith E. Sulivan, Christopher Tilley, Margaret E. Wedding, John D. West, Rose Ann Whittaker, Stephen Wilcoxson, Charles W. Wills, Sandra Wilson-Hypes, Kathleen A. Winter

Utah Pilot Participants

Brian Allred, Jamie Argyle, Loy Mitch Berkeley II, Jacquelyn Brooks, Stephen Brooks, Sue Campbell, Berni Carly, Les Chatelain, Neil Coker, Dennis O. Crezee, Craig Dixon, Kerry Easton, Daniel Evans, Philip L. Harris, Michael B. Hepworth, Jana Hicks, Stephen B. Hill, Carolyn Linford, Alan Matheson, Chris Morrison, Barbara Murdock, Launa M. Neilson, Kris Ollerton, Karynn Olsen, Christine O'Neil, Brooke Perkins, Marty Slack, Chris Stratford, Jenny Tuft, Don Wood

New Jersey Pilot Participants

Julie Aberger, Sonia F. Aguirre, Charles Angello, John Brophy, Tim Campbell, Steve Cohen, Harold L. Collins, II, Norman R. Deitch, Bob Dinetz, William Dougan, William Duffy, Fred Etting, William Faust, Joseph J. Gadoury, John Hansen, Judy L. Herrick, Frank V. Jasinski, Ed Kropniack, Jr., Ian Malik, Anthony F. Palmisaro, Robin Parker, Joseph Picone, Mario Pozo, Albert W. Rech, Jr., Bill Rosen, Henry Schleckser, Mary Ellen Schleckser, Barbara L. Service, Mary Ellen Smith, Susan Thomas, James Troisi, Stephanie H. Urbanowicz, Marianne Willis, Charles N. Zarelli, Linda L. Zarelli

Photographic Consultants

Jim Brown, MA, EMT-B
Maryland Institute for Emergency Medical Services Systems
Baltimore, Maryland

Jose V. Salazar, MPH, NREMT-P
Loudoun County Fire & Rescue
Leesburg, Virginia

Steven K. Frye, BS, NREMT-P
Anne Arundel County Fire Department Headquarters
Millersville, Maryland

Brian K. Slack, BA
Maryland Institute for Emergency Medical Services Systems
Baltimore, Maryland

We would also like to thank the following people for their collaboration on the photo shoots for this project. Their assistance was greatly appreciated.

Nancy J. Abramson, Public Relations Coordinator, Charlestown
Paul Brown, NREMT-P
Charles Chaney, CRT
Kim Chaney, EMT-B
Josh Clagett, EMT-B
Ethan Freyman, NREMT-P, CCI/OCV
Susan Hermann, CRT
Neil Holmes, CRT
Jennifer Hughes, EMT-P
Aaron Karvar, III, EMT-P
Brian Leenhouts, EMT-P
Michael McCabe, NREMT-P, CCI/OCV
Jenny Miller, NREMT-P
Beth Parrish, EMT-P
James L. Radcliffe, EMS Coordinator, University of Maryland Medical Center
Michael Shapiro, Bound Tree Medical Corporation
Sherman Spruell, EMT
Judy Sulivan, EMT-P
Kimberly Theden, EMT-P
Robert van Vugt, NREMT-P
Kathy Winter, EMT-P
P. Adam Zoltowski, EMT-P

Aging

LEARNING OBJECTIVES

1 Discuss aging in society today, including demographic trends.

2 Discuss geriatrics, gerontology, and the historical view of aging.

3 Discuss the social aspects of aging, including ageism, retirement, lifestyles, family, social roles, and the financial status of older people.

4 Demonstrate sensitivity to the negative stereotyping of older people and be able to educate others about stereotyping.

5 Describe living arrangements of older people.

6 Describe cultural differences in older people (ethnogeriatrics), particularly as they relate to the provision of medical care.

CHAPTER 1

Jeffrey T. Lindsey, MEd, MS, EMT-P

David R. Snyder, MA, NREMT-P

You have recently been hired by a large municipal EMS system. After your initial training, you are assigned to a district that contains a large older population. Included in your district are three nursing homes and several assisted-living facilities. You are eager to serve the population in your district.

How can you make a difference?

What should you do?

Aging

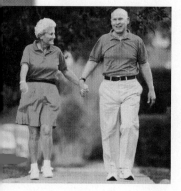

Older People and the EMS Provider

Everyone ages. As you sit reading this book, you are aging. If you haven't experienced it already, there will come a time when you and your loved ones are older and in need of emergency medical care. Would the EMS providers responding to your call be trained in how to care for your specific needs?

Attitude Tip

It is an honor to be involved in the life of an older person in any way.

Older persons are different from younger adults. Variability among individuals increases dramatically with age. Whereas most 50-year-old adults are quite similar to most other 50-year-old adults, an 85-year-old person is quite frequently very different from another 85-year-old. As a result of the aging process, many have one or several medical conditions. They are often taking one or more medications to treat these conditions. They are more easily affected by poor nutrition and changes in temperature. Older persons may suffer from a temporarily failing memory or from Alzheimer's disease. Their skin is more fragile. They experience grief from the death of loved ones, struggle with feelings of isolation, suffer a loss of independence, and experience depression.

These differences in older people complicate the emergency medical care delivered to them. If your patient experienced trauma, it may actually have been due to an underlying medical problem. Did the patient have a stroke while crossing the street, and then was hit by a car? Did the patient forget where they were, and walk in front of the car? Did they forget because they have Alzheimer's disease, or because they are grieving and are not eating properly? When you package the patient, how are you going to prevent their fragile skin from developing ulcers caused by the hard surface of the backboard? What if your patient is on a medication that cannot be mixed with what you would normally administer to treat their emergency? If a patient calls 9-1-1, but appears to have no real medical emergency, what could this mean? Will you know what questions to ask to discover the underlying problem?

The EMT-Basic course requires a minimum of 110 hours (more in some states). Of these 110 hours, approximately 1 hour pertains to the care of the older patient. The EMT-Paramedic course requires a minimum of 1,100 hours, of which 4 hours pertain to the care of the older patient. However, the number of older people is increasing. The latter half of the 20th century is often referred to as "the graying of America." As the Baby Boom generation approaches retirement age, the average age of Americans continues to rise. By the year 2000, the number of Americans over age 65 increased to 13% of the population (34.8 million). It is estimated that by the year 2030, those 65 and older will account for more than 20% of the overall population. As a result, patients over age 65 will continue to constitute a significant number of EMS transports and calls for service.

Why is it important for EMS providers to study how to care for older patients? The reasons are numerous. These patients make up an already significant and increasing number of EMS calls. Not knowing how to care for older patients can result in an insufficient level of care that does not treat the problem, may cause other problems, or even worsen the problem at hand.

Attitude Tip

Do you value and respect older people and their unique concerns and fears, whether they are clear minded and independent, frail and dependent, or demented and living in a nursing home?

The GEMS Diamond

In caring for older patients, it is important to remember certain key concepts. The **GEMS diamond** (▶ **Table 1-1**) was created to help you remember what is different about the older patient. The GEMS diamond is not intended to be a format for the approach to the older patient, nor is it intended to replace the ABCs of care. Instead it

TABLE 1-1   The GEMS Diamond

G Geriatric Patients

♦ Present atypically

♦ Deserve respect

♦ Experience normal changes with age

E Environmental Assessment

♦ Check the physical condition of the patient's home. Is the exterior of the home in need of repair? Is the home secure?

♦ Check for hazardous conditions that may be present (eg, poor wiring, rotten floors, unventilated gas heaters, broken window glass, clutter that prevents adequate egress).

♦ Are smoke detectors present and working?

♦ Is the home too hot or too cold?

♦ Is there a fecal or urine odor in the home?

♦ Are pets well cared for?

♦ Is food present in the home? Is it adequate and unspoiled?

♦ Are liquor bottles present (lying empty)?

♦ Is bedding soiled or urine soaked?

♦ Are there burn patterns on the walls, cabinets, or floors?

♦ If the patient has a disability, are appropriate assistive devices (eg, such as a wheelchair or walker) present?

♦ Does the patient have access to a telephone?

♦ Are medications out of date, unmarked, or from many physicians?

♦ If living with others, is the patient confined to one part of the home?

♦ If the patient is residing in a nursing facility, does the care appear to be adequate to meet the patient's needs?

M Medical Assessment

♦ Older patients tend to have a variety of medical problems, making assessment more complex. Keep this in mind in all cases—both trauma and medical. A trauma patient may have an underlying medical condition related to the emergency incident.

♦ Obtaining a medical history is very important in older patients, no matter what the primary complaint is.

♦ Initial assessment

♦ Ongoing assessment

S Social Assessment

♦ Assess ADLs
  ♦ Eating
  ♦ Dressing
  ♦ Bathing
  ♦ Toileting

♦ Are these activities being provided for the patient? If so, by whom?

♦ Are there delays in obtaining food, medication, or toileting? The patient may complain of this, or the environment may be suggestive of this.

♦ If in an institutional setting, is the patient able to feed him- or herself? If not, is food still sitting on the food tray? Has the patient been lying in his or her own urine or feces for prolonged periods of time?

♦ Does the patient have a social network? Does the patient have ways to interact socially with others on a daily basis?

serves as an acronym for the issues to be considered when assessing every older patient. The GEMS diamond will appear throughout the textbook whenever one of the four aspects of the diamond is being discussed.

"G" stands for geriatric. In other words, the first thing you should think of when you respond to an emergency involving an older patient is that older patients are different and may present atypically. You will need to remember the changes that occur with age. Just as important, remember that an older person is as human as a child or younger adult. Treat him or her with respect and dignity.

"E" stands for environmental assessment. The environment may contain clues to the cause of the emergency. Older people are more sensitive to temperature. Is the home too hot or too cold? Is the home well kept and secure? Are there hazardous conditions (poor lighting, throw rugs, poor wiring, broken windows)? These could be clues to elder abuse, neglect, an inability of the person to take care of himself or herself, depression, or a number of other problems.

"M" stands for medical assessment. Older patients tend to have a variety of medical problems and may be on numerous prescription, over-the-counter, and herbal medications. Obtaining a thorough medical history is very important in older patients.

"S" stands for social assessment. Older people may have less of a social network, due to the death of a spouse, family members, or friends. This can lead to depression. The older person may need additional help with **activities of daily living (ADLs)**, such as dressing and eating, but does not have anyone to help. You will need to find out if the patient has sufficient social support to care for both physical and emotional needs. Last but not least, a social assessment, like the environmental assessment, can help you uncover signs of elder abuse and neglect.

Remembering the components of the GEMS diamond will provide you with a concise way of remembering the important issues regarding older patients. Keep it in mind whenever you are involved with older people, and as you read this text. Using this concept will help you to make appropriate referrals, and as a result, you will help the older patient maintain his or her quality of life.

Attitude

Older people have unique health needs and problems that must be managed with skill and compassion. To care properly for older patients, you need to educate yourself about the clinical conditions associated with older patients, and you need to have the appropriate attitude when caring for an older patient ▼ **Figure 1-1** .

It is an honor to be involved in the life of an older person in any way. Your attitude as an EMS provider must reflect this. Just as it is your responsibility to manage the emotional needs of a pediatric patient, it is your responsibility to manage not only the emergency needs of older patients, but also their social, psychological, and environmental problems. With an attitude of compassion and caring, you can have a profound positive impact on the lives of older patients.

> ### Attitude Tip
>
> **With an attitude of compassion and caring, you can have a profound positive impact on the lives of older patients.**

Ageism

The term **ageism** was coined in 1969 by Dr. Robert Butler. Dr. Butler defined ageism as systematic stereotyping of, and discrimination

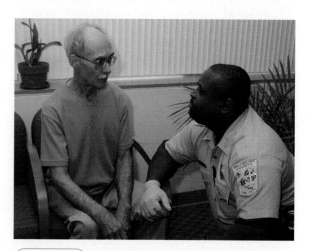

Figure 1-1   EMS providers need to be aware of the unique health needs and problems of older people.

against, people who are old. Ageism categorizes a person as senile, rigid in thought, comical, eccentric, stubborn, and unable to learn new things. Terms such as "geezer," "old hag," and "old goat" further perpetuate ageism. Referring to an older person as "honey" or "dear" or calling the older person by his or her first name are subtle forms of ageism.

It is never appropriate to refer to your older patients using these or similar terms, even if you think the patient cannot hear or understand you. The reality is that most older people are healthy, active, and continue to be engaged in society after retirement (▼ Figure 1-2). Using derogatory terms,

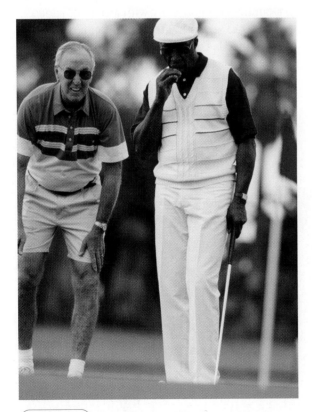

Figure 1-2 The majority of people are healthy, active, and continue to be engaged in society after retirement.

speaking in a condescending tone, and having a negative attitude toward older patients undermine the care you provide and will erode any trust you are trying to establish. There may be instances where you feel disgusted or disturbed by what you see on a call. This is no excuse for a negative attitude or a lower level of care. It unjustly punishes these patients simply for being old—something over which they have no control.

As human beings, we must understand and accept aging as part of the life cycle, and as a society, we must reverse the attitude that aging is an affliction. As professionals, we must understand the physiology and psychology of the aging process, how to manage the acute care needs of older patients, and educate older people about prevention techniques that promote and enhance the quality of life. Oftentimes, EMS is the entry point for the older person into the health care system. EMS providers should not treat older people with disdain and disgust, but rather with an understanding of their situations and needs and with the respect they have earned.

When thinking about older people, keep the following in mind: a person age 90 has experienced the Depression, two World Wars, the Korean and Vietnam conflicts, the Cold War, the civil rights movement, the women's liberation movement, the peace movement, the space age, and the computer age. Older people are unique individuals with a lifetime of experience. By example of a caring and compassionate attitude toward older patients, the EMS community can begin to win the battle against ageism.

The Older Population

To understand your older patients, you need to understand the demographics of the older population as a whole. This section provides a brief overview of the older population in the United States.

Geographic Distribution

Do you live in one of the five states with the largest percentage of people 65 and older (▼ **Figure 1-3**)? If so, you probably will have even more calls for older patients than the large number already experienced by your counterparts in other states. The percentages of senior citizens in the top five states are as follows:[1]

1. Florida—18.3%
2. Pennsylvania—15.4%
3. Iowa—15.3%
4. Rhode Island—15%
5. West Virginia—15%

People age 65 and older are less likely to live in metropolitan areas. It is estimated that 50% of older people live in suburbs, 27% live in cities, and 23% live outside of a metropolitan area.

Life Expectancy

People are living longer than ever before, increasing the number of older patients. Today, the average life expectancy of female Americans is 84 years. Men, on average, live for 81 years.

Rate of Aging

The number of people 65 and older has exploded over the last century. Take a look at (▶ **Table 1-2**). The 85-and-older age group is growing faster than the total number of people over the age of 65.

In 1999, there was a net increase of 200,000 older people. Two million people turned 65 and 1.8 million people over the age of 65 died in that year. This trend of growth in the older population is expected to continue in the future (▶ **Figure 1-4**).

Living Arrangements

Older people live in a variety of settings—with family, alone, and in institutions. Seventy percent live in a family setting, usually with a child or spouse.

In 1990, an estimated 9 million older people lived alone. It is believed that this number will

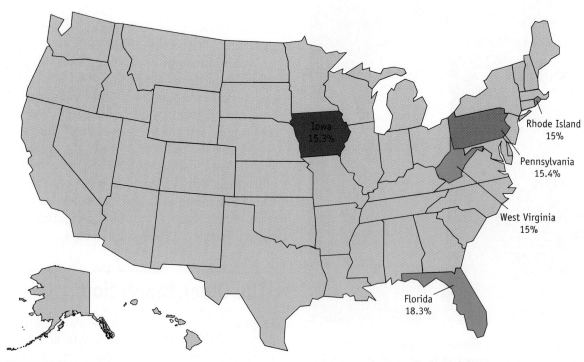

Iowa 15.3%
Rhode Island 15%
Pennsylvania 15.4%
West Virginia 15%
Florida 18.3%

Figure 1-3   The states with the largest populations of people over the age of 65 are highlighted on this map.

TABLE 1-2 Number of Older Adults in the United States in 2000		
Age	Number of People	Increase Since 1900
65–74	18.2 million	8 times more
75–84	12.1 million	32 times more
85 and older	4.2 million	32 times more

Source: http://www.aoa.dhhs.gov/aoa/STATS/Census2000/2000-1990-Pop.html

TABLE 1-3 Percentage of Older People Living in Institutions	
Age in Years	Percentage Living in Institutions
65–74	1.1%
75–84	4.5%
85 and older	19%

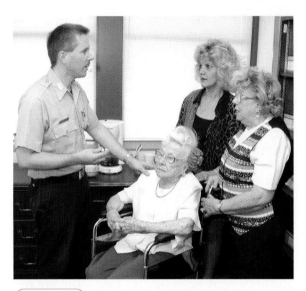

Figure 1-4 Over the past century, the life expectancy of United States citizens has increased significantly. As a result, the EMS provider needs to know how to care for older people.

increase to 13 million by the year 2010. Women are three times more likely to be widowed and live alone than are men. Individuals who live alone are more likely to use paid help as opposed to family caregivers.

Of all persons 65 years of age or older, 4.3% (1.6 million) live in an institutional setting. The rate of institutionalization increases with age ▶ **Table 1-3** .

Income and Poverty

Approximately 10.2% (3.4 million) of those 65 and older were below the poverty level in 2000. Another 6.7% (2.2 million) of older people were classified as "near poor." Older women are more likely to be impoverished than older men.[2] Income and poverty levels can affect the older person's eating habits, upkeep of their homes, and their health care, which can in some cases lead to emergencies.

On average, older patients spend more on health care than do other patients. The American population age 65 and older spends an average of 11% of their median income on health care costs, more than twice that spent by the entire population (5%). One third of health care costs in the United States is spent on persons age 65 and older. Public funds account for a major source of this spending.[3]

Overall Health

As people age, they may develop medical conditions. Chronic conditions limit 30% of people 65 to 74 years of age and 50.2% of those 75 years of age and older. The rate of disability increases with age. In people 65 to 69 years of age, 9% need help with activities of daily living (ADLs). In people 85 years and older, 45% need similar assistance.

The most frequently reported conditions in older patients are as follows:[4]

1. 40%—arthritis
2. 36%—hypertension
3. 30%—hearing impairment
4. 27%—heart disease
5. 18%—orthopaedic impairments
6. 17%—cataracts
7. 12%—sinusitis
8. 10%—diabetes

Use of Health Care Services

Individuals 65 years of age and older account for 36% of all hospital stays in the United States. People are receiving more of their care out of hospital, and with insurance issues, this trend will continue in the future. This population also has more contacts with doctors than those under 65 years of age.

The <u>old-age dependency ratio</u> depicts the dependency individuals place upon society as they age. It is defined as the number of older people for every 100 adults (potential caregivers) between the ages of 18 and 64. In 1990, there were 20 older people for every 100 "caregivers." By 2025, it is projected that there will be 32 older people for every 100 "caregivers." The supply of caregivers is not keeping pace with the growth of the older population. The need for caregivers is going to increase, and society is going to have difficulty keeping up with the demand for services as the population continues to age ▶ **Figure 1-5** .

As the older population grows, EMS providers will be required to offer services that are cost effective and efficient. Insurance regulations, costs associated with providing care, and facility issues will make cost a continuing concern.

Older People and the Health Care System

Older people are the largest single consumer of health care resources. People over 65 account for approximately 13% of the population, but they consume more than 30% of all prescription medications and outpatient resources, including EMS. Older people account for 20% of all emergency department visits.

The emergency department is an important means of access to health care by older people. Studies have concluded that the types of illness for which older people use the emergency department are distinct from those of younger adults. Younger adults typically are seen for surgical problems—mostly minor trauma—whereas older patients are seen in the emergency department for medical illnesses, many of which are serious or life threatening and require admission to the hospital.

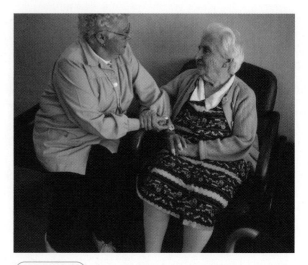

Figure 1-5   The supply of caregivers is not keeping pace with the growth of the older population.

Additionally, older patients, upon presentation to the emergency department, are more likely to be acutely ill and have several coexisting conditions at the time of admission. Older people living in rural areas use the emergency department less frequently than their urban counterparts, but tend to require ambulance transport more frequently.

The emergency department serves older patients in one of three ways: for treatment of emergency conditions; as a provider of primary care; and as an entry point into the long-term care system. Additionally, studies have shown that younger adults tend to use the emergency department after working hours, whereas older people tend to utilize the emergency department fairly consistently around the clock. Social and physical isolation also influence the older person's decision to utilize the emergency department. People who are single, widowed, or divorced are more likely to visit the emergency department, as these individuals live alone and have no immediate sources of help. The frequency of use of the emergency department by older patients has a direct impact on EMS. For increasing numbers of older people in society, the EMS provider is the only health care worker outside of the emergency department immediately available to assist the older person in crisis 24 hours a day, 7 days a week. The older a person is, the more likely he or she is to arrive in the emergency department by ambulance.

Types of Care Facilities for Older People

There are a variety of living facilities for older people that provide an array of care. The following sections describe these facilities. Some facilities are more prevalent in certain geographical locations, depending on the numbers of older people residing in the area, to meet the community's needs.

Active Adult Communities

Active adult communities have become very prevalent in the United States. They are also known as active adult living and active retirement communities. Fees are paid by private funds only. These communities offer age-restricted housing specifically created for seniors who enjoy participating in physical and social activities. The communities boast resort-type amenities, such as golf courses, tennis courts, pools, education classes, bike paths, and restaurants.

Independent Living in Senior Apartments

There are a number of rental developments that contain multiple units restricted to lease to those over the age of 55. Individuals who reside in these facilities may want additional physical or emotional security or prefer to live with other seniors.

Independent Living in Congregate Housing

Independent living in congregate housing may contain convenience services for the residents of the community. Some of the provisions may include meals, housekeeping services, transportation, or social events. Residents may have minor health

---

CASE STUDY 2

You are dispatched to the residence of a 75-year-old man who is unable to walk. Upon your arrival, a firefighter meets you outside of the patient's home with the following information: the patient was discharged yesterday from the hospital but has been unable to walk. The firefighter reports that the patient is conscious and his vital signs are stable: blood pressure is 140/90 mm Hg, pulse is 84 beats/min, and respirations are 16 breaths/min. Upon entering the patient's bedroom, you find the patient sitting on the edge of the bed conversing with firefighters. You learn that the patient was admitted to the hospital with congestive heart failure, and since returning home from the hospital yesterday by ambulance, has been unable to walk. The patient has significant swelling of both feet and ankles. The patient resides alone and has no family or neighbors for support. The patient states that he spoke to his family physician, who wants him returned to the hospital for possible re-admission. You learn from your dispatch center that the hospital to which the patient requires transport is on "bypass."

What are your concerns for this patient?

What actions should you take?

concerns. They may need the added security of having staff and other residents. They usually want and need access to health care. This type of housing is typically paid for on a monthly basis by private funds. Independent living is unlicensed, and thus the facilities and services may vary greatly.

Assisted Living

Assisted living is also known as residential care, board and care, and boarding house (▼ Figure 1-6). The residents need assistance with the activities of daily living (ADLs), such as bathing, dressing, and eating, or 24-hour supervision to maintain safety. Residents tend to need assistance with medication administration, but not more significant daily medical care. They enjoy the security of 24-hour staffing. Some facilities specialize in the care of Alzheimer's patients or those with other dementias.

The fees may be paid for with private funds, supplemental security incomes (SSI), long-term care insurance, or Medicaid. These facilities are typically licensed by each state, and licensing requirements vary by state.

Alzheimer's Care Facilities

Alzheimer's care facilities are specialized care facilities for those with signs of Alzheimer's disease or other dementias. The residents typically exhibit signs of impaired cognitive ability, forgetfulness, and/or wandering. The facility is designed and constructed to prevent residents from wandering off and to maintain safe activities. This may include features such as alarm systems on all doorways to prevent wandering outside and hallways that allow residents to wander in a continuous path without obstacles. Private funds, Medicaid, and long-term care insurance typically pay for the fees associated with Alzheimer's care facilities.

Nursing Homes

The term nursing home is the best known, and at times it is used generically for some of the other types of facilities. A nursing home is also known as skilled nursing facility, convalescent home, or long-term care facility. The residents require 24-hour nursing care and are unable to ambulate without the assistance of a wheelchair, walker, or another person in most instances. The resident cannot perform ADLs without assistance. The resident may need therapeutic or rehabilitative services including speech therapy, physical therapy, occupational therapy, respiratory therapy, or wound care.

These facilities are highly scrutinized by the government to ensure quality of care. Federal and state governments regulate staffing. There is a required number of staff to operate a nursing home, including an administrator on duty, registered nurses, licensed nurses, and nurses' aids. Private funds, long-term care insurance, Medicare, and Medicaid may pay for the fees associated with nursing home care.

Home Care

Home care allows the older person to remain in his or her own home and receive assistance from family, home care nurses, and other professionals delivered to them there. It is also known as home health care, personal care, and in-home care. With insurance regulations and restrictions in payment, home health care has become more economical, and hence, has seen an increase in popularity. More than 20,000 home care organizations deliver home care services to some 7.2 million individuals (roughly 2.7% of the United States population). Approximately 63% of the recipients are over the age of 65. Recipients of home care require services because of acute illness, long-term health conditions, permanent

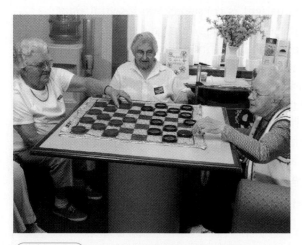

Figure 1-6   Assisted-living facilities aid older people with the activities of daily living.

disability, or terminal illness. Annual expenditures for home health care were estimated at $36 billion in 1999.

Most of these patients are home-bound (unable to leave the home to seek routine preventive health care), and many of them only see a physician when emergency situations arise and they must be transported to the hospital. Services offered include assistance with bathing, feeding, and exercising; administration of medication therapy; IV therapy; and chores (▼ **Figure 1-7**). Home health agencies are certified providers of skilled nursing care and are strictly regulated by state and federal laws. Private funds, long-term care insurance, private health insurance, Medicare, and Medicaid may pay for the fees.

Hospice Care

<u>Hospice care</u> is provided for those with terminal illnesses in their own home (▶ **Figure 1-8**). Hospice care allows for peace, comfort, and dignity. There are hospice services that provide in-patient care of the same type. Medicare identified 2,273 hospices in the United States in January 2001. There are also an estimated 200 volunteer hospices in the United States as well. As of February 1998, 44 states licensed hospices. In 1998, 76.2% of patients receiving hospice care were age 65 and older.[5]

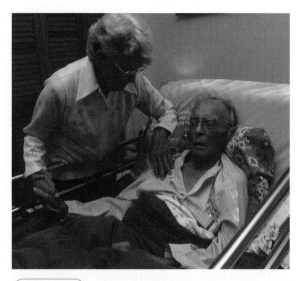

(**Figure 1-8**)   Hospice care allows people with terminal illnesses to receive palliative care in their own homes.

Hospice care focuses on **palliative care**, or relieving pain and controlling symptoms, as opposed to a primary focus on curative care (▼ **Table 1-4**). Hospice services include supportive medical, social, and spiritual services to the terminally ill, as well as support for the patient's family. Hospice and palliative care are discussed in more detail in Chapter 4. Health insurance, Medicare, or Medicaid typically cover the payment for hospice services.

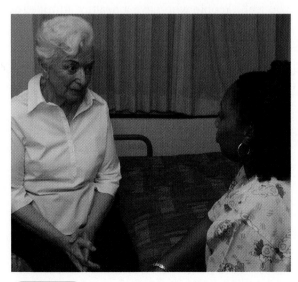

(**Figure 1-7**)   Home care covers a wide range of activities, and can be occasional or around-the-clock.

TABLE 1-4 New Hospice Enrollees by Primary Diagnosis in 1998			
All Cancer	57.4%	All Non-cancer	42.6%
Lung	16.1%	CHF	6.8%
Prostate	4.3%	COPD	4.4%
Colon	3.7%	Stroke	3.7%
Breast	3.6%	Alzheimer's disease	3.3%
Pancreatic	3.4%	"Ill-defined conditions"	22.3%
Other	26.3%		

Respite Care

Respite care provides temporary relief for caregivers, ranging from hours to days. This can be provided in the patient's own home or in nursing homes, assisted living facilities, or adult day care centers. The care ranges from assistance with ADLs to skilled nursing care, depending on the patient's typical level of care and need. In most instances, payment for respite care is from private funds.[6]

Historical View of Aging

In addition to understanding the demographics and living arrangements of older people, some background on the field of geriatrics will be useful. Gerontology is defined as the study of aging. Geriatrics is the branch of medicine concerned with the health of older people. The study of aging and the care of older people is not new. The Greek physician Galen in the first century A.D. used the term "gerocomy" for the care of older people. In 1903, at the Pasteur Institute in Paris, the term "gerontology" was invented. In 1909, Dr. Ignatius L. Nascher coined the term "geriatrics."

The advent of science in the 1600s led researchers and scientists to undertake a systematic study of the processes of aging. The 1930s laid the groundwork for many of the developments in gerontology. One of the concepts of this period is that aging is best studied in an interdisciplinary context. That is to say that aging is a *process* involving both physical and psychological changes.

Literature on aging generated between 1950 and 1960 equaled the production of the preceding 115 years. One thing to keep in mind when thinking about the history of aging is that in 1900, the average life expectancy was 49. In 2002, the average person can expect to live into their 80s. This represents a gain of over 30 years in just one century. This gain in life expectancy is unparalleled in the history of mankind.

What does the history of aging mean for EMS? The organized approach to EMS began with the passage of the Emergency Medical Services Systems Act of 1972 (Public Law 93-154). The original intent of EMS was to combat the growing number of highway traffic fatalities and out-of-hospital cardiac arrests. As EMS providers became proficient in providing emergency medical care,

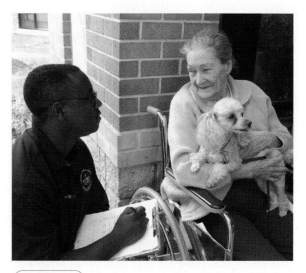

Figure 1-9   EMS providers are increasingly called on to care for the variety of needs of older people.

the scope of care and the number of patients served by the system increased. EMS providers now are increasingly called upon to care for the variety of needs of older people (▲ **Figure 1-9**).

Sociology of Aging

Lifespan Issues

How individuals perceive life as they grow older has a large effect on their aging process. There is a lot of truth to the adage "You are only as old as you feel." People who have a healthy attitude toward aging may be running marathons when they are 90 years old. People who fear growing older may feel useless and depressed.

Throughout the stages of life, people have emotional reactions to the aging process, especially during major life events. For example, parents who build their lives around their children may have difficulties when their children grow older. The difficulties they have in dealing with their new lifestyle as children grow can lead to uncertainty and depression, which will have an adverse effect on the aging process. On the other hand, if parents have a healthy attitude and enjoy watching their children grow into adulthood, they will see their role in their children's lives as evolving, not ending. Having a positive outlook on major life events can make the aging process smoother.

Later in life, women undergo **menopause**, and men undergo the lesser known "male menopause," or **andropause**—a time of lessening of testosterone and sexual hormone activity. Just as every individual is unique, these changes affect each individual differently. Individuals in some instances alter their social life style, which alters their aging process.

Views about retirement also have an effect on aging. People retire at different ages for different reasons. Economic reasons may influence the choice for some of when to retire. Once people stop working, they need to find another purpose in life. Those with hobbies and interests are better able to enjoy their retirements. Those who feel they have lost their purpose with retirement age more rapidly and with greater difficulty.

Attitude Tip

When errors are detected regarding the attitudes or approach of others toward older people, correct them with accurate information and your positive example.

The Self in Later Life

As aging occurs, coping with life's changes can be more difficult. How a person controls and copes with the aging process is an important factor in emotional reactions. The personality of the individual determines how well he or she reacts to the aging process. The individual's thought process aids in the emotional reaction to their aging process. How one expects the aging process to occur directly influences the individual's aging process.

End-of-Life Issues

There are several controversial issues with regard to ending one's life to honor the individual's modesty, dignity, self-esteem, and independence. Many people feel they should have the right to determine how and when they will die.

Late-life suicide often results from the loss of a spouse or the lack of wanting to continue to live with a terminal illness. Euthanasia has been legal-ized in a few states, but continues to be controversial. The right-to-die movement has focused on all the various issues; however, not all are accepted. **Do not resuscitate (DNR) orders** have assisted EMS providers in not implementing resuscitative efforts on a terminally ill patient who has no wish to continue living. A complete discussion of end-of-life care issues can be found in Chapter 4.

Controversy

EMS providers may encounter situations where the family does not want life support measures for their loved one. Most states have laws regarding resuscitation efforts, so it is important to research and understand the laws in your state regarding these situations.

Even though it is important to honor and respect the family's request, your first and foremost duty is to act in accordance with your responsibility as an EMS provider and within the confines of the law. It is also difficult to withhold treatment when the ability to provide resuscitative or life-saving care is what you are trained to do; however, it is just as important to honor a DNR should you be presented with one. Keep in mind, as an EMS provider, that the motives of others are not always known or may be taken out of context. Be respectful and follow the law and protocols governing your performance in these situations.

Influences in the Life Course

A variety of factors influence our process of aging. The following sections give an overview of some of these.

Social Class and Life History

The social class and the environment in which a person lives directly influence how that person deals with the aging process. Social institutions and their policies dictate how the issues of modesty, dignity, self-esteem, and independence are accepted within the institution's walls.

Race and Ethnicity

Our society is diverse in its ethnic culture. A person's race, ethnicity, and culture will influence how they deal with issues. In different cultures, the gender of an individual may alter the way the aging process is viewed in the culture. This subject is discussed in more detail later in the chapter.

Older Persons on Their Own

As they age, individuals want to maintain their independence as long as they possibly can. It is important to take an older person's wish for independence into consideration when faced with situations that could negatively impact independence.

Aging and the Family

The family needs to consider their responsibility to their aging members and take distance of the members into consideration (▶ **Figure 1-10**). The nuclear family is often extended miles apart, and younger family members may not be in close proximity to their aging members.

Crime and Older People

Older people become a prime target for a variety of scams if their awareness levels and cognitive abilities decrease. Phone schemes in which the scam artist gets bank account and credit card numbers from unsuspecting older people are common. Another scam is sweepstakes, in which

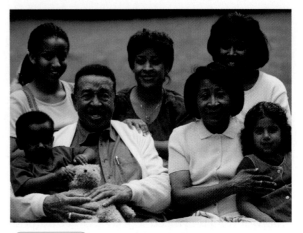

Figure 1-10   Families are an important resource for the older person.

forms are mailed to an older person with the intention of selling magazines and journals, and the older person often believes they must make a purchase in order to win.

Elder abuse has continued to climb as the demand to care for this population has increased. A complete discussion of elder abuse can be found in Chapter 14.

Older People Making Choices

The ability of the older person to make sane and rational decisions decreases as their mental capacity diminishes in those afflicted by certain ailments, such

CASE STUDY 3

You are dispatched to an intersection for a report of a struck pedestrian. Upon your arrival, you encounter an 82-year-old woman lying on the ground. She is bleeding from the right arm. Your assessment reveals that she is conscious and answers appropriately. Your examination reveals that she sustained a skin tear to the right arm. There appear to be no further injuries. You learn from the police officer present that the patient was attempting to cross the street with the light. The police officer states that the driver of the vehicle that struck the patient estimated the vehicle's speed to be approximately 15 mph. The police officer remarks that this is the third time this month that an older pedestrian has been struck at this intersection. Your scene assessment reveals a newly opened senior apartment building on one side of the street and a grocery store on the other side of the street.

What are your thoughts?

What are your intervention decisions?

as dementia. When older people make bad decisions, it may cause financial and health problems. Consideration of decision-making ability with regard to health care issues is vital in the prehospital setting.

Psychology of Aging

As a person ages, his or her status in society decreases. The individual's roles in work, the community, and the family diminish because society does not recognize the older person's role as valuable. People believe that the older person cannot contribute what he or she once could to society. Also, after retirement, people tend to disengage from society and decrease the number of activities in which they are involved.

How a person sees himself or herself has a direct effect on psychological well-being. As a person ages, the likelihood of experiencing depression increases. Keeping active helps older people to be happier (▼ **Figure 1-11**). Becoming involved in the community, church, or the work force may help older people to remain happy and decrease the risk of depression.

Ethnogeriatrics

Ethnogeriatrics is defined as health care for older people from diverse ethnic populations. Why is it important for EMS providers to study ethnogeriatrics? Demographic projections indicate that the number of ethnic older people in the United States is rapidly increasing and will continue to do so (▼ **Table 1-5**).

Racial and ethnic influences impact the prevalence, morbidity, and mortality of diseases and access to hospital and community services (▼ **Figure 1-12**). Studies indicate that on average, older persons from most ethnic minority populations use formal health care services less than their white counterparts. Exceptions to this are emergency services and acute care. This has a direct impact on EMS and the emergent care of ethnic older people. Listed in (▶ **Table 1-6**) are the leading causes of death based on ethnicity.

You are encouraged to learn about the needs of the ethnic older people within the communities you serve.

TABLE 1-5 Percent Change in Population 65 and Older, 1990–2030	
African Americans	131%
American Indians, Eskimos, and Aleuts	147%
Asian and Pacific Islanders	285%
Hispanics	328%
Whites	81%

Source: American Geriatrics Society Ethnogeriatrics Curriculum.

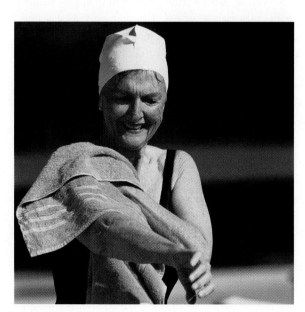

Figure 1-11   Older people who have hobbies and activities are happier and healthier than those who disengage from society.

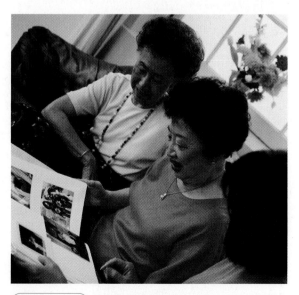

Figure 1-12   Racial and ethnic influences impact the prevalence, morbidity, and mortality of diseases and access to hospital and community services.

TABLE 1-6	Leading Causes of Death for Persons of Different Ethnicities Age 65 and Over			
White	African American	American Indian	Asian or Pacific Islander	Hispanic
Heart disease	Heart disease	Heart disease	Heart disease	Heart disease
Cancer	Cancer	Cancer	Cancer	Cancer
Stroke	Stroke	Diabetes	Stroke	Stroke
COPD	Diabetes	Stroke	Pneumonia/ Influenza	COPD
Pneumonia/ Influenza	Pneumonia/ Influenza	COPD	COPD	Pneumonia/ Influenza

Source: American Geriatrics Society Ethnogeriatrics Curriculum.

Providing Care to Other Ethnic Groups

EMS providers must have an understanding of the wide degree of variation among traditional minority groups in the United States as well as the differences between older adults born in the United States and those born abroad. Providers who do not have experience working with older patients of other ethnicities may have a tendency to prejudge them based on hearsay and emotions. In order to overcome this tendency:

♦ Examine your own cultural attitudes and values that could affect interactions.

♦ Have adequate knowledge of ethnic groups in your community.

♦ Develop the appropriate skills necessary to manage the needs of older people of different ethnicities. For example, learn the appropriate ways of showing respect and acknowledging the older person's health beliefs.

Being a health care professional means being a student as well as a provider. Take the time to learn about the ethnic groups you serve. Not only do intergenerational differences exist, but cultural differences exist as well. Getting to know the culture you serve will allow you to understand how the older population perceives and utilizes health care. This, in turn, will help you to provide professional and compassionate care. One way to do this is to interview an older person of a different ethnicity in the community who is willing to share his or her cultural values and beliefs. Another way is to invite a community leader from another ethnic group to become part of the training process. This will allow community cultural values to be incorporated into educational programs.

Communication Tip

Get to know the various cultures you serve in order to understand how the older population perceives and utilizes health care.

While some older people may speak English well, others may speak English only as a second language. Additionally, many older people read English, but may wish to discuss complicated issues in their native language with family. Allow the older person the time to do this, as others in the family may not speak English. It may also have a calming effect on the family.

Communication Tip

Allow an older patient the time to discuss complicated issues in their native language with family if he or she desires to do so.

There may be times when the older patient does not speak English and you must rely on a family member or interpreter. The following are general guidelines to be employed when using interpreters:

♦ Ask short questions.

♦ Avoid technical terminology, abbreviations, and jargon.

♦ Avoid colloquialisms, abstractions, idiomatic expressions, slang, similes, and metaphors.

♦ Encourage the interpreter to translate the patient's own words as much as possible. This will allow for a better grasp of the patient's understanding and emotional state.

♦ During the interaction, look at and speak directly to the patient.

♦ Listen to the patient, even though you do not understand. Be alert for nonverbal clues. Obvious or subtle body language is present in all cultures. If you observe particular body language cues that appear significant, take note, and attempt to learn their significance.

There are many differences in the explanations of disease and treatment that are based on the older person's culture. Some older people may rely on beliefs such as nature, balance, and spiritual interventions to explain physical states. All of these beliefs have an impact on how the older person defines wellness, illness, and decision-making regarding health care.

Physical Examination

The following are general points when conducting a physical examination on an older person of another ethnicity:

♦ Cross-gender examinations (a male provider examining a female patient, or vice versa) are unacceptable in many cultures. However, do not delay care in these circumstances. The preservation of life is most important.

♦ Ask the patient for preference of the presence of family during the physical examination. Again, the severity of the situation will determine if time allows for this.

♦ Symptom recognition, meaning, and how ethnic older people report these vary culturally. For example, "air heavy" or "air not right" may mean dyspnea for some Native American older people. "Heavy heart" may indicate depression among Chinese Americans.

♦ Dementia and depression are considered mental illnesses in some cultures, and are therefore highly stigmatized. In others, dementia is seen as part of aging and is defined as a minimal problem.

♦ Talking about death is considered inappropriate in some cultures, such as Chinese and Navajo.

Attitude Tip

An informed mind and a positive attitude toward the older population will result in a higher interest level, improved communication and assessment, and more effective care and management of older patients.

Summary

The premise of geriatric EMS is clear: care for every older patient in every sense of the word. By taking the time to study geriatrics, you are extending your knowledge beyond that of initial certification and preparing yourself to properly manage the diverse needs of the older patient. Most importantly, however, you embrace the older population you are caring for. Remember, aging is a process, and older patients are people.

One day, you and your parents, siblings, friends, and extended family will be part of the older population, perhaps living in a facility and in need of emergency care. The measures you take to improve the emergency care of the older population today will shape the emergency care you receive tomorrow. By being aware of opportunities for prevention, you can have a positive impact on the health of the population that is served.

Attitude Tip

"The diseases of the aged are worthy of the most careful study. Let us not dismiss his ailments with the facile diagnosis: 'you are old.'"
—I. L. Nascher

Case Study Summaries

CASE STUDY 1 SUMMARY

Wanting to make a difference with the population you serve is the first step. Given that you have a large number of older people in your district, including three nursing facilities and several assisted living facilities, there are several things that you (and your department) can do to have a positive impact on the care you provide to your older patients. One of the things that can be done is to visit each nursing facility. This will give the staff at those facilities an opportunity to meet you and for you to meet them. This can result in developing a positive rapport. EMS providers are part of a multidisciplinary team of health care professionals who care for older patients. Expectations can also be established from these visits— what expectations do you have from the nursing facility when called? Similarly, what can the nurs

ing facility expect from you? The goal in establishing such relationships is improved patient care. Additionally, such visits allow you to "preplan" the facility should a fire or other large-scale incident occur. The same can be said for assisted living facilities. If your department or agency is equipped with a computer-aided dispatch (CAD) system, identify these facilities in your CAD system as high-risk, so that other responders are aware of their existence. Most important is that these relationships are ongoing—one visit will not suffice. If there are senior centers in your district, visit them. The EMS system should become part of senior center fairs. The older people in the community need to know that the EMS system is there for them and how to access it.

CASE STUDY 2 SUMMARY

Your first concern should be that this patient is not able to walk, and therefore not able to provide for himself. You realize that the patient should be transported to the emergency department, but the emergency department to which you wish to transport is on "bypass." Do you transport to another hospital? It is ideal that the patient be returned to the hospital from which he was recently discharged, under the care of his own physician. One way of meeting this patient's

needs and honoring the hospital code status is to telephone the emergency department to make them aware of your situation. Perhaps admission arrangements have already been made, and the patient will not have to remain in the emergency department. Often, these situations can be worked out by taking the time to make the right calls. This does require more time, but by doing so, you will be providing for the best interest of the patient, which is the goal of prehospital care.

CASE STUDY 3 SUMMARY

Your first concerns are to treat the injuries to the patient. In this case, there are no life-threatening injuries. Given the patient's age and the mechanism of injury, the patient should be appropriately immobilized and transported to the emer-

gency department. Your other concern is that the police officer informed you that this was the third time in a month an older pedestrian had been struck at this intersection. Your scene observations revealed a newly opened senior apartment complex on one side of the street and a grocery store on the other side of the street. This should arouse your suspicion that perhaps the traffic light at the intersection is not long enough to allow the older pedestrian to cross, or that there may be obstructions to motorists. Injury prevention must become part of the EMS provider's responsibilities and routine. In this case, there is an excellent opportunity to possibly prevent a serious or fatal pedestrian accident from occurring. Contact the local or state bureau of highways so that an evaluation of the intersection can be made. The solution may be as simple as extending the time allowed in the crosswalk.

Endnotes

1. http://www.census.gov. Accessed 07/23/02.
2. U.S. Department of Health and Human Services Administration on Aging. *A Profile of Older Americans: 2001*. http://www.aoa.gov/aoa/stats/profile/2001/8.html. Accessed 5/6/02.
3. http://www.aoa.dhhs.gov/aoa/stats/profile/2001/12.html. Accessed 5/6/02.
4. Administration on Aging. A Profile of Older Americans: 2001. http://www.aoa.gov/aoa/stats/profile/2001/12.html. Accessed 11/13/02.
5. National Association for Home Care website. http://www.nahc.org. Accessed 11/13/02.
6. http://www.springstreet.com/seniors/kyo/ccrc.jhtml. Accessed 5/6/02.

Bibliography

Cunningham WR, Brookbank JW. *Gerontology, the Psychology, Biology, and Sociology of Aging*. New York: Harper & Row; 1988.

Gubrium JF, Holstein JA. *Aging and Everyday Life*. Blackwell, MA: Malden; 2000.

Hardy MA. *Studying Aging and Social Change: Conceptual and Methodological Issues*. Thousand Oaks, CA: Sage; 1997.

Hatch LR. *Beyond Gender Differences: Adaptation to Aging in Life Course Perspective*. Amityville, NY: Baywood; 2000.

Kenyon GM, Randall WL. *Ordinary Wisdom: Biographical Aging and the Journey of Life*. Westport, CT: Praeger; 2001.

Maddox GL, Lawton MP. *Focus on Kinship, Aging, and Social Change*. New York: Springer; 1993.

Matcha DA. *The Sociology of Aging: A Social Problems Perspective*. Boston: Allyn and Bacon; 1997.

Matras J. *Dependency, Obligations, and Entitlements: A New Sociology of Aging, the Life Course, and the Elderly*. Englewood Cliffs, NJ: Prentice Hall; 1990.

Qualls SH, Abeles N. *Psychology and the Aging Revolution: How We Adapt to Longer Life*. Washington, DC: American Psychological Association; 2000.

U.S. Bureau of the Census.

U.S. Department of Health and Human Services, Administration on Aging: "Profile of Older Americans."

U.S. Department of Health and Human Services, Centers for Disease Control and Prevention, National Center of Health Statistics.

U.S. Department of Health and Human Services, Centers for Medicare and Medicaid Services.

U.S. Department of Labor, Bureau of Labor Statistics.

Normal Changes with Age

LEARNING OBJECTIVES

1 Define the factors that cause older people to be at risk for increased medical care.

2 Identify the general decline in organ systems in older people.

3 List the major diseases and disorders common to older people.

4 Explain why the special needs of older people and the changes that the aging process brings about in physical structure, body composition, and organ function provide a fundamental knowledge base for maintenance of life support functions.

5 Define normal psychological changes affecting older people.

CHAPTER 2

Michael D. Panté, NREMT-P

CASE STUDY 1

You are assigned to a local health fair to staff a booth with information about your service and to provide blood pressure screenings. An 82-year-old woman asks to have her blood pressure taken. You take it and report a blood pressure of 136/88 mm Hg. She begins to explain to you that when she was younger her pressure was always 100/60 mm Hg, but over the last 20 years it has gradually increased. She asks if this is normal.

Is it?

What should your response be?

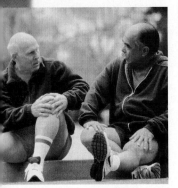

Introduction

The human body has the ability to age to around 115 years. In the body's everyday process of replacing dead cells with new ones, the ability to regenerate cells is surpassed by the amount of cell death. This large amount of cell death leads to tissue death, organ death, and finally death of the body. The top causes of death in older patients include heart disease, cancer, and cardiovascular accident (CVA). (▼ Table 2-1) lists the top ten causes. Aging of body systems makes the older person prone to the effects of these disease states.

With advancing age, everyday activities take on new requirements. Activities of daily living (ADLs) include basic everyday functions needed to sustain life, such as feeding oneself, walking, dressing, and getting up from a chair. **Instrumental activities of daily living (IADLs)** include basic everyday activities that require a higher level of function, such as going shopping, making a meal, cleaning up, or using the telephone. As a person ages, ADLs and IADLs may take more planning or may require additional help that was not needed in

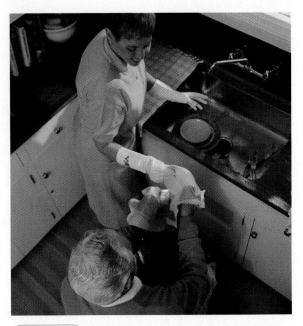

(**Figure 2-1**)   For older adults, activities of daily living may require help or added planning.

younger years (▲ **Figure 2-1**). For instance, a decrease in muscle mass can mean that only lighter loads of groceries can be carried from the store, making additional or more frequent trips necessary. Deterioration in eyesight, hearing, and peripheral nervous system response makes driving more difficult. Older drivers often compensate for these deficiencies by taking commonly traveled routes or making three right turns in order to avoid one left turn. They may also develop medical complaints upon overexertion.

Seemingly minor ailments can be excessively burdensome to an already compromised older person. An upper respiratory infection can make the patient weaker, which then keeps the patient from getting up and having meals or drinking appropriate amounts. This leads to dehydration, which makes the patient's symptoms worse. Because the older person does not have the reserves that a younger person might, he or she may have a harder time compensating for illness and is often forced to seek medical care. This is also very common when a patient has a chronic condition, such as chronic obstructive pulmonary disease (COPD), and it flares up.

Multiple health conditions combine to make assessing and caring for the older person difficult. Conditions affecting one system can produce problems that affect another. For example, the patient who has congestive heart failure (CHF)

TABLE 2-1 Top Ten Causes of Death for Persons Age 65 and Over	
1. Diseases of the heart	605,673
2. Cancer	384,186
3. CVA	139,144
4. COPD	97,896
5. Pneumonia	82,989
6. Diabetes	48,974
7. Trauma	32,975
8. Nephritis	24,830
9. Alzheimer's disease	22,416
10. Septicemia	19,012

Source: National Vital Statistics Reports. July 24, 2000; 48 (11).

and COPD will have a build-up of fluid from the CHF that can worsen the COPD, making assessment and management more difficult.

With changes in anatomy and physiology can come an increase in patient complaints. One becomes short of breath more easily with decreases in normal lung function, or may trip because of a reduction in the muscle mass needed to move around. These changes in the body also make it harder to communicate with and assess older patients. This chapter looks at some of these changes, system by system.

Attitude Tip

Realize that growing old *does not* naturally or normally include confusion, dementia, delirium, depression ("blues"), falls, weakness, syncope, and other conditions related to disease processes.

Integumentary System

Wrinkling and loss of resiliency of the skin (the integumentary system) are the most visible signs of aging. Wrinkling occurs because the skin becomes thinner, drier, less elastic, and more fragile. Subcutaneous fat becomes thinner, making a loosened outer cover for the body. **Elastin**, the substance that makes the skin pliable, and **collagen**, the substance that makes the skin strong, both decrease with age. Skin tears or injuries from what is considered light contact or bumps occur frequently. Attempts to establish an intravenous (IV) line can be more difficult because the thinner skin tears during insertion of the catheter, or while holding the patient still when making the attempt.

The tightened skin of youth allows subcutaneous injuries to **tamponade**, or close and stop bleeding, easily (▼ **Figure 2-2a**); however, with aging skin, bleeding may go unnoticed or uncontrolled, producing large hematomas underneath the skin (▼ **Figure 2-2b**). Injuries to the skin are slow to heal because of diminished capillary blood flow. Pressure ulcers, also called decubitus ulcers or pressure sores, occur when an older patient remains stationary, allowing the weight of the body to compress the already thinned skin. With little blood flow to regenerate the cells damaged by the pressure, tissue dies and a sore results. Sebaceous glands produce less oil, making for dryer skin. Sweat gland activity also decreases, hindering the body's ability to sweat and help regulate heat.

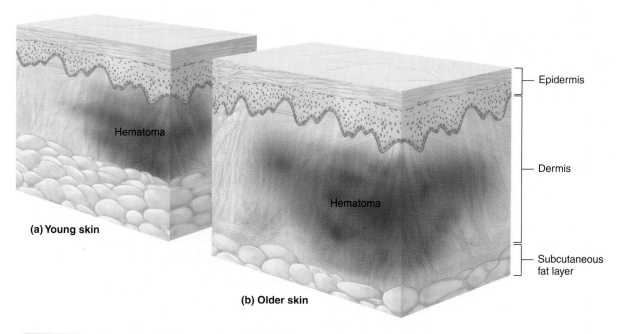

(a) Young skin

(b) Older skin

— Epidermis

— Dermis

— Subcutaneous fat layer

Hematoma

Hematoma

Figure 2-2 **A.** In young skin, the tight interface between skin and the subcutaneous fat layer tends to control bleeding in subcutaneous injuries. **B.** The looser connection between skin and fat in older skin exerts less control on bleeding and may result in larger hematomas.

With aging, hair follicles produce less **melanin**, which is a pigment that provides color to the skin and hair. The lowered production of melanin results in less color in the hair. Without color, the hair is gray. In addition, hair becomes thinner. A hair strand has a life expectancy of 4 to 5 years. Many hair follicles stop producing hair as they age (more common in men) and the follicles will produce thinner, smaller hair during the aging process.

Respiratory System

The respiratory system sees many changes throughout life. All parts of the respiratory system are affected by aging. Age-related changes in the respiratory system result in a predisposition to respiratory illness. Normal activity can produce shortness of breath that necessitates resting. A minor respiratory infection may propel the older patient into a life-endangering episode.

Musculature of the upper airway weakens with age. This may allow the tongue and soft tissue of the oropharynx to close in easily, narrowing the airway when the patient becomes overtaxed or less responsive. Changes in bones and teeth can alter the shape of the face and mouth, making an airway harder to maintain when attempting to ventilate these patients.

Many older patients require dentures or dental appliances to eat. Improperly fitted or loose plates are an airway obstruction waiting to happen. Dentures are also associated with food-related obstructions due to the loss of sensation of the hard palate (roof of the mouth). A denture made for the upper jaw has a plastic connection that covers the hard palate, an area that provides sensory information required for determination of food particle size. When the denture blocks this sensation, the patient may attempt to swallow a larger piece of food than is tolerable. (You may be familiar with the same risk caused by alcohol intoxication.)

The loss of mechanisms that protect the upper airway is a concern in older adults. These can include a decreased ability to clear secretions, as well as decreased cough and gag reflexes. The cilia that line the airways lessen as we age, and the innervation of the structures in the airway provides less sensation. Without the ability to maintain the upper airway, aspiration and obstruction are more likely.

The smooth muscle of the lower airway also weakens with age. When a younger patient inhales, the airway maintains its shape, allowing air to enter (▼ **Figure 2-3a**). As these muscles weaken with age, strong inhalation can make the walls of the airway collapse inward and cause inspiratory wheezing. Conversely, strong exhalation can cause expiratory wheezing (▼ **Figure 2-3b**). The collapsing airways result in low flow rates because less air can move through the smaller airways, and air trapping because air does not completely exit the alveoli (incomplete expiration).

By age 75, the **vital capacity** (volume of air moved during the deepest inspiration and expiration) can drop to 50% of what it was in young adulthood. This occurs because of the loss in respiratory muscle mass, increases in the stiffness of the thoracic cage, and decreases in the available surface area for the exchange of air.

Physiologically, vital capacity decreases and **residual volume**, which is the amount of air left in the lungs after the maximum possible amount of air has been expired, increases with age. This leaves stagnant air resting in the alveoli and hampers good gas exchange, which can produce a relative **hypercarbia** (increased carbon dioxide in the bloodstream) and related acidosis, even at rest.

The spine, ribs, breastbone, and muscles work together to pump air in and out the lungs (**ventilation**). Aging adversely affects ventilatory function. The muscles of the chest wall and the

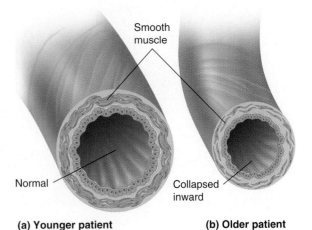

(a) Younger patient   (b) Older patient

Figure 2-3   **A.** Healthy muscle in the younger patient's airway helps maintain the open airway during the pressures of inhalation. **B.** Muscle weakening with age can lead to airway collapse that may produce wheezes.

diaphragm weaken with age. In addition, **kyphosis**, the exaggeration of the curvature of the upper spine, can further reduce the body's ability to compensate during respiratory distress.

The brain's processing of sensory input from the nervous system is the most often overlooked aspect of the respiratory system affected by age. **Chemoreceptors** located in the aortic arch sense carbon dioxide and oxygen concentrations in the blood and signal the brainstem to trigger each breath (▼ Figure 2-4). Aging produces a decrease in sensitivity in these receptors. Nerve impulse transmission from the brainstem through the phrenic nerve (which controls the diaphragm) and intercostal nerves slows, which can produce a sluggish response to signals from the chemoreceptors. This will produce a lowering of arterial oxygen concentration of approximately 1 mm Hg/year from

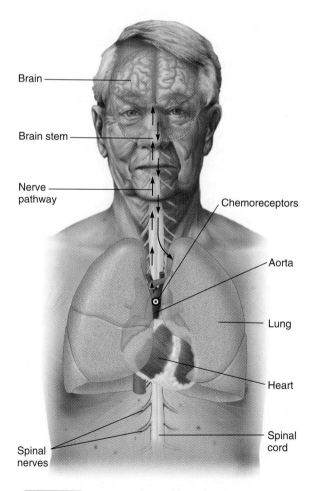

Brain

Brain stem

Nerve pathway

Chemoreceptors

Aorta

Lung

Heart

Spinal cord

Spinal nerves

Figure 2-4 Age-related deterioration of chemoreceptor sensitivity in the aortic arch and nerve signal transmission can slow signals to and from the brainstem that control ventilation.

age 65 to 80. A pulse oximetry reading of 93% to 95% may be normal because of these changes.

Cardiovascular System

Cardiac function declines with age consequent to anatomic and physiologic changes that are largely related to the high incidence of coronary disease caused by **atherosclerosis**. In this disorder, cholesterol and calcium build up inside the walls of the blood vessels, forming plaque. The accumulation of plaque eventually leads to partial or complete blockage of blood flow. Age-related changes typically include a decrease in heart rate, a fall in **cardiac output** (the amount of blood pumped out of the heart in one minute) secondary to lowered **stroke volume** (the amount of blood pumped out of the heart in one beat), and the inability to elevate cardiac output to match the demands of the body.

Arrhythmias, or irregular or abnormal heart rhythms, are common as aging alters the heart's electrical system. The number of cells in the sinoatrial (SA) node will decrease 90% by age 75. Because this is the origin of the normal heart beat, the loss hinders the heart's ability to produce a normal sinus rhythm. The SA and atrioventricular (AV) nodes both see a decline in pacemaker cells. Fibrosis and fatty deposits along the electrical pathway add to the risk of aberrancy. There is also a progressive loss of bundle branch fibers, leading to aberrant conduction syndromes. Common cardiac arrhythmias such as atrial fibrillation and junctional rhythms lack the coordinated filling of the ventricles by the atria, referred to as "atrial kick," which accounts for 30% of the total stroke volume. As the atria fibrillate, they pool small amounts of blood that can clot. If these clots flow into the system (embolize), they can plug up small vessels and cause ischemia to the tissues supplied by those vessels. Thus atrial fibrillation increases the risk of **pulmonary embolus** (a blood clot that breaks off from a large vein and travels to the blood vessels of the lung, causing obstruction of blood flow), myocardial infarction, infarction of the extremities, and strokes.

With age, the vascular system becomes stiff, resulting in increases in the systolic blood pressure. As the pressure of systole increases with age, the left ventricle works harder and becomes thicker, similar to what happens to a muscle when it is trained. The muscle also loses its elasticity in this process. The thickening and stiffening of this muscle decreases filling in the ventricle, thus decreasing the cardiac output. This stiffening also occurs in the heart valves, which may impede normal blood flow into and out of the heart. As the blood passes through these stiffened valves, a heart murmur may be heard, even in the absence of disease.

Older patients are prone to a 20 mm Hg drop in systolic blood pressure when moving from a sitting to a standing position. This is called **orthostatic hypotension**, or postural hypotension, and occurs because the **baroreceptors** in the aortic arch and carotid sinus become less sensitive to changes in blood volume. These receptors sense the change in blood pressures and send a signal to the adrenal glands to secrete hormones to alter blood pressure. The heart's response to epinephrine and norepinephrine decreases with age (▼ **Figure 2-5**). The aging heart takes longer to speed up and then return to normal when the adrenal glands secrete these hormones. The body is thus less able to compensate quickly for low perfusion states or rapid postural changes.

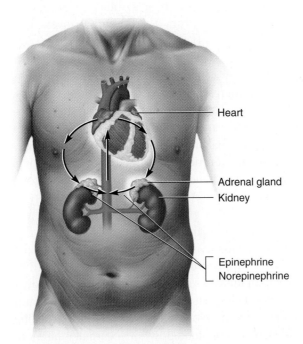

(**Figure 2-5**) As aging slows the heart's response to epinephrine and norepinephrine from the adrenal glands, it takes longer for the heart to speed up and then slow again in response to the demands of the body.

Blood vessels become stiff with age because of decreased elastin and collagen in the vessel walls. This reduces the peripheral vessels' elasticity by as much as 70%. Compensation for blood pressure changes will be hampered by the lessened distensibility and contractibility of the peripheral vessels.

Atherosclerotic disease affects more than 60% of people over age 65. The process begins in the early teens and progresses throughout life. The coronary vessels are most commonly associated with this disease. Atherosclerosis, however, presents problems throughout the circulatory system. Atherosclerosis, or narrowing of the blood vessels, means the vessel is unable to increase the supply of blood when there is an increased demand. Further, atherosclerosis can contribute to development of an **aneurysm**, or weakening and bulging of the blood vessel wall, with risk of rupture if subjected to high stretching forces.

Nervous System

Nervous system changes can result in the most debilitating of age-related ailments. The central and peripheral nervous systems see significant changes during life. The brain weight will shrink 10% to 20% by age 80. There is a selective loss of 5% to 50% of **neurons**—the cells that make up nerve tissue and receive and transmit impulses—and the remaining neurons shrink in size. The frontal lobe will lose up to 20% of its **synapses**, the junctions between neurons, throughout life. Motor and sensory neural networks become slower and less responsive. The metabolic rate in the older brain does not change, and oxygen consumption remains constant throughout life.

Sandwiched between the meninges that surround it, the brain takes up almost all of the space provided for it in the skull. Protection of the brain inside these membranes is provided by cerebrospinal fluid (CSF). Age-related shrinkage (**atrophy**) produces a void between the brain and the outermost layer. This provides room for the brain to move when stressed. The shrinkage also produces stretching of the bridging veins that return blood from inside the brain to the dura mater. If trauma moves the brain forcibly, the bridging veins can tear and bleed (▶ **Figure 2-6**). Bleeding can

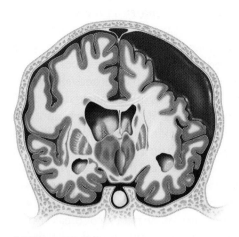
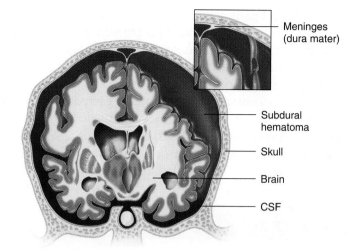

(a) Younger adult   **(b) Older adult**

Meninges (dura mater)
Subdural hematoma
Skull
Brain
CSF

Figure 2-6   Brain atrophy with age can make tearing of the bridging veins more likely with trauma, as well as creating a space into which bleeding can occur without producing immediate signs of increased intracranial pressure.

empty into this void, resulting in a **subdural hematoma**, and go unnoticed for some time. Increased intracranial pressure (ICP) is required in order for signs of head trauma to be present; the ICP will not rise, and thus its signs will not be present, until the void has been filled and pressurized.

Peripheral nerve function slows with aging. Sensation becomes diminished and misinterpreted. This makes for slow reflexes, a contributing cause of trauma. Nerve endings deteriorate, and the ability of the skin to sense the surroundings becomes hindered. Therefore, hot, cold, sharp, and wet items can all become dangerous because the body cannot sense them quickly enough. We rely on the sensation of pain to treat a patient's illness or injury. Pain from an injured area may not be felt in the affected tissue, but rather in the surrounding areas. This can alter the classical presentation of disease states. Pain from a cardiac event, such as angina, may present only as neck or jaw pain in the older person, and chest pain or pressure, which is normally associated with cardiac problems, may be absent or lessened. Some older patients may not experience any pain at all despite a cardiac problem.

Sensory Changes

Pupillary reaction and ocular movements become more restricted with age. The pupils are generally smaller in older patients, and opacity of the eye's lens lowers visual acuity and makes the pupils sluggish to respond to light. Visual distortions are also common in older people. Thickening of the lens makes it harder for the eye to focus, especially at close range. During eye exams in the field, upward gaze may be limited in many normal older patients because of degenerative changes in the elevator muscles. Peripheral fields of vision become narrower and there is a greater sensitivity to glare, which leads to a constricted visual field. These patients may become disoriented and anxious when they cannot adjust to the surroundings. Make every effort to allow the patient to wear eyeglasses and adjust the light to reduce this stress   ▼ **Figure 2-7** .

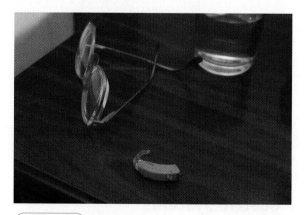

Figure 2-7   Ensuring that an older patient who has eyeglasses or a hearing aid is using it may reduce the patient's disorientation and stress, and will likely improve your communication with the patient during assessment.

Hearing loss is about four times more common than loss of vision. Older people often have the greatest loss at high frequencies. With age, changes in several structures of hearing produce loss of high-frequency hearing, or even deafness. If an older patient uses a hearing aid for everyday activity, it is best to keep it in place to provide for better communication and assessment—during your assessment, and for transport to the hospital where there will be further medical evaluation.

Attitude Tip

Avoid assumptions or thoughts like "They're just old—what do you expect?" or "He's supposed to be confused/demented/delirious—look at his age!" Always rule out medical problems (eg, head trauma, infection, metabolic problems, depression) before concluding that an older patient is demented.

Psychological Changes

Often, older adults find themselves dealing with medical illness, physical limitation, and social loss. Psychological problems of this age group often involve depression, anxiety, and adjustment disorders. These conditions are found quite commonly, but they are by no means a normal part of the changes that occur with aging. (Chapter 11 discusses these subjects in more detail.) Depression and anxiety can be associated with medical conditions such as heart disease or diabetes, and with medication use. These factors may contribute to excessive demanding and controlling behavior on the part of the older adult, and may cause family members or caregivers to be resistant, frustrated, or angry, making the situation more difficult to handle.

Renal, Hepatic, and Gastric Systems

In the kidneys, both structural and functional changes occur. Their filtration function, for example, falls an average of 50% between the ages of 20 and 90. Kidney mass decreases by 20% and there is a loss of **nephrons**, the basic filtering units in the kidneys, between the ages of 30 and 80. Aging kidneys respond less efficiently to stress relating to the circulation of blood, or **hemodynamic** stress, and to fluid and electrolyte imbalances. Many drugs are eliminated by renal excretion, including some used in common cardiac conditions (digoxin, procainamide, disopyramide) and psychiatric disorders (lithium), as well as most antibiotics. Thus, underlying renal dysfunction is the cause of many drug interactions and problems in older patients.

The liver's use of enzymes to break drugs down into more water-soluble compounds, or **hepatic metabolism**, diminishes with age for two reasons: hepatic blood flow decreases, and the production and function of metabolic enzymes decline. In addition, environmental stresses—such as tobacco smoke, alcohol, and drugs—hinder the liver's ability to produce metabolizing enzymes. The body uses these enzymes to metabolize drugs into more water-soluble compounds, making it possible to use and dispose of these drugs ▼ **Figure 2-8**). Impaired liver enzyme activity or impaired blood flow to the liver results in accumulation of the drug at higher, possibly toxic, levels.

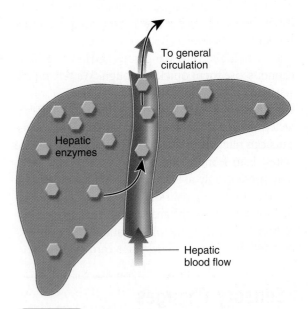

Figure 2-8 The ability of the liver to break some medications down into forms the body can use and dispose of depends on hepatic blood flow and on production and functioning of metabolizing enzymes. Both diminish with age.

Changes in gastric and intestinal function may inhibit nutritional intake and utilization. Taste bud sensitivity to salty and sweet sensation decreases. Saliva secretion decreases, which lowers the body's ability to process complex carbohydrates. Gastric motility slows with age because of the loss of intestinal tract neurons. This can lead many patients to feel constipated or not hungry. There is a decrease in the gastric acid secretion. Blood flow in the **mesenteries**, or membranes that connect organs to the abdominal wall, may drop by as much as 50%, decreasing the ability to extract nutrients from the intestines. Gallstones are increasingly common with age, and anal sphincter changes reduce elasticity and can produce fecal incontinence.

The condition of the oral cavity has important implications for eating. Loose-fitting dentures can cause pain when chewing. When combined with gastrointestinal changes, the patient may experience poor oral intake and loss of appetite, leading to weight loss and loss of body protein stores. This form of malnutrition may affect medications that are protein bound, such as warfarin or phenytoin. Changes in gastric function may alter absorption of medications administered orally. For these reasons, medications may pass through the GI tract without being completely absorbed, or may be stored and accumulated, leading to increased medication levels and actions.

Medication Tip

Malnutrition and renal, hepatic, and gastrointestinal changes can cause medications either not to be absorbed properly, or to accumulate in the body at abnormally high levels.

Musculoskeletal System

Changes in physical abilities can affect older adults' confidence in their mobility. The muscle system atrophies and weakens with age. Muscle fibers become smaller and fewer, motor neurons decline in number, and strength declines, but most older people maintain the ability to carry out daily activities. The ligaments and cartilage of the joints lose their elasticity. Cartilage also goes through degenerative changes with aging, contributing to arthritis.

Muscle mass decreases over time and is replaced by fat. This increase in fat also alters the body's capacity to use some drugs. Diazepam, for instance, is distributed in the patient's fat. The more fat, the greater the spread of the drug and the lower the concentration, but the longer it is stored in the body. Alcohol is distributed in lean tissue. Because there is less lean tissue in older adults, the blood level rises more quickly.

The stooped posture of older people comes from atrophy of the supporting structures of the body. Two out of three older patients will show some degree of kyphosis, commonly called "humpback," "hunchback," or "Potts curvature" (▼ **Figure 2-9**). Lost height in older adults generally results from compression in the spinal column, first in the disks and then from the process of **osteoporosis** in the vertebral bodies. (Osteoporosis is the generalized loss of bone mass caused when bone reabsorption exceeds new bone production.) This change in shape affects how older patients are positioned for opening airways and spinal immobilization.

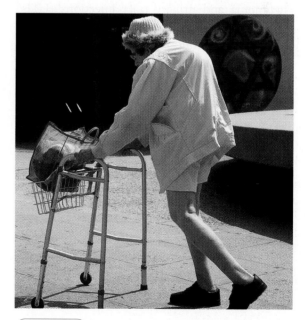

Figure 2-9   Kyphosis, seen to some degree in two thirds of older adults, affects how you should position the patient when you open the airway or immobilize the spine.

CASE STUDY 2

After completing your shift, you stop at your grandfather's apartment on the way home to see how he is doing. You notice that he appears to be having some trouble getting around. He says that it is just arthritis and jokingly tells you not to get old.

Will every older person experience the effects of arthritis?

Can these aches and pains be a sign of something more serious?

Osteoporosis occurs as the skeleton ages. Postmenopausal osteoporosis is by far the most common form. Clinically significant postmenopausal osteoporosis, present in one third of older women, is the basic cause of vertebral body collapse, hip fractures, and forearm fractures in this group.

Immune System

Because they are more prone to infection and less able to fight it, older patients often present with some type of infection. Systemic and cellular immune responses become less effective. Pneumonia and urinary tract infections (UTIs) are common in bed-bound patients. There is also an increase in abnormal immune system substances in the aging body, which has been correlated with an increased incidence of infection.

Summary

From birth to old age, the body undergoes many changes. As we get older, these changes alter the ways that the body can compensate for the stress of illness or injury. It is important to understand the physiology of normal aging in order to anticipate an older person's response to changing conditions. Activities that were done easily as a younger person may become more difficult or impossible, requiring additional help or changes in the task. Physical changes take place in every system of the body. Different communication methods must often be used to compensate for sensory deterioration. Physical and psychological changes require the EMS provider to be able to assess and differentiate complicated medical conditions. Treatment choices may require changes to match the aging body's decreased responses.

Attitude Tip

Remember that "growing old does not mean becoming worthless and waiting for death," but that "growing old is simply a process that all living things begin on the day they are born." [1]

Case Study Summaries

CASE STUDY 1 SUMMARY

An increasing blood pressure is normal during the aging process. However, there are many factors involved in evaluating blood pressure. Your answer should be based on your system's programmed response (that may be to just give the numbers and not to advise) or to have her follow up with her personal physician. Because blood pressure is made from a combination of cardiac output and systemic vascular resistance, issues related to hypertension can affect multiple areas within the body. Common organs affected by hypertension include the heart, lungs, kidneys, brain, and the vessels throughout the body.

CASE STUDY 2 SUMMARY

Not every person will experience the pain of arthritis. During the aging process, pain in the joints can be a sign of arthritis, muscle fatigue, swelling from any number of causes, or referred pain from something more serious. Often, older people do not feel chest pain from cardiac muscle ischemia or infarction. The first clue may be an ache in the neck, back, or arm. Older patients often misinterpret these signs for something much less serious.

Endnotes

1. Garbin E Jr. Ageism in Modern Society. 1998; May 11. Online at http://www.eng.udf.edu/~garbin/ageism.htm.

Bibliography

Bosker G, editor-in-chief. *Geriatric Emergency Medicine*. St. Louis: Mosby; 1990.

Cassel CK, ed. *Geriatric Medicine*. 2nd ed. New York: Springer-Verlag; 1990.

Cotman CW. Stealing time: Precious memory [online article]. June 10, 1999. Available at: http://www.pbs.org/stealingtime/living/memory.htm

Duthie EH, Katz PR, eds. *Practice of Geriatrics*. 3rd ed. Philadelphia: WB Saunders; 1998.

Freeman JT. *Aging's History and Literature*. New York: Human Sciences Press; 1979.

Judd RL, Warner CG, Shaffer MA. *Geriatric Emergencies*. Rockville, MD: Aspen Publishers; 1986.

Lonergan, ET, ed. *Geriatrics*. Stamford, CT: Appleton & Lange; 1996.

Masoro EJ, Bertrand H, Liepa G, Yu BP. Analysis and exploration of age-related changes in mammalian structure and function. *Fed Proc.* 1979; 38(6):1956-1960.

MEDLINEplus Medical Encyclopedia. Aging changes in skin [online article]. May 29, 2002. Available at: http://www.nlm.nih.gov/medlineplus/ency/article/004014.htm

The Merck Manual of Geriatrics [online]. March 7, 1999. Available at: http://www.merck.com/pubs/mm_geriatrics

Sanders AB, [ed]. *Emergency Care of the Elder Person*. Beverly Cracom Publications; 1996.

Schrier RW, [ed]. *Geriatric Medicine*. Philadelphia: WB Saunders; 1990.

Vreeken A, Hall BL. Emergency care and the geriatric population. *Emergency Care Quarterly*. 1990;6(1): 27-34.

Walshe TM. *Manual of Clinical Problems in Geriatric Medicine*. Boston: Little Brown; 1985.

Communicating with Older People and Their Caregivers

LEARNING OBJECTIVES

1 Discuss and recognize communication challenges in the older person, including visual, hearing, and speech.

2 Describe principles that should be employed when assessing and communicating with an older patient.

3 Describe communication strategies used to provide psychological support.

4 Recognize the emotional need for independence in older people.

5 Recognize and appreciate the physical and emotional difficulties associated with being a caregiver of an impaired older person.

6 Demonstrate appropriate attitudes toward all members of the health care community.

CHAPTER 3

Barbara Dodge, BA, NREMT

David R. Snyder, MA, NREMT-P

CASE STUDY 1

At 2:00 a.m., you are dispatched for a patient injured in a fall. You arrive at the home in a BLS ambulance and find a 78-year-old woman lying on the floor by her bed. Her husband states that she was on her way to the bathroom when she fell. He was unable to pick her up, so he called 9-1-1. He tells you that he thinks she has hurt her hip. The patient is facing away from you, on the floor between the bed and the wall. Though you were speaking to her as you approached, she was startled when you touched her. She doesn't answer until you raise your voice.

How should you communicate with this patient?

What questions should you ask her husband?

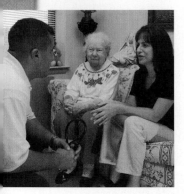

Communication and the Older Adult

Education, training, and experience are the foundations for successful assessment and treatment of any patient. The key to making your knowledge work for you and your patient is **communication**. Communication allows us to receive information that keeps us alive and healthy. For older people, the ability to communicate is crucial to living effectively in new or changing environments. For the healthy older person, communication may be the central skill in negotiating the right to remain independent. For older people with disabilities, communication is important to maintain in order to prevent further deterioration, isolation, and dependence.

Older people have a greater need for good human relations than younger adults. Older people need ties to family and to friends to counterbalance the forces of aging. Good communication skills will help you to gain more information in your assessment. When your patients trust you, it is easier for them to explain the problem and answer your questions. With trust, the patient is more willing to listen to you and work with you. Without good communication skills, you could frighten, alienate, insult, anger, or perhaps even harm your patients. No matter how difficult the situation, EMS providers can find effective ways to enhance communication with older patients, and thus make the patient care experience a positive one.

Communication is not just talking; it is also listening. Your first communication sets the tone with your patient. How you speak may enhance or detract from what you say.

As an EMS provider, when you step onto a scene to care for an older patient, you are being asked to take control. People called you because

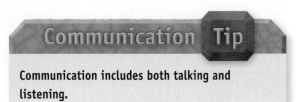

Communication Tip

Communication includes both talking and listening.

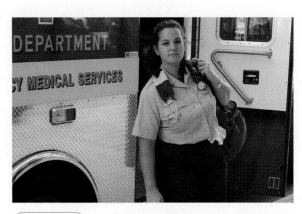

Figure 3-1   It is important that you present yourself as competent, confident, and concerned.

they needed help. Whether that call was for emergent or nonemergent care, they called you to do something they could not do themselves. What you say and how you say it can determine the success or failure of the call.

It is important, from the very beginning, that you present yourself as competent, confident, and concerned (▲ **Figure 3-1**). You must take charge of the situation, but do so with compassion. You are there to listen, then act on what you learn.

Attitude Tip

Be patient when interviewing older people, recognizing physical, intellectual, and psychosocial barriers that slow or interfere with effective communication.

Age-related Communication Changes

Communication disorders constitute the nation's number one handicapping disability. Studies indicate that more people suffer from hearing, speech, and language impairment than from heart disease, venereal disease, paralysis, epilepsy, blindness, cerebral palsy, tuberculosis, muscular dystrophy, and multiple sclerosis combined. Conditions such as stroke, cancer, degenerative neurological diseases, and trauma can affect the older person's ability to communicate. The aging process brings about changes in vision, hearing, taste, smell, and touch. Also, there are changes in communication abilities that accompany aging, dementia, and other diseases. Advanced age can make a person's voice tremulous, weak, hoarse, and higher or lower pitched than it was in middle age. Older people may say, "My voice tires." These symptoms may be bothersome, but they are considered a normal consequence of aging (in the absence of any clinical conditions that might be causing them).

The sections that follow discuss those changes that primarily affect patient and provider interactions.

Types of Communication Skills

Verbal and Nonverbal Communication

Of the two types of communication, nonverbal communication is just as important as the verbal type. **Verbal communication** includes words and the volume, pitch, inflection, and tone of the voice. **Nonverbal communication** includes eye contact, hand gestures, body position, facial expressions, and touch. Touch can be important to the seriously ill or confused older patient. Touch can often calm and reassure, and can increase attention and nonverbal communication in the confused older person. Take the older patient by the hand, or touch the patient on the arm. Be aware, however, that some patients prefer not to be touched. Cultural belief may prohibit touching as well. Some older female patients may feel uncomfortable when touched by a male EMS provider. EMS providers should respect a patient's wishes not to be touched.

Be sure that your words, facial expressions, and body language are consistent with each other. Patients can sense inconsistencies and insincerity, which will undermine the trust you are trying to establish.

Listening

Listening is a vital communication skill. When asking questions of older people, be sure to wait for their answers. They may need a little more time to process your question, and may speak

slowly when responding (▼ **Figure 3-2**). Unless the need to treat and move is urgent, take time to listen patiently for answers to your questions. Make sure your patients can hear and understand you. Check comprehension by asking the patient to demonstrate that he or she has understood you, by stating, "In your own words, tell me what you understood from what I just told you," or other similar queries. Often this brings to light misunderstandings or hearing problems that the patient was too embarrassed to mention. Effective listening allows the EMS provider the opportunity to comfort and calm the patient if the patient's tone conveys fear or confusion.

Attitude Tip

Take adequate time to listen and talk with your stable older patients. Don't limit your assessment to the obvious problem. Oftentimes, older patients who express that they are not well or who are overly concerned about their health or general condition are at risk for a serious decline in their physical, emotional, or psychological state!

EMS providers also need to listen to more than just the words of the patients. Listen to the way they say the words. Their tone may convey fear or confusion. They may be afraid to tell you the truth about their situation. Listen and look around. Be aware of the surroundings. If you suspect abuse, you may want to interview the patient

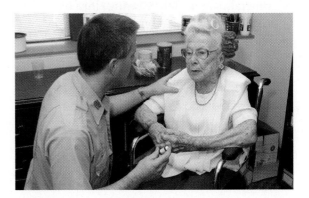

Figure 3-2 Older patients may need a little more time to process your question and may speak slowly when responding.

separately from the caregiver. Elder abuse and neglect are discussed in Chapter 14.

> **Communication Tip**
>
> Pay attention to both the verbal and nonverbal communication of your patients. You will receive better information about their condition if you listen to more than just their words.

Communication Techniques

Your first words can gain the patient's trust. Speak respectfully when you introduce yourself. If you know the patient's name, use it: "Mrs. Johnson, my name is Barb. I am an EMS provider and I am here to help you." Older people may be insulted if you use their first name. Don't take that chance. If they suggest that you call them by their first name, it is fine to do so. If you do not know their name, use "Sir" or "Ma'am." Do not use "Hon," "Dearie," or "Grandma." Use short words, and ask only one question at a time.

> **Attitude Tip**
>
> Call a patient by first name only if the patient suggests it. Using the full name shows respect.

In general, when interviewing the older patient, the following techniques should be employed[1]:

♦ Identify yourself. Do not assume the older patient knows who you are.

♦ Be aware of how you present yourself. Frustration and impatience can be portrayed through body language.

♦ Look directly at the patient.

♦ Speak slowly and distinctly.

♦ Explain what you are going to do before you do it. Use simple terms to explain the use of medical equipment and procedures, avoiding medical jargon or slang.

♦ Listen to the answer the patient gives you.

♦ Show the patient respect. Never use the patient's first name without his or her permission. Refer to the patient as Mr., Mrs., or Miss.

♦ Do not assume that all older patients are hard of hearing. Ask the patient if he or she can hear you, and double check by asking him or her to tell you his or her understanding of what you just said.

♦ Do not talk about the patient in front of him or her; to do so gives the impression that the patient has no say in any decision making. This is easy to forget when the patient has impaired cognitive (thought) processes or has difficulty communicating.

♦ Be patient.

As is true in patients of any age, older patients have more difficulty communicating clearly when they are stressed by an emergency or personal crisis. The National Victim Center has identified several useful techniques for communicating with older adults in stress situations (▶ **Table 3-1**).[2]

Communication Challenges

The first source of information is obviously the patient. However, in some cases, the patient may not be able to provide complete or accurate information about his or her injury or illness. You may need to consult a caregiver or bystander.

It is important to be sure that your patients can understand you and that you understand them. Older patients may have some significant challenges to communication, such as problems with vision or hearing, speaking difficulties, language or cultural barriers, and underlying fears. The next sections discuss each challenge in more detail.

Vision Impairments

Diseases of the eye, such as cataracts, glaucoma, **macular degeneration** (deterioration of the cen-

TABLE 3-1   Techniques for Communicating with Older Patients in Stress Situations

- ◆ Do not assume that an older adult has a sensory or cognitive impairment; be sensitive to the individual's particular needs.

- ◆ If possible and applicable, choose an environment that encourages communication (▼ **Figure 3-3**). Eliminate factors that interfere with effective listening, such as the television or radio, and minimize any distractions. This may involve moving the patient to the ambulance where one-on-one interaction can take place.

- ◆ If the patient's story appears rehearsed, be aware that the patient could be experiencing abuse.

- ◆ If the patient appears fearful while relating facts, listen carefully. Ask further questions. There could be several different underlying reasons for their fears. Additionally, the older person in crisis may not readily volunteer information.

- ◆ Try to position the patient so light is not shining in his or her eyes.

- ◆ Position yourself about an arm's length away from the patient. Sit or stand facing the patient at the patient's eye level, so that your eyes and mouth are clearly visible. Be sure you have the patient's attention before speaking.

- ◆ Keep interactions short and simple.

- ◆ Have one provider conduct the interview, rather than multiple providers asking different questions.

- ◆ Keep your voice and mannerisms calm.

- ◆ Do not shout. If necessary, speak slightly louder without shouting or yelling. (Extremely loud tones are not heard as well as normal tones by people with hearing aids.)

- ◆ Show a willingness to listen through effective nonverbal communication. Be attentive.

- ◆ Ask questions to clarify confusion, but ask only one question at a time. Wait for a response to one question before asking another.

- ◆ Allow time for hearing and comprehending.

- ◆ Be especially sensitive to the patient who is tired and not feeling well. Tired or ill people are less able to understand or remember what is asked or said.

- ◆ Observe closely for nonverbal clues to see that the patient has understood you. (For example, are you receiving a blank stare, or are the patient's eyes squinting?)

- ◆ If the patient misunderstands, rephrase the question rather than repeating the same words.

- ◆ Don't interrupt. It discourages free speaking, and the interruption may cause the patient to forget what he or she was going to say.

Source: National Center for Victims of Crime.

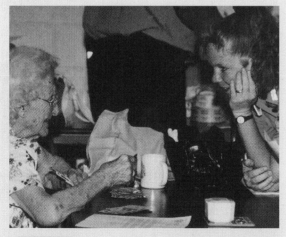

Figure 3-3   Try to find a quiet environment that encourages communication.

tral portion of the retina), and visual problems secondary to stroke or diabetes are more common in the older population. Fifteen percent of all adults over the age of 65 have serious visual impairments. Any time you are called to an older patient who is not wearing glasses, you should ask if he or she has glasses. If the patient says yes, ask where the glasses are kept and if you can get them. Carefully help the patient put the glasses on. If there is a glasses case, remember to put it in his or her bag or purse for transport.

The EMS provider should be aware of visual changes when assessing and transferring patients. Particularly when transferring the patient, make sure to support the patient to prevent the patient from falling.

If the patient is blind, be sure to tell him or her everything you are doing. You may need to put his or her hand on your stethoscope and cuff to show what equipment you are using (▼ Figure 3-4). Do not assume that a patient who is blind is also deaf.

Communication Tip

For patients who have some degree of hearing loss, don't yell! Lean closer to them and speak into their ear. Also remember that those with limited vision are *not* necessarily hard of hearing.

Hearing Impairments

Hearing loss is the most common communication disorder in the older population, and is the third most prevalent chronic condition in this group. About 28 million people in the United States have some degree of hearing difficulty. Of this number, 80% have irreversible hearing loss. Of the population over the age of 65, 54% have hearing loss.

Hearing loss as a result of aging is called **presbycusis**. Presbycusis is progressive in nature with high-frequency sounds being affected first. Although the process begins after age 20, it is often between ages 55 and 65 that high-frequency sounds are affected.

If your patient does not respond to your verbal questions, try speaking more loudly. Position yourself approximately 18 inches directly in front of the patient. People who are hearing impaired have probably learned to use body language, such as hand gestures and lip reading. Also, hearing-impaired patients have more difficulty hearing higher-frequency sounds. Thus, a lower-pitched voice may be easier to hear than a higher-pitched voice. If your patient seems to be having difficulty hearing you, don't just speak louder; try lowering the pitch of your voice.

Ask if your patient has a hearing aid. If not, you could facilitate hearing by the "reverse stethoscope" technique: Put the ear pieces of your stethoscope in the patient's ears and speak softly into the diaphragm of the stethoscope (▼ Figure 3-5). This will amplify your voice. (▶ Table 3-2) offers more ideas on communicating with hearing-impaired patients.

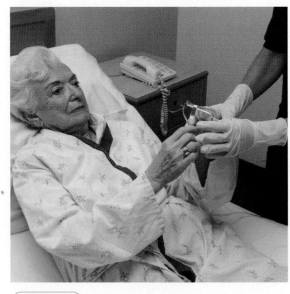

Figure 3-4   If your patient is blind, you may want to have him or her touch the equipment you are using.

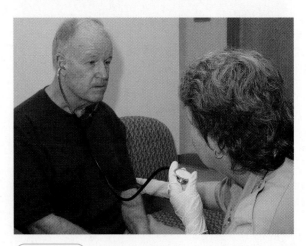

Figure 3-5   If a hearing-impaired patient does not have a hearing aid, you can amplify your voice with a "reverse stethoscope" technique.

TABLE 3-2 Tips for Communicating with Hearing-Impaired Patients

1. Ask if the patient has a hearing aid and would like to use it.	7. Speak *slightly* louder than normal, but do not shout. Use a lower pitch.
2. Stand at a distance of approximately 18 inches from the patient.	8. Always face the hearing-impaired patient, and let your facial expression reflect your meaning.
3. Reduce background noise, such as television or radio.	9. Never speak from another room or out of the sight of a hearing-impaired patient.
4. Arrange to have light on your face, not behind you, if possible.	10. Use short sentences.
5. Position yourself at the visual level of the listener.	11. Rephrase misunderstood sentences.
6. Speak at a natural rate, unless you see signs of incomprehension.	12. Remember that the hearing-impaired person will not hear and understand as well when tired or sick.

Hearing Aids

Basics

A hearing aid is essentially a device that makes sound louder. Hearing aids cannot restore hearing to normal, just as glasses cannot cure vision problems. Hearing aids provide a benefit in that they improve hearing and listening ability, which ultimately improves the quality of life.

Types of Hearing Aids

Your patient's hearing aid will be one of these types (▼ **Figure 3-6**):

♦ *In-the-canal* and *completely-in-the-canal:* These hearing aids are contained in a tiny case that fits partly or completely into the ear canal.

♦ *In-the-ear:* All parts of the hearing aid are contained in a shell that fits in the outer part of the ear. This type of hearing aid is generally larger than the canal-type hearing aids.

♦ *Behind-the-ear:* All parts of this hearing aid are contained in a small plastic case that rests behind the ear. The case is connected to an ear-mold by a piece of clear tubing.

♦ *Conventional body type:* This type of hearing aid is an older style that is generally worn by people with profound hearing loss. It is usually worn on the chest, either in a shirt or coat pocket or in a harness. The microphone, amplifier, and battery are contained within the case of the hearing aid. A cord carries the electrical signal to the receiver, which is attached to the ear-mold placed in the external ear.

Special Features

Many hearing aids have optional features that can be built in to assist in different communication situations. Two of the more common options are directional microphones and telephone switches.

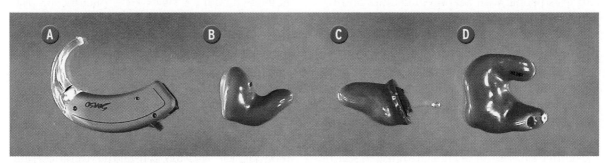

Figure 3-6 Different types of hearing aids. **A.** Behind-the-ear type. **B.** Conventional body type. **C.** In-the-canal type. **D.** In-the-ear type.

Some hearing aids have a switch to activate a microphone that responds to sound coming from a specific direction, as occurs in face-to-face conversation. This changes from the normal nondirectional mode (picks up sound almost equally from any direction) to focus on sound coming from the area in front of the person; sound coming from behind is reduced. A telephone switch changes from the normal microphone to a setting that eliminates environmental noise; the person can only pick up sounds from the telephone in this mode of operation.

Helping with Hearing Aids

If the patient has a hearing aid, ask if you can assist with inserting it. Use hand gestures to signify putting a hearing aid in your ear. If the patient says yes, ask where they are and assist the patient in putting the hearing aids in. Hearing aids are often kept in a small box or case. The box may be the size of a small cellular phone, or as large as a 4- by 5-inch gift box.

When you find the hearing aid, check to see if the batteries are in. Often, hearing aid users disconnect the batteries when the aids are not needed, to prolong the life of the batteries. If the back of the hearing aid is open and the battery is in the little "door," just snap the door closed. If the battery is loose in the box, you will need to insert it into the hearing aid. Some hearing aids have a preset volume; others will need to be turned on and the volume set. If you have to turn it on, be sure to set the volume at midrange. It can always be adjusted later, but you don't want to scare the patient with a loud burst of sound. The hearing aid with the red dot always goes in the right ear. Remember: Red-Right.

There are a few basic things you can do to solve hearing aid problems (▶ **Table 3-3**). If necessary, assist the patient with contacting an **audiologist** (a health care professional who evaluates and tests people with hearing difficulties and rehabilitates those whose impaired hearing cannot be improved medically or surgically). If the patient is transported to the emergency department, find out if an audiologist is available to see the patient in the hospital and evaluate the hearing aid.

To insert the hearing aid, follow the natural shape of the ear. It needs to fit snugly without forcing. If you hear a whistling sound, it could mean that the hearing aid is not in far enough to create a seal, or that the volume is up too loud. Try repositioning it,

or remove it and turn the volume down. If you can't get the hearing aid in with two tries, put it in the box and take it with you. Be sure to document the transport and transfer of hearing aids to hospital personnel. Never try to clean hearing aids, and never get them wet! Water will damage a hearing aid. However, the mold can be cleaned if separated from the rest of the hearing aid.

Speech Impairment

Physiological Causes

For many older people, it is difficult to produce speech that is loud enough, clear, and well spaced. Weakness, paralysis, poor hearing, or brain damage can damage the delicate functions that make these abilities possible.

Dentures

Although dentures may not be thought of as a communication concern, they do help the person who wears them to communicate. Without dentures, a patient's speech may be slurred or mumbled. He or she may be embarrassed to try to talk. Ask if your patient wears dentures. If the answer is yes, offer to get them. Usually the dentures will be in the bathroom or on a bedside stand. Remember that dentures kept in a soaking solution need to be rinsed before inserting.

Ask if the patient can put the dentures in. If the patient can insert the dentures, you should hand him or her the top plate first, just the way it would fit in the mouth (▶ **Figure 3-7**). After the top plate is inserted, hand the patient the bottom denture in the same manner. If the patient cannot insert the dentures and wants you to, insert the top plate first, holding it securely with your thumb. Then lay the bottom denture carefully along the bottom ridge. Ask the patient if the dentures are comfortable.

For patients who are wearing dentures and require transportation in the supine position, monitor the airway constantly. Dentures can come loose and create an airway obstruction.

TABLE 3-3   Troubleshooting Problems with Hearing Aids

If the hearing aid will not work at all:

♦ Be sure the hearing aid is turned on.

♦ Try a fresh battery.

♦ Check the tubing to make sure it is not twisted or bent.

♦ Check the switch to make sure it is on M (microphone), not T (telephone).

♦ Try a spare cord (for a body aid). The old cord may be broken or shorted.

♦ Check the ear mold to make sure it is not plugged with wax.

If sound from the hearing aid is weaker than usual:

♦ Try a fresh battery.

♦ Check tubing for bends and ear mold for wax or dirt.

♦ If the hearing aid has been exposed to extreme cold, it may not work until it is at room temperature.

♦ There may be excessive wax in the ear. The patient should consult the physician.

If the hearing aid goes on and off or sounds scratchy:

♦ Work the switches and dials back and forth, as lint or dust will interfere with electrical contacts.

♦ On body hearing aids, try changing cords.

If the hearing aid whistles continuously:

♦ A new ear mold or new tubing may be needed. The patient should see the audiologist.

Additional things that can be done include the following:

♦ If excessive dirt or wax collects on the mold, it can be washed in warm water using mild soap. *The mold must be removed from the hearing aid prior to washing.* Never allow the hearing aid to become wet; however, the mold can be washed if removed from the hearing aid. Wipe excess water from the mold, blow to clear any moisture from the tube, and allow the hearing aid to dry overnight.

♦ Discard any batteries that appear to be leaking. Clean the battery case.

Hearing aids must be handled with care. Here are things to avoid:

♦ Never attempt to remove wax from any opening of an in-the-ear hearing aid.

♦ Never expose a hearing aid to excessive heat.

♦ Never allow a hearing aid to become wet. Should a hearing aid become wet:

Remove the batteries at once.

Wipe the exterior of the case with a dry absorbent cloth.

Place the hearing aid in a warm place. The low heat setting of a hair dryer can be used for drying.

♦ Never take a hearing aid apart to examine the insides. This may void warranties.

♦ Do not wash the ear mold in alcohol, acetone, cleaning fluid, or extremely hot water. The use of chemicals may dissolve the plastic material of the ear mold. Hot water may soften the plastic and allow the ear mold to change shape.

For older trauma patients with hearing aids, where there is a possibility that the hearing aid could become dislodged or blood soaked, remove the hearing aid, place it in a plastic bag, and transport it with the patient to ensure that the hearing aid is not damaged or lost.

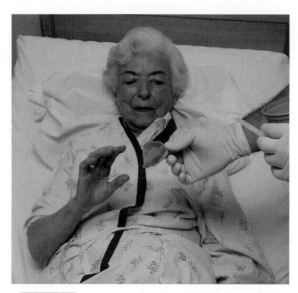

Figure 3-7 Hand dentures to a patient the way the dentures would fit in the mouth, with the top plate first.

Aphasia

Aphasia is an impairment of language that affects the production or understanding of speech and the ability to read or write. Aphasia is always due to injury to the brain, most commonly from a stroke. Aphasia can range from being very mild to making communication with the patient almost impossible. Aphasia may affect mainly a single aspect of language use, such as the ability to recall the names of objects, to put words into sentences, or to read. There are several types of aphasia, which are listed in ▶ **Table 3-4**. Approximately one million people in the United States are affected by aphasia. ▶ **Table 3-5** lists ideas to help you communicate with an aphasic patient.

Dementia

Dementia affects the patient's ability to communicate. Language difficulties common in dementia patients affect the ability to name things or say what they want to say. In fact, this is an early indication of the disease. Other characteristics of patients with dementia include an appearance of frustration, withdrawal, suspiciousness, paranoia, delusions, hallucinations, irritability, and restlessness—all of which affect the communication process.

Dementia patients also become very concrete or literal; they can no longer think in abstractions. There is also a delayed reaction time in conversation. Those with dementia may forget what was just said to them, or what they were in the middle of saying. As the disease progresses, language difficulties become more severe. Symptoms may also worsen in the evening. ▶ **Table 3-6** offers ideas on how to communicate with patients with dementia. (Dementia as a clinical condition is covered in detail in Chapter 11.)

Other Disorders Affecting Communication

Apraxia

Apraxia is an impairment in carrying out purposeful movements. Commonly, patients with apraxia will show you something in their wallet, or lead you to show you something, but this is the extent of their nonverbal communication. These patients are unable to perform common expressive gestures on request (such as waving good-bye). Apraxia may also primarily affect oral, non-

TABLE 3-4	Types of Aphasia
◆ **Global aphasia:** The most severe form of aphasia; may be seen immediately after the patient has suffered a stroke, and may improve rapidly if the damage has not been too extensive. The patient with global aphasia is the most difficult to communicate with, because they can produce few recognizable words and understand little or no spoken language.
◆ **Broca's aphasia:** Often referred to as nonfluent aphasia because speech output is severely reduced to short sentences of less than four words. Vocabulary is limited, and the formulation of sounds is often laborious and clumsy for the patient.
◆ **Wernicke's aphasia:** Often referred to as fluent aphasia because speech output is not affected, while comprehension is affected. Patients with Wernicke's aphasia tend to produce sentences incorporating irrelevant words.
◆ **Anomic aphasia:** Applied to patients who have a persistent inability to find specific words in their vocabularies. However, patients with anomic aphasia understand speech well.

TABLE 3-5   Communicating with an Aphasic Patient

1. Ask the family member or caretaker if the patient has difficulty with listening or talking. If the difficulty is with listening, use an environmental "show me" approach. If the difficulty is with talking, use multiple-choice questions.

2. Talk to the patient with aphasia as an adult, and not as a child. Avoid talking down to the patient.

3. Avoid open-ended questions. Use focused questions instead.

4. During conversation, minimize background noise.

5. Make sure you have the patient's attention before communicating.

6. Praise all attempts to speak. Encourage the use of all modes of communication.

7. Give the patient time to talk, and a reasonable amount of time to respond. If the patient takes too long to answer, ask the patient to repeat the question to see if he or she comprehended it. Accept all communication attempts (speech, writing, gesture) rather than demanding speech. Avoid insisting that each word be produced perfectly.

8. Keep your own communication simple, but adult. Simplify sentence structure and reduce your own rate of speech. Keep your voice at a normal volume and emphasize key words.

9. Augment speech with gestures and visual aids whenever possible. Repeat a statement when necessary.

TABLE 3-6   Communicating with the Dementia Patient

1. Use clear, concrete, familiar language.

2. Convey only one idea at a time, speaking simply and not too fast.

3. Do not use medical jargon.

4. Use short sentences. If the patient does not understand, repeat exactly what was just said. This allows time for the patient's brain to process the information. If the words are varied, this requires greater effort from the patient. If the patient still cannot understand, repeat using different words.

5. Accompany your words with gestures.

6. If the patient is frightened or distracted, it may help to touch the patient gently on the arm to maintain his or her attention and convey concern (▶ **Figure 3-8**).

7. If the patient tries to answer, but loses the train of thought, repeat back the last few words the patient said as a reminder.

8. Do not give lengthy explanations as to why something is being done; the patient may not understand.

9. Use nouns instead of pronouns. The patient with dementia may lose track of whom the pronouns are referring to. Don't say, "Your husband is here, may I ask him some questions about you?" Instead, say, "Your husband is here, may I ask your husband some questions about you?"

10. Avoid using the word "don't." Dementia patients sometimes cannot understand this commonly used contraction.

speech movements, such as pretending to blow out a candle. Apraxia can manifest as a speech impairment, with the inability to produce speech with the correct rhythm and timing. The speech of a person with apraxia is characterized by highly inconsistent errors.

People with severe apraxia are usually limited in explaining themselves by pantomime or gesture, except for expressions of emotion. Apraxia may even prevent the patient from being able to manipulate objects.

Dysarthria

<u>Dysarthria</u> refers to a group of speech disorders resulting from weakness, slowness, or uncoordination of the speech mechanism due to damage to the nervous system. Dysarthria is a disorder of speech production, not language. Unlike apraxia

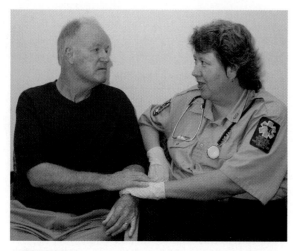

Figure 3-8 It may be useful to touch an older patient who is anxious or confused.

of speech, the speech errors that occur in dysarthria are highly consistent from one occasion to the next.

Parkinson's Disease

In patients with Parkinson's disease, there may be decreased facial expression. Also, the mouth may become soft and speech may become monotonal.

> **Attitude Tip**
>
> To improve the communication among (and care provided by) members of the interdisciplinary team, actively participate in seminars, workshops, and other continuing education programs attended by providers from the various disciplines responsible for the out-of-hospital care of older patients. Professional relationships can be strengthened, and standard protocols reviewed and shared.

Underlying Fears

The patient may have concerns that lead to decreased communication. Being aware of common fears will help you communicate in a caring and compassionate manner. It is natural for older people to want to stay in their own homes or in a home-type situation as long as possible. Some may stay longer than is safe for them because they do not want to give up their independence, cannot afford other care, or do not realize that their condition has deteriorated beyond the point where they can safely care for themselves. It is important that EMS providers be respectful of older patients' need for independence and the emotional attachment they may have for their homes. Older patients may fear that when they leave their home to go in an ambulance, they will be moved to a nursing home or even worse, never leave the hospital.

With this in mind, there are a few steps that you can take to make the patient more comfortable. If the patient seems fearful, ask specifically what he or she is nervous about; simply vocalizing these concerns may help this patient establish a sense of trust in your care. Your patient could also be concerned about a longtime companion; **separation anxiety**, a well-known problem in children, is also common in older people. Either transport the patient's loved one in the front of the ambulance, or suggest that a friend or neighbor drive the companion to the medical facility. Pets can also be a source of anxiety for the patient. A patient who lives alone may not want to go to the hospital and abandon a pet. If there is no family present, ask a neighbor or friend to watch the pet.

Money can also be a concern. Health care is expensive, and many older people are on budgets. Be aware that your patient could be deeply concerned that hospitalization will cause the loss of savings and even the home. Listen to your patient's fears with compassion, and acknowledge their importance to the patient.

Additional Challenges

In addition to the communication challenges of vision, hearing, speech, and underlying fears, there may be other considerations that make it difficult for an older person to tell you about his or her condition. The patient may take several medications, some of which may mask symptoms. He or she may have been in pain for a prolonged time, and not notice a gradual worsening of symptoms, or could have dementia, delirium, stroke, psychiatric disorders, or other illnesses that affect the ability to communicate thoughts. In these circumstances, it is very useful not only to collect information from the patient, but also to confirm this information with another source such as a caregiver, family member, or bystander. Finally, the patient who comes from an ethnic or cultural background different from yours may communicate differently.

Attitude Tip

Though your patient's fears and anxieties may not seem important to you, they are very real and important to the patient. By acknowledging the concerns and making it clear—with your words and your actions—that you understand their importance, you will do much to calm and reassure.

Attitude Tip

Improving your attitude toward, and communication skills with, professional caregivers in nursing homes, long-term care facilities, skilled nursing facilities, and home-health care will improve the continuum of care received by older patients from the interdisciplinary team.

Communicating with Home Care or Hospice Caregivers

If a home-care patient's condition worsens, the caretaker may need to call for EMS. The change in condition may be sudden, such as an injury from a fall, or may be a gradual worsening of an ongoing problem, such as prolonged diarrhea or breathing difficulties. A caregiver may be able to offer additional details about the patient's health history and recent changes that have led to the need to call you. In addition to the patient, the caregiver may provide critical and reliable information.

Full-time care of an impaired older person can be very stressful. If the patient is confused, demanding, irritable, depressed, or resistant to assistance, it can make the work of the caregivers extremely difficult. For family members to watch someone they care about slipping away may be almost unbearable. Caregivers may be tired and seem frustrated, nervous, or even angry. This is known as "caregiver burnout" and may have contributed to the reason for the call for help. Be sensitive to the caregiver's emotions. Listen carefully and document what they tell you. Be respectful and nonjudgmental, but don't forget to be alert for signs of abuse or neglect.

CASE STUDY 2

You are dispatched to the home of a 76-year-old man for a change in mental status.

You are greeted at the door by the patient's wife, who tells you that her husband has been acting very strange over the past several weeks. Attempts to get the patient to see his private physician have failed. As you inquire about what is specifically wrong with the patient, the wife tells you that lately the patient has become withdrawn, irritable, and suspicious. Finally, the wife tells you that the patient does not know that EMS has been called.

You enter the room and identify yourselves as EMS providers. The patient looks at you but does not respond. The wife yells to the patient that you are EMS providers. The patient seems to understand, but does not know why you are there. Your partner takes the wife into the next room and closes the door. You sit down next to the patient, and tell him that his wife is concerned about him. You ask how the patient is feeling. The patient tells you that he is feeling fine. As the patient is talking, you notice that he is speaking very loudly. You ask if the patient has any trouble hearing. The patient becomes teary eyed and tells you that he fears he is going deaf. The patient explains that he has been having increasing difficulty hearing his family, and cannot speak on the telephone.

What is your impression?

What is your course of action?

Communicating with Patients in Care Facilities

Many patients who reside in nursing facilities, group homes, or assisted-living facilities have dementia and other illnesses that may make communication with the patient challenging. As with any situation, it is important to collect information from the patient initially, but also to note whether the patient seems confused, and confirm the information with others as needed. Particularly in nursing homes, the nursing staff and nurses aides often know each patient very well, and can provide valuable information about what the patient is usually like, the sequence of the events that led up to the call for help, and detailed medical information that the patient may not be able to provide (▼ Figure 3-9). Be sure to get the name and phone number of a contact person at the facility in case further information is needed later.

> **Attitude Tip**
>
> Be sensitive to a caregiver's emotions. Caring for an older person can be very stressful and tiring.

Communicating with Bystanders

Occasionally, you will be called to care for an older patient in a location where bystanders are present who can provide useful information. Listen carefully to what is said. Bystanders can provide key information, and they may be your only source of information if the patient is unconscious, confused, or extremely ill (▼ Figure 3-10). Ask them to describe what they saw and heard. Ask questions about time, such as "How long has it been since you saw her fall?" "Did she lose consciousness?" or "Did you (or anyone else) do anything to assist her?" Ask if there has been any change since they have been with the patient.

Also ask bystanders if they observed the patient prior to the injury or illness, and what happened in the minutes preceding the injury or illness. Lastly, ask if the older person is known to any of the bystanders. If so, attempt to get an address or telephone number. The police can be of assistance by contacting the patient's residence to inform family that the patient was transported to the hospital. Be sure to document the information as having been offered by bystanders.

Communicating with Other Health Care Professionals

Many members of the health care community are involved in the care of the older patient, all of whom play a vital role in the health of the patient. These health care workers can be nursing home staff, adult day care center personnel, social workers, assisted-living home workers, or the patient's own health nurse. Above all, maintain a respectful demeanor with other members of the health care community who are involved in the care of the older patient.

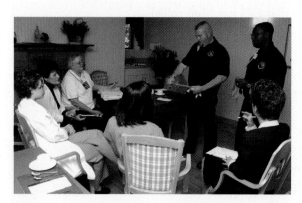

Figure 3-9   Staff members in nursing homes often know each patient very well, and can provide valuable information about the patient.

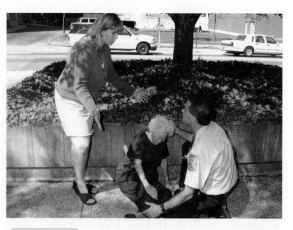

Figure 3-10   Bystanders may be your only source of information.

CASE STUDY 3

You are dispatched to a local coffee shop for an 82-year-old man with shortness of breath. You respond in a BLS ambulance. An advanced life support (ALS) paramedic ambulance is 20 minutes behind you.

First responders are administering oxygen via a nonrebreathing mask. A bystander tells you that the man said he was feeling a little under the weather when he came in to have coffee with some of his buddies. The man started "breathing heavy," so the bystander walked him to a table and waited for him to feel better. He was unable to talk and seemed to be getting worse. The bystander asked someone to call 9-1-1. Another bystander claiming to be an old friend of the man states, "George had a heart attack a few years ago and still has some heart problems. I think last time he did this, they put him on a ventilator."

What should you ask the bystander in this situation?

What treatment should you provide based on this information?

For the most part, those who care for older patients every day will be able to provide information about the patient. There are instances when a health care worker responsible for an older patient may not have the information you need. This can be frustrating, especially when the patient's condition is critical and information is needed quickly. When this occurs, try other methods of obtaining the information needed. If the patient resides in a long-term care facility or assisted-living facility, or is in an adult day care program, there will be a chart containing information. If adequate information cannot be gathered from a chart, ascertain whether a caretaker or family member can be contacted. Obtain the name and telephone number of this person. Upon arrival at the emergency department, this information can then be given to the hospital staff. Above all, maintain a respectful demeanor with other members of the health care community who are involved in the care of older patients.

Summary

Good communication is essential to successful assessment and treatment of older patients. There are many things that make communicating with older patients challenging. Keep in mind the age-

Attitude Tip

As an advocate for your older patients, in addition to evaluating their clinical presentation, gather information about their physical environment and psychosocial status from observations made at the residence, including their baseline functional status or activities of daily living (ADLs). Then, clearly report those observations and your related concerns to the receiving staff at the emergency department (ED) or other facility.

related changes in the older person, disease processes affecting communication, and differing cultural values. Be aware not only of what you say, but also how you say it.

Communication consists both of gathering and providing information. Listen and observe. You can learn a lot about your patient by being aware of potential vision impairments, hearing impairments, and underlying fears. A few seconds spent enhancing communication with your patient is time very well spent. An extra measure of patience may be in order when dealing with older patients and their caregivers. Our oldest and most vulnerable patients deserve nothing but the kindest and most sensitive care.

Case Study Summaries

CASE STUDY 1 SUMMARY

Upon arrival at the scene, make sure it is safe and that you utilize body substance isolation (BSI) appropriate to the situation. You note a frail older woman in some distress. She is alert with some response, not all of which is appropriate. There are no signs of spinal injury. Her airway and breathing are normal and there are no signs of distress. Upon focused history and physical exam, the patient looks frightened and says, "What? What?" You then ask her husband if she has a hearing impairment. He states that she does, and that her hearing aids are in the drawer behind you. Her husband states that he usually helps her put them in, but he is shaking and asks you if you will do it. You put her hearing aids in. She smiles and thanks you.

You continue with your focused history. The patient states that she has a history of arthritis, heart failure, and high blood pressure. She takes many different medications. She tells you that she was on her way to the bathroom and found herself on the floor. The patient does not know why she fell. She complains of severe pain in her left hip and of being cold. She has no other complaints.

She has pain on palpation of her left hip. Sensation and pulse are present in her left foot. She cannot move her left leg, and it is rotated outward. There are no other obvious injuries. Her vital signs are a respiratory rate of 16 breaths/min, an irregular pulse of 112 beats/min, and a blood pressure of 168/98 mm Hg.

Your treatment starts with administering oxygen via nonrebreathing mask. Immobilize the patient using pillows and a long backboard or orthopaedic frame. Cover the patient with blankets to keep her warm. Then, move her to the ambulance and begin transportation.

A detailed physical exam reveals unequal pupils and a small contusion to the left elbow. The patient continues to deny pain to any other area. There is no tenderness to the spine or back. In your ongoing assessment, the patient's status remains unchanged. She complains of pain to her left hip. You notify the receiving hospital via radio and take a second set of vital signs, which are a respiratory rate of 18 breaths/min, an irregular pulse of 102 beats/min, and a blood pressure of 156/94 mm Hg.

CASE STUDY 2 SUMMARY

You have encountered a 76-year-old male patient who states he has been having increased difficulty hearing over the past several weeks. The patient's wife had previously informed you that the patient has been withdrawn, irritable, and suspicious. You learn from the patient that he suffers only from mild high blood pressure and high cholesterol. Your assessment does not reveal anything remarkable, and the patient denies any recent trauma. The patient's vital signs are a

blood pressure of 150/90 mm Hg, a pulse of 82 beats/min, and respirations of 16 breaths/min.

You explain to the patient that he may be suffering from hearing loss, but recommend evaluation in the emergency department to rule out any other cause. You further tell the patient that if he is suffering from a decline in hearing, a hearing aid custom fitted for the patient may greatly improve his hearing. The patient agrees to be transported to the emergency department.

Because the patient's condition is stable, no further intervention is necessary.

The symptoms the patient is experiencing are typical reactions to hearing loss. The patient withdraws because communication has become frustrating and unsatisfying. People who are hard of hearing become irritable because they cannot understand those who are speaking to them. Two of the most common consequences of hearing impairment in older people are depression and withdrawal. Patients may be thought to have dementia when they are really suffering hearing loss. Additionally, a hearing loss can strain family relations. In this case study, the patient's wife turned to the EMS system for help.

CASE STUDY 3 SUMMARY

As always, your scene size-up starts with ensuring that it is safe, and you utilize BSI appropriate to the situation. You note a 65-year-old man with acute respiratory distress. He is alert and responds with nods. A check of ABCs indicates an open airway, very deep and labored breathing, and a fast and irregular radial pulse.

Your initial treatment is to assure oxygen administration, prepare for transport, and arrange rendezvous of ALS. Your focused history and physical exam reveal lung congestion that could be heard without a stethoscope. Ankle swelling and engorged neck veins are evident. The patient is unable to answer questions with words, but nods "yes" or shakes his head "no" appropriately. Vitals are a respiratory rate of 32 breaths/min, an irregular pulse of 162 beats/min, and a blood pressure of 204/112 mm Hg.

Further treatment is to continue administering oxygen via nonrebreathing mask. You initiate emergency transportation in semi-sitting position, assure the patient's comfort, and arrange a rendezvous with ALS. In the ongoing assessment, the patient remains acutely short of breath. He denies chest pain. After 10 minutes, the patient is transferred to the ALS ambulance, where he is treated with medications and transported to the hospital. A second set of vitals reveals a respiratory rate of 24 breaths/min, an irregular pulse of 140 beats/min, and a blood pressure of 200/110 mm Hg. A third set of vitals is also taken, which finds a respiratory rate of 26 breaths/min, an irregular pulse of 142 beats/min, and a blood pressure of 190/98 mm Hg.

Bibliography

Hogan T. *Geriatric Emergencies: An EMT Teaching Manual.* Turlock, CA: MedicAlert; 1996.

National Aphasia Association. *Communicating with People Who Have Aphasia.* New York: Author; 1988.

End-of-Life Care Issues

LEARNING OBJECTIVES

1 State the leading causes of death in the older population (distinguish between trauma and medical).

2 Define palliative and hospice care programs.

3 Discuss what to do when signs of impending death are present.

4 Discuss do not resuscitate (DNR) orders, living wills, and other legal considerations as they relate to the care of the older patient.

5 Discuss considerations when treating the older patient with a terminal disease.

6 Discuss grief and loss as they relate to the older patient, the care provider, the patient's family, and the EMS provider.

CHAPTER 4

Jennifer Kapo, MD

Jack Schwartz, JD

CASE STUDY 1

Mrs. Z is a 78-year-old woman with metastatic lung cancer who is enrolled in a home hospice program, and has completed a DNR order, which has been signed by her primary care physician. She had been doing well with adequate symptom management for the past month; however, over the last 24 hours she has become increasingly withdrawn, her urine output has diminished, and she is now making gurgling noises when she breathes. Although she was told to call hospice if symptoms worsened, her daughter panics and calls 9-1-1.

When you arrive at the scene, you find Mrs. Z bradycardic, hypothermic, and lethargic. Although her respiratory rate is low, a choking noise is coming from her throat with each breath.

What is your impression?

Is there anything you can do?

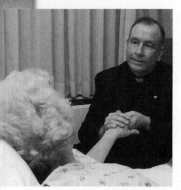

Epidemiology of Death in Older Patients

Approximately three fourths of all deaths in the United States occur in persons over the age of 65. In the past, people commonly died suddenly from trauma or infectious diseases. As shown previously in Table 2-1, during the 1990s, the leading cause of death in older persons was chronic diseases, such as cardiovascular disease and cancer. Other leading causes of death include chronic obstructive pulmonary disease, pneumonia, dementing illness such as Alzheimer's disease, and complications from diabetes. Alzheimer's disease is the 10th leading cause of death in Caucasians; however, it is not as common in other racial groups. This changing pattern has resulted in a longer length of time spent at the "end of life" and, therefore, the growing need for health care provider expertise in caring for dying patients.

Older Americans die in different settings, and under diverse circumstances. A report published in 1994 states that 55% of all Americans died in the hospital, 21% died at home, and 19% in nursing homes. The aggressiveness of treatments at the end of life varies widely as well. A national study reviewing care of all dying patients in intensive care units (ICUs) at university-affiliated and community hospitals revealed that 23% received full ICU care including CPR, while 22% had full ICU care without CPR, 10% had life support withheld, and 38% had life support withdrawn.

Research has revealed that during hospitalization, some patients and their families make decisions to withdraw or forgo life-sustaining treatments at the end of life. These decisions are often made in a step-wise pattern (▶ **Figure 4-1**). Relatively invasive treatments such as ventilation, resuscitation, and vasopressors are withheld early in the course of a terminal illness, while other treatments such as antibiotics, enteral, and/or parenteral feedings are continued until later in the illness course or until death occurs.

Attitude **Tip**

Remember that "DNR" *does not* mean "do not treat!"

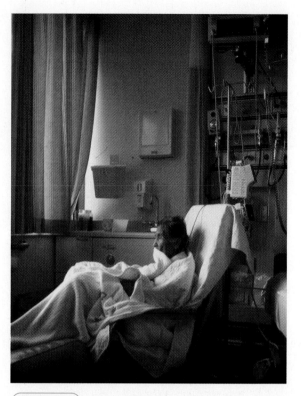

Figure 4-1   The decision to withdraw life-sustaining treatments is often made in a step-wise pattern.

What Constitutes a Good Death?

Controversy

The meaning of a "good death" can vary from person to person.

Although the goal of end-of-life care is to provide patients with a meaningful, dignified, and comfortable death, there is a surprising lack of data describing what patients and their families believe constitutes a "good death." While some patients with terminal illness choose to have as aggressive care as possible, others have a goal of comfort rather than cure or prolongation of life. Researchers have had difficulty answering the question of what constitutes a "good death." In one survey, seriously ill patients identified specific characteristics as being important. These included:

TABLE 4-1	Components of a Good Death
Pain and symptom management	
Clear decision making	
Preparation for death	
Completion	
Contributing to others	
Affirmation of the whole person	

Source: Steinhauser KE, et al. In search of a good death: Observations of patients, families, and providers. *Annals of Internal Medicine.* 2000; 132(10):827.

♦ Pain and symptom management

♦ Preparation for death

♦ Achieving sense of completion

♦ Being treated as a whole person

♦ Being mentally aware

♦ Having funeral arrangements made

♦ Not being a burden

♦ Helping others

♦ Coming to peace with God

Another research group identified six themes constituting a good death, shown in ▲ **Table 4-1**. Patients also want to avoid prolongation of suffering and to strengthen relationships with family members. The researchers discovered that psychosocial and spiritual issues are as important as physical symptom management to patients with terminal illness.

Hospice and Palliative Care

While some patients continue to receive aggressive treatment until their death, others choose hospice care, forgoing curative therapy for comfort measures alone. In 1990, the World Health Organization defined **palliative care** as the "active total care of patients whose disease is not responsive to curative treatment." It further defines palliative care as:

♦ Affirming life and regarding dying as a normal process

♦ Neither hastening nor prolonging death

♦ Providing relief from pain and other distressing symptoms

♦ Integrating psychological and spiritual aspects of patient care

♦ Offering a support system to help the family cope during the patient's illness and in his or her own bereavement

In 1983, the Medicare Hospice Benefit was created to enable terminally ill Americans and their families to receive comprehensive end-of-life care. Hospice care provides pain and symptom management and addresses the psychosocial, emotional, and spiritual needs of patients. The care can be delivered in freestanding hospice facilities, hospitals, nursing homes, and patients' homes. Hospice care is available 24 hours a day, seven days a week by a team consisting of the patient's family/caregiver, patient's physician, hospice physician, nurses, home health aides, social workers, clergy, trained volunteers, and occupational and physical therapists ▼ **Figure 4-2**.

Patients are eligible for the hospice benefit if they are certified by a physician as having a life expectancy of six months or less and sign a state-

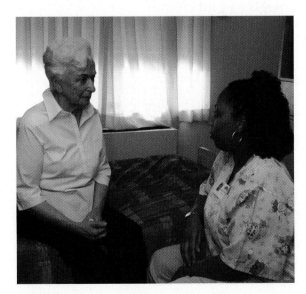

Figure 4-2 A patient in hospice care receives visits from physicians, nurses, home health aides, social workers, clergy, and therapists.

ment stating that they choose hospice care rather than curative care. The benefit covers care related to the terminal illness including physician visits, home visits by nurses, home health aides, clergy visits, social work visits, bereavement counseling, medical supplies and equipment, drugs for symptom and pain management, volunteer visits, and occupational therapy/physical therapy. The benefit will also cover general inpatient care if an acute crisis in symptom management occurs. Caregivers responsible for taking care of hospice patients are offered respite by placing patients in a freestanding hospice or nursing home temporarily.

Any patient has the right to stop hospice care at any time and return to curative care. A patient also can elect to return to hospice care at any time if a physician certifies that his or her life expectancy remains six months or less.

Impending Death

The patient described in Case Study 1 is showing signs of impending death. These include[1]:

♦ Decreased intake of food and drink

♦ Decreased orientation

♦ Increased time spent sleeping and becoming more difficult to arouse

♦ Cool extremities with the development of a lacy patterned rash

♦ Decreased urine output

♦ Decreased ability to hear and see

♦ Irregular breathing pattern

♦ Difficulty clearing respiratory secretions accompanied by development of the "death rattle"

♦ Hypothermia or hyperthermia

♦ Bradycardia or tachycardia

EMS providers can recognize these signs and help to reassure the family. If the patient has a valid **do not resuscitate (DNR) order**, CPR is not indicated or appropriate if his or her heart stops and/or he or she stops breathing. If you have any question regarding the validity of a DNR or the description of the level of interventions the patient wants, resuscitation should be started while contacting medical control for further instructions. When no resuscitative measures are attempted, aggressive comfort measures are needed (▼ Figure 4-3). These include oxygen delivered by nasal cannula or face mask, breathing treatments with albuterol, and morphine as needed for pain and respiratory distress per local protocol. The patient should be placed in a comfortable position.

There are times when EMS is called to the scene of a dying patient with a valid DNR order. Although the decision for a DNR order had already been made, family members may not understand what to do, and may not be ready to face the death of a loved one.

If you are called to the scene where death is imminent, the actions you take will have a lasting impact on the family. This is a time when compassion, understanding, and sensitivity are most needed. Ascertain the family's wishes with regard to having the patient remain in the home or be transported to the hospital. If the family wishes the patient to be transported, their request should be honored. During transport, contact medical control, and advise the receiving hospital of the situation. If a family member requests to accompany the patient, he or she should be allowed to do so.

If the family wishes the patient to remain at home, this request should be honored as long as it is in accordance with your local or state protocol. For many patients and their families, dying at home in a familiar place is preferable. If you can do so, remain with the family until death has oc-

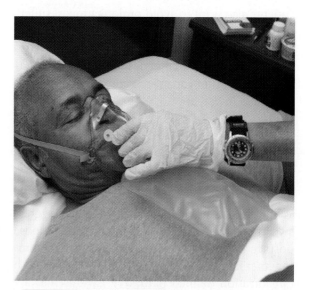

Figure 4-3   If the patient has a clear DNR order signed by a physician, aggressive comfort measures should be taken.

curred if possible. While this may take time and be stressful for some EMS providers, remember that you will be providing comfort at a time when it is most needed. This is particularly true when the loved one is alone. Find out from the family if there is anyone that the family would like called.

Attitude Tip

Remember that "no CPR" does not mean "no caring."

Controversy

The rule of double effect is an ethical principle used to justify certain treatment decisions made by health care providers at the end of life. The rule of double effect means that it is morally acceptable to give a treatment that hastens death if the main intention is to provide relief of suffering. A common example of this is a practitioner escalating the dose of morphine with the knowledge that it may hasten death through respiratory depression, but with the intention of relieving pain and suffering.

Local protocols for handling the death of a patient vary. You must learn your local or state regulations. Check your protocol to learn if the coroner needs to be called to report the death, and if so, who is responsible for contacting the coroner. Also check whether a pronouncement of death is required, and if so, who makes it. You may offer to call the funeral home for the family, although this is not universally accepted as the EMS provider's responsibility.

EMS providers are trained to preserve life. If there is no DNR order, they are responsible for starting resuscitation if there is any chance that a patient can be revived. However, many local health systems have protocols stating that when death is obvious, attempts at resuscitation are not necessary. These may include decapitation, rigor mortis without hypothermia, obvious mortal wounds without signs of life, and decomposition.

Controversy

There may be situations when the family disagrees with the DNR and the patient is unable to speak for himself or herself. The patient's wishes should be respected in regard to resuscitation. If a family wants CPR started, but there is a DNR order stating otherwise, attempt to convince the family to honor the patient's wishes. If the disagreement continues, begin resuscitation while contacting medical control for assistance.

In some states, the DNR order can be revoked. A patient can revoke the order verbally or by physically destroying the directive. In some states, the legal spokesperson for the patient, known as the surrogate decision maker, can revoke the order by stating that they are expressing the patient's wishes. You will need to learn your local or state law and protocol.

Ethical and Legal Issues

This section discusses a patient's ethical and legal right to refuse unwanted care, including CPR. The discussion covers living wills, other advance directives, and DNR orders. It then relates these legal tools for care in the EMS setting.

Most people agree that people are entitled to make their own decisions about health care as long as they can understand the consequences of the decisions they are contemplating. This ethical principle is often called autonomy. **Autonomy** is the right of an individual to make choices freely, in accordance with the individual's own goals and values.

The ethical principle of autonomy is recognized legally in various ways. In every state, patients who are capable of thinking clearly (also known as having decision-making capacity) may give consent to receive or refuse proposed treatments. The **informed consent doctrine**, which was developed by the courts, allows a patient to decide against unwanted medical interventions. Even if an intervention would probably prolong a patient's life, the patient may refuse it. The right

CASE STUDY 2

Harry, a 70-year-old man and longtime smoker, has stage III lung cancer. Although his prognosis is grim, Harry is still well enough to live at home with his wife Joan. One morning, while Harry is at his back fence chatting with a neighbor, he grimaces, clutches at his chest, and collapses. The neighbor immediately calls 9-1-1, and says that Harry looks like he might have had a heart attack.

You and your partner arrive at the scene and begin resuscitation efforts under protocol. Meanwhile, hearing the siren, Harry's wife Joan, who had been inside the house, rushes out. Seeing what you are doing, Joan shouts, "Stop! Harry has a living will and doesn't want this. Just keep him comfortable." Joan then runs back into the house and returns to the back yard with a legal document. "This is Harry's living will," she shouts. "Look right here, it says he doesn't want CPR."

What should you do?

---

to refuse life-sustaining treatment is also protected under the U.S. Constitution and the constitutions of some states.

Controversy

Advocates of physician-assisted suicide argue that it too should be recognized as a legal right. Today, only Oregon recognizes physician-assisted suicide as a legal right. In other states, assisting a suicide is a criminal offense. In every state, however, withholding or withdrawing treatment to carry out a patient's wishes is not considered assisting a suicide.

The right to refuse life-sustaining treatment applies to resuscitation efforts. Thus, if a patient with intact capacity decides against attempted CPR in the event of cardiac or respiratory arrest, CPR should not be attempted. Instead, the patient's decision should result in the creation of a DNR order.

Though this right exists, it is sometimes difficult to know the wishes of an individual patient. The problem comes down to one of communication: How does a patient who has decided against CPR and other forms of life-sustaining treatment communicate this decision effectively?

Effective communication of patient decisions depends on the setting and the time period to be covered. A hospital inpatient, for example, who is asked about code status during a hospital stay can simply decide in response to the question. Even though CPR is normally what the hospital physician does when a patient has a cardiopulmonary arrest, a patient has the right, under the informed consent doctrine, to decline this intervention. If a patient does so, the attending physician's in-hospital DNR order becomes the means of communication about the patient's decision to health care practitioners within the hospital.

Some people, however, have an opinion about resuscitation and other forms of life-sustaining treatment beyond the short time span of a hospital stay. In other words, they want to make plans about their health care in case of future events. The means of expressing their decisions is called an **advance directive**.

Every state has enacted a law allowing people to give directions about end-of-life care in advance of need—hence, the term "advance directive." Although these laws grant rights to all adults, older people as a group are more willing than younger people to recognize the importance of this way of anticipating future health care issues.

One kind of advance directive names a future decision maker. This advance directive anticipates a future situation in which decisions about CPR and other forms of life-sustaining treatment must be made, but the patient is unable at that time to make them. The patient uses the advance directive to name a decision maker of the patient's choosing. This type of document is variously called a **durable power of attorney** for health care, health care proxy, or a health care agent.

The other kind of advance directive (which can be done together with appointing a decision maker, or alone) documents decisions about particular end-of-life treatments in particular situations. Depending on the law in each state, it can cover CPR and other forms of life-sustaining treatment in the event of terminal condition, permanent unconsciousness, and fatal illness prior to the terminal phase. This type of document is called either a **living will** or an instructional directive (▼ **Figure 4-4**). Because it is impossible to anticipate all of the particular decisions to be made at the end of life, these documents must be read carefully to be sure they apply to the situation the pa-

tient is facing at that time. In contrast, a surrogate decision maker may be able to make various decisions as long as he or she acts in accordance with what he or she thinks the patient would want in that situation.

Most people do not have any formal type of advance directive. Every state has its own procedures for how family members can make decisions about end-of-life care on behalf of an incapacitated patient. Many states have laws and guidelines on surrogate decision making, spelling out who can make decisions and under what circumstances. In other states, family decision-making rights are decided by the court. Sometimes the only way a decision can be made is by a court-appointed guardian or conservator.

Surrogate Refusal of Life-sustaining Medical Treatment

The most famous court cases on the so-called right to die have involved efforts by families to withdraw life-sustaining treatment that they were sure a loved one would not want. For example, the family of

---

INSTRUCTIONS

FLORIDA LIVING WILL

PRINT THE DATE
PRINT YOUR NAME

Declaration made this __ day of _____ , 20 __ .

I, _____ willfully
and voluntarily make known my desire that my dying not be artificially prolonged under the circumstances set forth below, and I do hereby declare:

If at any time I have a terminal condition and if my attending or treating physician and another consulting physician have determined that there is no medical probability of my recovery from such condition, I direct that life-prolonging procedures be withheld or withdrawn when the application of such procedures would serve only to prolong artificially the process of dying, and that I be permitted to die naturally with only the administration of medication or the performance of any medical procedure deemed necessary to provide me with comfort care or to alleviate pain.

It is my intention that this declaration be honored by my family and physician as the final expression of my legal right to refuse medical or surgical treatment and to accept the consequences of such refusal.

In the event that I have been determined to be unable to provide express and informed consent regarding the withholding, withdrawal, or continuation of life-prolonging procedures, I wish to designate, as my surrogate to carry out the provisions of this declaration:

PRINT THE NAME, HOME ADDRESS AND TELEPHONE NUMBER OF YOUR SURROGATE

Name: _____

Address: _____

_____ Zip Code: _____

Phone: _____

© 1996
CHOICE IN DYING, INC.

FLORIDA LIVING WILL—PAGE 2 of 2

I wish to designate the following person as my alternative surrogate, to carry out the provisions of this declaration should my surrogate be unwilling or unable to act on my behalf:

PRINT NAME, HOME ADDRESS AND TELEPHONE NUMBER OF YOUR ALTERNATIVE SURROGATE

Name: _____

Address: _____

_____ Zip Code: _____

Phone: _____

ADD PERSONAL INSTRUCTIONS (IF ANY)

Additional instructions (optional): _____

_____

_____

I understand the full import of this declaration, and I am emotionally and mentally competent to make this declaration.

SIGN THE DOCUMENT

Signed: _____

WITNESSING PROCEDURE

Witness 1:

TWO WITNESSES MUST SIGN AND PRINT THEIR ADDRESSES

Signed: _____

Address: _____

Witness 2:

Signed: _____

Address: _____

© 1996
CHOICE IN DYING, INC.

Courtesy of Choice In Dying, Inc.
200 Varick Street, New York, NY 10014 212-366-5540

Figure 4-4 A living will or similar advance directive is used to express wishes about end-of-life care for particular situations.

Karen Ann Quinlan, who was in a persistent vegetative state (PVS), successfully sued a New Jersey hospital for the right to remove her ventilator. The family of Nancy Beth Cruzan, also a PVS victim, sued for the right to remove her feeding tube, but lost in the U.S. Supreme Court because they did not present enough evidence of what Nancy would have wanted. Later, after additional evidence was brought forward, a trial judge in Missouri allowed the removal of the tube. In many states, surrogate decision making is now authorized by law.

Any one of these mechanisms—a patient's right to accept or refuse treatments, a health care proxy's decision, an instruction in a living will, or a surrogate's or guardian's decision—can result in a decision to forgo attempted CPR in favor of comfort care alone. When a patient is in a health care facility, the facility is responsible for documenting these decisions, including the entry of in-facility DNR orders.

Increasingly, however, patients with DNR status are in the community. Many are at home, often receiving care from a hospice program. Others, whether under hospice care or not, are in nursing homes or assisted-living facilities. For a variety of reasons, EMS providers might be called to a scene at which the patient, based on a prior decision, has DNR status.

Given that EMS providers must react swiftly and decisively when they arrive on a scene, communicating DNR status in a practical way poses special challenges. The patient who is in the midst of cardiac arrest is hardly likely to be able to articulate a reasoned decision about CPR. Furthermore, an EMS provider cannot be expected to interpret a legal document or decide whether a civilian on the scene is legally authorized to direct that CPR not be attempted.

Consequently, procedures have been created allowing a prior, legally recognized decision to forgo CPR to be translated into a form of communication that EMS providers can honor: an order specifically authorizing DNR/comfort care procedures in the community setting. This kind of order has different names in different states, including prehospital DNR, out-of-hospital DNR, CPR directive, comfort care DNR order, Comfort One order, and DNR order. In the discussion that follows, the last term, DNR order, is used to refer to any order that tells EMS providers not to follow the usual CPR protocol but instead to provide comfort care measures only.

The Law Governing DNR Orders

The most important legal fact about DNR orders is that no single, national law applies. Instead, DNR orders are governed by state law and by state or local protocols. It is important to find out what law and protocol procedures apply in your state and region. More than 40 states have adopted laws and protocols on this subject. Although no two are identical, many have elements in common.

One common element is that DNR/comfort care procedures are to be followed only if a specially designed identification is on or near the patient. In most states, the special DNR order itself serves as the authorizing signal for DNR/comfort care procedures. Other documents, like a living will, do not. Become familiar with your local protocol regarding which document(s) authorize EMS providers to provide only DNR/comfort care **▼ Figure 4-5**).

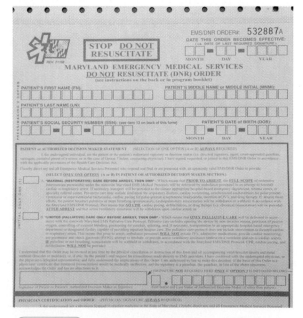

Figure 4-5   A DNR form is commonly used to identify a patient with a do not resuscitate status.

Validity of DNR Order

Another issue is the validity of the order form. In some but not all states, a physician must certify on the DNR order form that the patient has a medical condition that state law identifies as qualifying for the order. Usually, this is a terminal condition, but in a few states other conditions qualify as well. If a state requires a physician's signature on the form (and nearly all do), the form is not valid without it. Some states require a patient's or proxy's signature as well. Check protocol for the steps that EMS providers are to take to verify that a DNR order is valid.

Controversy

Is a DNR order from a state other than yours valid? It depends on the law of your state. About a dozen states recognize out-of-state DNR orders.

If the DNR order or other identifying device appears to be valid, it is to be honored. What exactly that means depends on the specific requirements of state law and applicable protocol. Typically, it means that if the patient has no pulse or is not breathing, then CPR is not to be performed. Many protocols go into detail about what is to be done, and not done, if a patient has a DNR order. The Maryland DNR protocol, for example, labels as "inappropriate" CPR, cardiac monitoring, intubation, and the use of a pneumatic anti-shock garment. Instead, supportive care is to be provided, including noninvasive means to open the airway and positioning for comfort.

Immunity

The final legal issue to be discussed is __immunity__. Immunity provisions are meant to protect EMS providers from the risk of being sued under certain circumstances. In most states, the law that authorizes a DNR order also explicitly provides that EMS providers who give comfort care based on an order cannot be sued for failing to provide CPR. In other states, EMS providers who carry out a DNR order are protected by more general immunity provisions in the EMS law or by "Good Samaritan" laws. Immunity usually protects against both being sued and disciplinary action by a licensing or certification agency.

Immunity issues also can arise when an EMS provider performs CPR despite the existence of a DNR order. Although generalizations are difficult to make because of great variation in wording from one state law to the next, an EMS provider will surely not be sued for performing CPR when unaware of a DNR order. Similarly, the law of most states would protect an EMS provider who performed CPR because he or she had decided, in good faith, that a DNR order was not valid or had been revoked.

Communication with Families and Friends

Health care providers are traditionally uncomfortable discussing death and dying with patients. Proposed reasons for this include the notion that health care providers should maintain professional distance, the sense that they are

---

CASE STUDY 3

Lilly, an 86-year-old woman with advanced Alzheimer's disease, is a resident at a nursing home. When you arrive at the nursing home, you find Lilly without a pulse or respiration. You see a bracelet on her wrist indicating DNR status.

What should you do?

admitting failure, and lastly, the general lack of experience in end-of-life communication.

One of the most difficult tasks for which an EMS provider is responsible is communication with the family and friends of a patient who has just died. It is important to recognize that every family and circumstance is unique. In general, recognize that once the patient dies, the family becomes your patient (▼ Figure 4-6).

Before initiating a conversation with friends and family, gather as much information regarding the case as possible to convey a clear description of the death. Be aware of the importance of nonverbal communication. Maintain good eye contact. If possible, find a nearby quiet location away from what may be a chaotic situation, and find a place where the bereaved and the informant can sit and face each other. Listen to their concerns. Expect any reaction! The death of a loved one can be one of the most stressful experiences of a person's life. Allow the bereaved person time to express grief.

Statements such as "You have my sincere sympathy" are more effective than stating, "I am sorry." It is possible that grieving people may interpret the statement "I am sorry" as the EMS provider admitting to blame for wrongdoing, or for poor care of the patient. Ask if there are any questions, use the word "died" rather than euphemisms such as "passed away," and be truthful with responses.

Offer to call a neighbor, another family member, and/or clergy to assist with the acute grief associated with the death. In surveys of family members

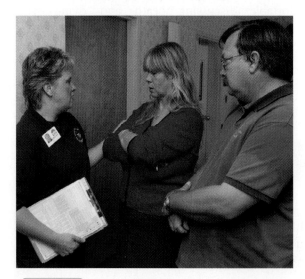

Figure 4-6 If a patient dies, the family becomes your patient.

who just experienced a death in the family, one of the most distressing experiences was the feeling that they were abandoned. If possible, attempt to convey a sense that they will not be left alone.

Bereavement

Health care providers need to develop a basic understanding of grief and bereavement. **Bereavement** occurs in the time after a loss during which grief is experienced, and includes the adaptation to that loss. This time period can be extremely stressful, as well as potentially life threatening to the bereaved. It increases the risk of sleep disorders, suicide attempts, substance abuse (including alcohol, tobacco, and illicit drugs), and overall mortality. (▼ Table 4-2) lists risk factors for poor outcome of the bereaved.

TABLE 4-2   Risk Factors for Poor Outcome of Bereavement
Ambivalent or dependent relationship
Older age
Female gender
Death of child
Sudden and unexpected death (especially if associated with violence, suicide, or substance abuse)
Having cared for the deceased for more than 6 months
Deaths with stigma, such as death due to AIDS or suicide
Lack of social contacts

After: Sheldon F. ABC of palliative care: Bereavement. *BMJ.* 1998; 316(7129):456–458.

Communication Tip

You should develop an understanding of grief and bereavement to better communicate with family members when a patient dies.

Attitude Tip

When at the scene of a recent death, you may witness a person suffer an acute grief reaction. Signs and symptoms of acute grief may include intense crying spells, denial, sense of derealization, and somatic or body complaints. One of the most valuable interventions is simply to remain present and offer a few moments for the expression of grief.

The tasks of successful bereavement involve searching for the meaning in the death and finding hope for the future. Writers have described stages of grief, such as the famous Kübler-Ross stages that include denial and isolation, anger, bargaining, depression, and acceptance. Others discuss grief in terms of initial shock, pangs of grief, despair, and adjustment. A common understanding of bereavement is that humans do not necessarily experience the stages in any particular order or schedule. Although no intervention has been proven effective to help all bereaved individuals, those identified as being at high risk for complicated bereavement may benefit from group and/or individualized counseling, and possibly antidepressant drug therapy.

Critical Incident Stress Debriefing

Caring for dying patients can be incredibly rewarding; however, it can also be considerably stressful for families, as well as for health care providers. EMS providers are at risk for developing guilt for not "saving" the patient, and suffering from their own sense of loss regarding the death of patients. Many health care organizations have **critical incident stress debriefing (CISD)** in place for EMS providers and other health care providers who deal with death on a regular basis (▶ **Figure 4-7**). CISD is a process instituted to help prevent **posttraumatic stress disorder (PTSD)** in workers exposed to a critical incident, such as a natural or manmade disaster or a sudden death, that could overwhelm the coping skills of an individual health care worker. Manifestations of PTSD can include difficulty with sleep, recurrent nightmares, detailed "flashbacks," and depression.

During CISD, the team involved in the critical incident meets with peer counselors and mental health professionals to discuss the incident and to develop coping strategies. CISD has been proven to decrease the number of EMS providers

CASE STUDY 4

A 72-year-old man with a history of high cholesterol, hypertension, and diabetes, collapses to the ground outside a busy shopping mall. Upon arrival, you find him to be asystolic with fixed pupils and no blood pressure. Despite best attempts at resuscitation, he has not been revived, and after communication with medical control, CPR has been discontinued. The newly widowed wife has arrived at the scene.

How do you tell her what happened?

What can you offer her?

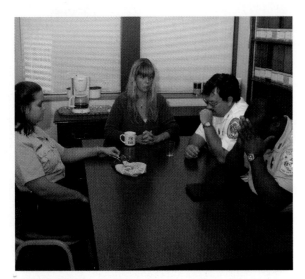

Figure 4-7 Critical incident stress debriefing may help EMS providers deal with the stress of their job.

Attitude Tip

Always support and respect the DNR patient's wishes not to be resuscitated, permitting them to die with dignity, and always supporting and reassuring family members at the scene.

who develop professional "burnout" resulting from the burdens and stresses of the field of emergency medicine. ▶ Table 4-3 lists warning signs of burnout to be aware of in yourself and in colleagues.

Summary

Honoring a patient's wishes about end-of-life care is important both legally and ethically. Sometimes a patient, or someone else authorized by law to speak on the patient's behalf, has made a decision against attempted CPR in the event of cardiac or pulmonary arrest. In the community setting, this decision can be documented in a DNR order. It is essential that EMS providers be aware of the legal requirements for a DNR order in their state, look for the order or other authorized identification of a DNR patient, and then follow protocol accordingly. When they do, they are protected by legal immunity. If any doubt exists as to the validity of the DNR order, err on the side of resuscitation.

TABLE 4-3 Warning Signs for Burnout
Physical
◆ Weight loss or gain
◆ Frequent headaches
◆ GI disturbances
◆ Insomnia, muscle tension
◆ Loss of libido
◆ Increased smoking or drinking
◆ Accidents
Anxiety
◆ Anger, irritability
◆ Frustration, "scapegoating"
◆ Feeling stretched, overwhelmed
◆ Judgment errors
◆ Changing moods
◆ Dulled emotions, depression
◆ Excessive dedication
◆ Looking too busy
Interpersonal
◆ Enjoying life at work more than at home
◆ Power struggle with others
◆ Critical of coworkers
◆ Unconsciously replicating old family problems with staff, eg, sibling rivalries or parent–child roles
◆ Distancing coworkers, family
◆ Depersonalization of patients
◆ Intellectualization
◆ Family resents long hours at work
Nonacceptance
◆ Helplessness
◆ Inadequacy, insecurity
◆ Depression, guilt
◆ No way to cope with mistakes, bad outcomes, losses at home, losses at work, death
◆ Loss of meaning or purpose

After: American Academy of Hospice and Palliative Medicine. Storey P. (ed.). *Primer of Palliative Care.* 2nd ed. Dubuque, IA: Kendall/Hunt Publishing; 1996:29.

As an EMS provider, you will be faced with situations that involve the death of a patient. In these difficult cases, your communication with family and friends of the patient can make a profound difference in their grieving process. Be sensitive and caring in your interactions. Also, take care of yourself and your coworkers by allowing yourself to grieve, by seeking critical incidence stress debriefing when applicable, and by being attentive to the signs of burnout.

CASE STUDY 5

Mr. D is a 68-year-old man with a history of metastatic colon cancer that has continued to spread despite optimal therapy. His physician has recommended hospice care. His wife called 9-1-1 when he developed increasing abdominal pain. When you arrive, they ask you about hospice care.

What can you tell them about it?

Case Study Summaries

CASE STUDY **1** SUMMARY

The patient is exhibiting signs of possible impending death with bradycardia, hypothermia, and diminished respiratory rate. First, verify the DNR order and explain your findings with the family. Explain that the choking noise from the patient is common at the end of life and likely is the result of "pooling secretions" that the patient is unable to clear. Assure the family that the patient is unlikely to be suffering from these secretions. Physicians can treat the sensation of "air hunger" with opiate medications, such as morphine, as well as decrease the volume of secretions with the use of anticholinergic medications. Oxygen can be given via nasal cannula without significant invasion. Determine if the family or patient wishes the patient to be transported to the hospital for further care, or if he/she wishes to remain at home. The key in this situation is to provide care to make the patient as comfortable as possible, and to comfort the family. Sensitivity and compassion are paramount.

CASE STUDY **2** SUMMARY

Under the law and protocols of most states, you do not have the authority to stop CPR when the patient's wife produces a living will. The patient was not identified as a DNR patient by any recognized sign. Follow standard protocol or the instructions of the EMS command and control physician. You would have legal immunity for your good-faith actions. Try to calm the patient's wife as best you can, and tell her to bring the living will with her to the emergency department.

CASE STUDY **3** SUMMARY

Under the law and protocols of most states, you should forgo CPR and instead initiate comfort care procedures for this properly identified DNR patient. You would have legal immunity for your good-faith actions.

CASE STUDY SUMMARY

If at all possible, find a quiet place where you can sit with the widow to deliver the news of her husband's death. Remember to speak calmly and clearly and maintain good eye contact. Use clear terms that a person without medical training will understand, not medical jargon, and avoid the use of euphemisms.

Expect any reaction of grief. It is important to allow the bereaved to express himself or herself. Another service you can offer to a family, if time allows, is to help the bereaved contact family members or other social supports so that they are not left alone.

CASE STUDY 5 SUMMARY

Know the basic components of hospice care. Know that palliative care is defined as the active total care of a patient whose disease has progressed to the point that curative treatments are unlikely to be of benefit. Explain that the patient and family may be eligible for comprehensive

care (including physician care, nursing care, chaplains, medicines, and durable medical equipment) under the Medicare Hospice benefit if their doctor determines the patient's prognosis to be 6 months or less due to terminal illness.

Endnotes

1. Enck RT. The last few days. *American Journal of Hospice and Palliative Care.* 1992;9:11–16.

2. Koenig KL, Tamkin GW. Do-not-resuscitate orders. Where are they in the prehospital setting? *Prehospital Disaster Med.* 1993;8:51–54.

3. Sabatino CP. *Survey of State EMS-DNR Laws and Protocols.* Washington, DC: Commission on Legal Problems of the Elderly, American Bar Association; 1999.

Suggested Educational Resources

Bruena E, Portenoy RK. *Topics in Palliative Care.* New York: Oxford University Press; 1998.

Assessment of the Older Patient

1 Compare the assessment of the older patient with that of a younger adult patient.

2 Describe normal and abnormal findings in assessment of older patients.

3 Recognize common emotional and psychological reactions to aging.

4 Recognize normal and disease states in older patients.

5 Describe common complaints of the older patient, including shortness of breath; chest pain; altered mental status; abdominal pain; dizziness or weakness; trauma; generalized pain; falls; and nausea, vomiting, and diarrhea.

Teresita M. Hogan, Lead Editor, MD, FACEP

Heather Davis, MS, NREMT-P

Michael O'Keefe, MS, NREMT-P

James D. Upchurch, MD, NREMT-P

CASE STUDY 1

You are dispatched to Loving Care Nursing Home at 1:40 p.m. for an older woman who is confused. En route to the call, you begin to consider the possibilities that you will discover on scene, such as stroke, fever, drug overdose, medication interaction, diabetic emergency, and so on. You arrive in 5 minutes and bring all of your portable equipment into the facility with you.

You are directed to the patient's room, where you find a family member at the bedside of an awake older woman. You send someone to find the attending nurse.

Your first impression is that the room is very cold, the TV is loud, and there is a strong odor of urine. You greet the family member, who introduces herself as the patient's daughter, and proceed to the bedside of the patient. The patient appears very thin and is cold to the touch as you feel her pulse. She is not aware of your presence until you speak to her. She responds verbally, but you cannot understand her. With further questioning, her speech improves a little. Several more questions reveal that she does know her name, but not her age, the time, place, or current events.

What are the possible problems this patient could be experiencing?

What can you ask in your history and look for in your physical exam that would narrow down the possibilities and lead to the best assessment?

Assessment of the Older Patient

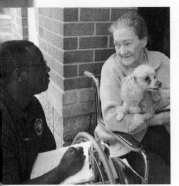

PART I: ASSESSMENT FACTORS SPECIFIC TO OLDER PATIENTS

Introduction

Normal assessment findings in an older patient are different from those of a younger patient due to physiologic and anatomic changes that occur with age. Several factors, including genetic makeup, chronic diseases, and lifestyle choices, affect how well a person ages. The 70-year-old individual whose chronic disease, such as hypertension or diabetes, started at age 40 is likely to have more organ damage than the 70-year-old person whose hypertension or diabetes started at age 60. A 70-year-old marathoner will have maintained better overall health status than the individual who has accelerated the aging process through the use of tobacco and alcohol, overeating, overexposure to sunlight, or lack of activity (▼ **Figure 5-1**). It is important to think of the older patient not only in terms of age, but also medication use, lifestyle choices, and the duration of chronic disease(s).

Assessment is the primary building block for management of any patient in the field. To treat any patient, an EMS provider must be able to detect abnormal findings and distinguish them from normal findings, and distinguish acute changes from chronic changes. This is especially important in older patients whose aging process can add to the complexity of assessment.

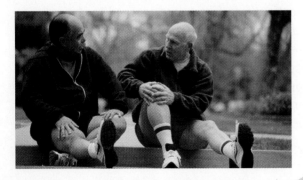

(**Figure 5-1**) Several factors affect how well a person ages. An older person who remains athletic, for instance, will have better overall health than one who has made unhealthy lifestyle choices.

Assessment of the older patient follows the same approach used in younger adults (▶ **Figure 5-2**). The EMS provider needs to conduct a scene size-up, and an initial assessment of the patient in all cases. Findings in the initial assessment as well as the patient's overall condition will dictate how the assessment proceeds.

Trauma patients with a significant mechanism of injury as well as unresponsive medical patients must receive a rapid assessment in order to further identify and manage immediate life threats. Conversely, patients with non-significant mechanisms of injury and responsive medical patients should receive a focused history and physical exam that is based upon their chief complaint.

The decision to perform a detailed physical examination is also guided by the patient's condition. Generally speaking, if the patient is in need of a rapid assessment (medical or trauma) at the scene, they will need a detailed physical examination while en route to the hospital.

Scene Size-Up

Assessment begins with the scene size-up. During scene size-up, we gain access to the patient and assess the general condition of the patient's surroundings, including factors related to your own safety and that of the patient. Access to the older patient may be limited and assistance may be required. If the patient has fallen and is unable to come to the door, you may need to find other routes of access, possibly requiring the fire department or police to assist. Residential care or nursing homes may pose access issues. You may be delayed by a front desk or admitting person, or need direction from the staff to the patient. It is common to have to summon the nurse from another patient's room in order to give you a report or answer your questions. However, you do need to question nursing home caregivers who know your patient about what is going on. They are often the best source of information on these patients and are a resource to use routinely.

In addition to your normal scene size-up, on calls with older patients be sure to assess the environment for hazards. Is the environment well maintained? Is there concern over environmental hazards:

Patient Assessment

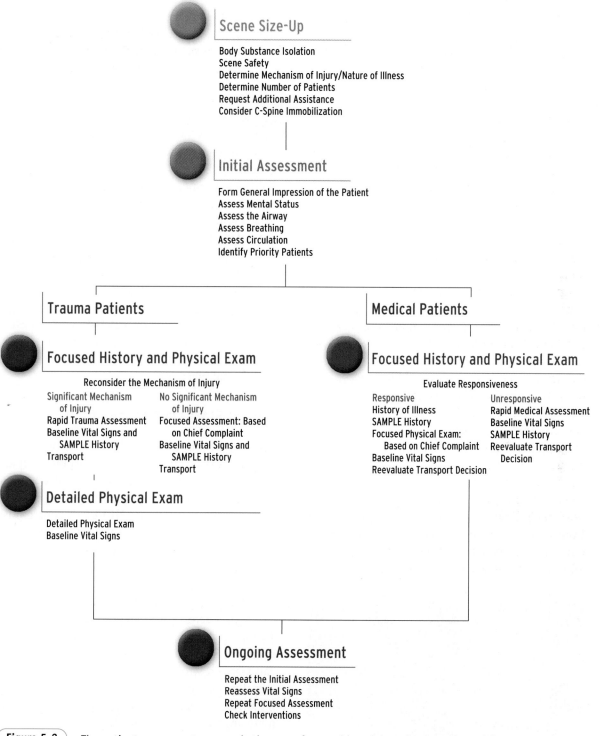

Scene Size-Up

Body Substance Isolation
Scene Safety
Determine Mechanism of Injury/Nature of Illness
Determine Number of Patients
Request Additional Assistance
Consider C-Spine Immobilization

Initial Assessment

Form General Impression of the Patient
Assess Mental Status
Assess the Airway
Assess Breathing
Assess Circulation
Identify Priority Patients

Trauma Patients

Focused History and Physical Exam

Reconsider the Mechanism of Injury

Significant Mechanism of Injury	No Significant Mechanism of Injury
Rapid Trauma Assessment	Focused Assessment: Based on Chief Complaint
Baseline Vital Signs and SAMPLE History	Baseline Vital Signs and SAMPLE History
Transport	Transport

Detailed Physical Exam

Detailed Physical Exam
Baseline Vital Signs

Medical Patients

Focused History and Physical Exam

Evaluate Responsiveness

Responsive	Unresponsive
History of Illness	Rapid Medical Assessment
SAMPLE History	Baseline Vital Signs
Focused Physical Exam: Based on Chief Complaint	SAMPLE History
Baseline Vital Signs	Reevaluate Transport Decision
Reevaluate Transport Decision	

Ongoing Assessment

Repeat the Initial Assessment
Reassess Vital Signs
Repeat Focused Assessment
Check Interventions

Figure 5-2 The patient assessment process is the same for an older adult as for a younger adult.

too cold, too warm, exposure to carbon monoxide or other toxins (▼ **Figure 5-3**)? The EMS provider alone has access to this vital information that may be critical to the ongoing care of the patient.

Personal protection for the EMS provider is important. Residents in long-term care facilities have an increased chance of being infected with resistant bacteria and tuberculosis. After you secure your own personal safety, do the same for your patient. Because older patients often have weakened immune systems, your simple cold or flu could cause a serious health problem if you pass these germs on to them. If you are ill, wear a mask and gloves to keep from contaminating the frail older patient. Better yet, stay home until you are well.

Initial Assessment

The goals of the initial assessment are to detect and treat immediate threats to life and determine the priority of care for the patient. It is based on your immediate assessment of the environment and the patient's chief complaint. The initial assessment of the older patient differs from that of the young in many ways. Some of the most critical differences are detailed below.

In addition to patient assessment, there are additional elements of assessing the scene that occur during this phase:

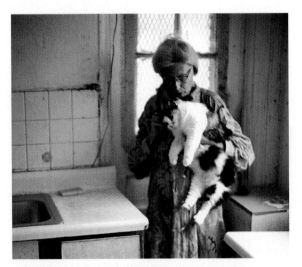

Figure 5-3 During scene size-up, observe the environment for signs of toxic exposure or danger to yourself and the patient. An oven being used for heating after the patient's electricity was shut off could indicate toxic gas presence or explosion danger—and should also make you wonder about a hypothermic patient.

◆ Is the home or institution clean or dirty? Is there food in the house? What medications are in the house? Bring the medication bottles into the emergency department.

◆ Is the patient at risk of abuse or neglect? Is there evidence of drugs, alcohol, or altered mental status?

As you assess the older patient, take note of the patient's general appearance. Once again, the environment may give you valuable clues. If you notice a hospital bed in the living room, absorbent pads, suction equipment, or bandaging materials, it is a good bet that the patient has serious or chronic health issues. You might find alcohol bottles but not a lot of food in the kitchen. Home oxygen connected to a patient will enlighten you about his chronic pulmonary problems. But, the ashtray next to his chair will tell you he still uses tobacco, an equally important finding.

Often, you are the only person with access to this critical information, so be sure to gather scene-specific information. You are the only link to this vital piece of the puzzle.

Mental Status Assessment

Aging by itself does not cause mental status changes. Mental status impairment, confusion, delirium, and dementia are all caused by pathologic or disease processes. You should NEVER accept confusion as "normal." You need to identify what disease caused the mental status change and when the change began. Do this for every confused older patient, every time.

Older patients may have chronic mental status impairment as well as new or acute changes. The difference between old and new will determine the seriousness of the call. A new change can signal a stroke, meningitis, many other serious illnesses, or polypharmacy. You may miss a life threat if you don't distinguish chronic impairment from acute impairment. Only by establishing the patient's baseline mental status can you evaluate if there is a change from this baseline.

Just as you depend on the parent to give you a history for a young child, you need to find a responsible person to give you the history of a confused older patient. Always interview the patient first, but don't forget to listen to the patient's caregiver. Recognize and report the caregiver's concerns about the patient, as well as any noticeable signs of caregiver stress or frustration related to their continuous caring for the patient. They may also be in need of help.

> ## Attitude Tip
>
> Listen to the patient's caregiver, recognize and report concerns expressed about the patient, and note any signs of caregiver stress or frustration. Caregivers often need help, too.

Typically in the initial assessment, a basic alert, verbal, painful, unresponsive (AVPU) assessment will suffice. Determination of orientation to person, place, time, and event may also be useful. Only the most severely altered will not be able to recall his or her own name. Ask if the patient knows where he or she is right now. At home, at work, in the street, in an ambulance—would all be acceptable answers. Asking the day of the week is a common way to determine orientation to time. However, many institutionalized patients may not know the day of the week. Asking the time of day (morning, noon, or night) may be more useful because even nursing home patients have a routine that may help them recall the time of day.

Lastly, orientation to the event can be determined by asking the patient what happened today to cause the call for EMS. After this type of mental status assessment, it will be necessary to ask family or caregivers about the patient's usual ability to recall the elements of person, place, time, and event. You then can determine the reliability of the history gathered from the patient himself once you know his baseline mental status. Use family, caregivers, and the patient's chart to recover important facts about medical history when the patient is an unreliable historian.

In early stages of dementia, older patients are aware of and often embarrassed by the loss of their cognitive abilities. They will often attempt to cover up or make light of their confusion. Do not be fooled! Do not accept answers like "Of course I know what day it is. Don't bother me with stupid questions when I am in pain." You don't need to be rude to get a straight answer, but you may have to be patient (▶ **Figure 5-4**). Obtain complete answers that are needed to distin-

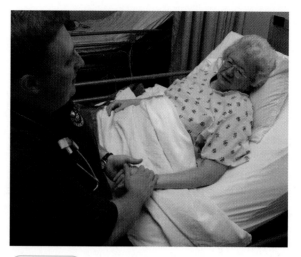

Figure 5-4 You may have to be patient, but you don't need to be rude to get the complete answers needed to distinguish old from new mental status changes.

guish old from new mental status changes through firm, but kind, repeated questioning.

> ## Attitude Tip
>
> Patients in the early stages of dementia may be embarrassed by the loss of their cognitive abilities. If the patient resists your questioning, don't be rude in an effort to get a straight answer, but do further question the patient gently, explaining that you are there to help.

Often the answer to "old versus new?" is found in nursing home records, or learned from nursing home personnel or friends and family. You *must* take the time to question these sources and establish the baseline. Then ask the critical questions of what is new today or what has changed.

Airway Assessment

Airway management in the older adult can be compromised by several anatomic changes common with age. Dentures are commonly used, and can help or hinder airway patency. If you need to assist ventilations with a bag-valve-mask device, try to leave dentures in place. When attempting to get a good seal, dentures will help to support the soft tissues of the face so they do not collapse inward.

If you need to intubate patients, removal of dentures is suggested. This prevents damage to the patient's mouth, as well as the possibility of fracturing the denture and risking aspiration or ingestion of the fragments.

An older patient's ability to protect his or her own airway may be compromised by prior disease. Prior strokes or severe dementia can result in loss of gag reflex and loss of normal swallowing mechanisms. These patients are often on soft or liquid diets. This fact should alert you to the possibility of airway compromise and risk of **aspiration pneumonia**.

In assessing the effectiveness of breathing in older patients, recall that their normal range for respiratory rate is the same as in the young adult—12 to 20 breaths/min. Chest rise may be more difficult to assess due to increased chest wall stiffness. It is important to expose part of the chest to ensure adequate chest expansion. You may need a stethoscope to assess rate and depth of respiration (▼ **Figure 5-5**). The astute EMS provider knows that a more involved exam is often necessary in the older patient. Be sure you take the time to perform it.

Bony changes also occur in the jaw and cervical spine. The jaw-thrust maneuver, and especially the head tilt-chin lift maneuver, can be difficult to accomplish and should be performed gently to prevent damage. Be more suspicious of potential cervical spine injury when evaluating the airway of any older patient. Older bones can be more brittle and more subject to injury, so take precautions accordingly. The jaw thrust results in the least amount of cervical spine motion. In contrast, a head tilt-chin lift results in a large amount of motion, which can damage an injured spinal cord. The stiffness and exaggerated curvature seen in the cervical spines of some older patients make positioning a challenge. You need to meet this challenge with appropriate pads to ensure airway patency and patient comfort. This is true with all older people, even when there is no concern of cervical trauma.

Circulatory Assessment

Circulation is produced by the cardiac output, which depends on the volume of blood pumped out of the left ventricle with each heart beat. The normally aging adult heart is less responsive to stimulation from the nerves that adjust the heart rate and strength of contraction. This can result in a lower heart rate and weaker pulse than expected in the younger adult. Always check pulses on both sides (bilaterally) to confirm that your findings are due to reduced heart function and not a blockage of flow to a specific extremity. An irregular pulse is also more common in the older patient. A history of **arrhythmias** and other problems is important when assessing circulatory status in any older patient.

The pulse check may need to be adjusted in older patients. Peripheral pulses can be difficult to feel due to vascular changes and poor circulation. Do not assume that the patient does not have a pulse because you cannot feel the radial pulse. Gently use the pulse of one of the carotid arteries for older patients when you cannot feel a peripheral pulse. Also, you can auscultate an apical pulse by listening to the heart with your stethoscope on the left chest. You can at least determine heart rate and rhythm with this technique.

Heart rate, blood pressure, capillary refill, and mental status are all indicators of circulatory status. In older patients, heart rate may be affected by medications commonly taken by older people, especially **beta blockers**. You should be familiar with these

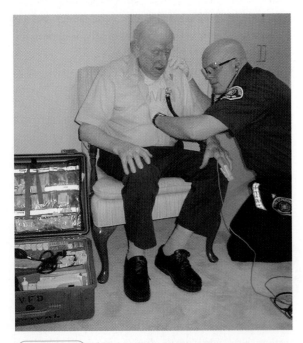

Figure 5-5 Assess the chest for adequate expansion. This may require exposing the chest or using a stethoscope.

medications and take extra care in the assessment of patients who are taking these drugs. A patient who is volume depleted from blood loss or dehydration usually increases heart rate to compensate. Patients taking beta blockers are unable to increase their heart rates in these situations because of the effect of the medication. You can miss shock in these cases if you are misled by a normal heart rate.

> ### Medication Tip
>
> **In older patients, heart rate may be affected by medications, especially beta blockers. Patients taking beta blockers may not be able to compensate for blood loss or dehydration by increasing the heart rate.**

Low blood pressure is an indicator of hypoperfusion. However, if patients have a very high baseline blood pressure, then a blood pressure that would be considered normal in a younger patient could indicate shock in the older patient. Again, establishing a baseline is crucial (▼ **Figure 5-6**). The change from this baseline will be your best indictor of a problem. Similarly, very high blood pressure may signal impending stroke or other problems.

Older patients may have chronic skin conditions that decrease the ability to assess capillary

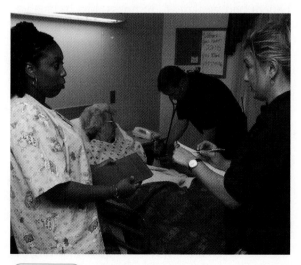

(**Figure 5-6**) Establishing a baseline blood pressure is crucial. Change from this baseline is the best indicator of a problem, and a "normal" pressure may not be adequate if the baseline is very high.

refill. Alternate sites for evaluation of perfusion include the lips and the conjunctiva, the inner lining of the eyes. Use these alternate sites and see if they give you better information. Again, establish the patient's baseline and determine if there is a recent change. Poor perfusion is serious. Patients who begin with circulation already compromised will deteriorate more quickly because their reserve is at a lower level. Provide supplemental oxygen generously. You may also want to give IV fluids earlier if no contraindications exist.

The assessment of volume status, or dehydration, is different in the older patient as well. Look for signs of dehydration, such as dull eyes, poor urine output, low blood pressure, and dry mucous membranes, which help to establish an accurate picture of dehydration. Only with the combined findings would you formulate a treatment plan around aggressive **fluid boluses**.

Patient Medications

People with chronic diseases are generally also taking medications, and may be taking several. Because older people use more prescription medications than their younger counterparts, their chance of experiencing side effects is increased. A thorough medication history in older patients is essential. Also keep in mind that older people tend to use more over-the-counter medications and herbal remedies, so don't forget to ask patients about these. Be careful to question whether there are any medications the patient is supposed to be taking, but is not. **Nonadherence** with medications can often cause deterioration of the patient's condition. The same is true for any other nonadherence, such as failure to comply with diet for diabetes, causing hyperglycemia, or failure to restrict salt intake, causing worsened congestive heart failure. It is especially important to determine if there is a new medication, either prescription or nonprescription, or a recent change in dose of a medication that may have contributed to the reason for the call.

> ### Medication Tip
>
> **As people age, they tend to use more over-the-counter medications and herbal remedies. Don't forget to ask patients about these.**

> ## Medication Tip
>
> While interacting with older patients, you have an opportunity that many health care providers do not—you observe the patient first hand. If the patient is not transported to the emergency department, you may be the only person who interacts with him or her. You can affect how well older patients keep track of their medications by distributing the medication diary found in Appendix B. This measure takes only a minute, but may save a life.

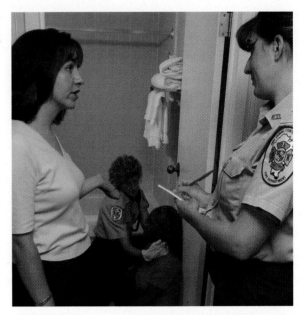

Figure 5-7   Determining both mechanism *and* cause of injury in an older patient involves asking more questions than you do with patients in other age groups.

Trauma and Medical Assessment

Mechanism of Injury and Nature of Illness

At the scene, you must determine whether the patient is injured, ill, or both. This requires you to determine any applicable mechanism of injury and/or nature of illness. Be cognizant of the fact that the patient's injury may be secondary to a medical problem. Conversely, medical conditions can be exacerbated by an injury.

Determining the mechanism of injury involves asking more questions than you do with patients in other age groups (▶ **Figure 5-7**). For example, when an older patient falls, it is very important that you determine the *cause* of the fall. Falls caused by weakness, dizziness, or palpitations most likely have a very dangerous underlying cause. You need to be a master at separating these causes. In the older patient, falls are NOT a simple trauma call. When a medical cause exists for a fall, it is often more important and life threatening than the injury from the fall itself.

In every "trip and fall" call, you must establish three things:

1. Was there really a trip and fall?
2. Is there, in fact, a medical cause of the fall?
3. If there was a trip and fall, is there an environmental hazard that can be fixed?

Many older patients will say they tripped, even if they did not, for fear of being labeled "frail." The expert EMS provider evaluates to see if the mechanism stated is plausible. If the patient reports a broken sidewalk, is the sidewalk in fact broken? Is there some hidden hazard, such as a poorly lighted hallway or a loose area rug? When you identify hidden hazards, you may be saving the patient from a future injury. Be aware of potential causes of falls in the environment of older patients. See Chapter 6 for more details about evaluating falls.

If the mechanism reported does not sound plausible, then specifically question whether the patient had weakness, dizziness, loss of balance, difficulty walking, chest pain, shortness of breath, or palpitations. Any of these can signal a serious medical condition requiring ALS care. It is better to doubt the story and discover a serious medical problem, than be unaware and miss a potential life threat.

Be especially suspicious of single-vehicle collisions. The patient may have lost control of the car due to syncope prior to the collision. Is there a chance the patient had syncope prior to the fall or the collision? Even if the patient answers "no," he or she may have had syncope but cannot remember clearly. When a person passes out, blood flow to the brain is shut off. The memory of passing out is not recorded. You need to be the detective who questions, "What is the last thing you remember?" Was there a period of time when the patient experienced decreased mental alertness, making the patient unaware that time has passed? Do not miss a life-threatening syncope because you are unaware of this common lack of recall.

Immobilization Concerns

Immobilize the spine earlier and for lesser indications than in the young. Older patients, especially those with arthritis, may sustain spinal injury with a lesser mechanism than a younger, more flexible patient. With older patients, you must be more aware to pad the areas behind the head and neck. If a patient's spine is <u>kyphotic</u> (has an exaggerated angle or curvature), modify your immobilization technique to prevent motion and maintain patient comfort. It is quite a challenge to immobilize older patients. Because their risk of injury is greater, practice is important to develop good skills with these techniques.

The older patient has thin skin that can quickly be damaged simply by the weight of the body on a hard surface (▼ **Figure 5-8**). In the areas of pressure contact with the backboard, place folded towels, wash cloths, or other soft padding material to prevent the formation of a pressure ulcer, or worsening of one that is already there (▶ **Figure 5-9**). Note specifically the mid-back, shoulders, sacrum, heels, and occiput. Ensure that these areas are cushioned. Commercial backboards with padding are now available from various manufacturers. If you routinely transport many older patients on a backboard, your service should consider investing in these boards. Ask your patient about areas where they feel pressure, and slip pads in as needed. Make this a priority. In addition to areas of contact, pay special attention to areas where arthritis or curva-

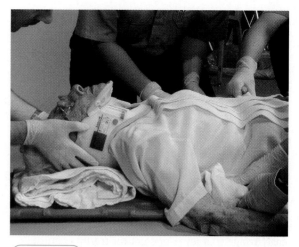

Figure 5-9   Provide padding at bony prominences to prevent damage by backboard pressure on fragile skin.

ture of the spine, frequently seen in older patients, creates a space between the patient's body and the backboard. Make sure to fill in this space with towels or blankets so the patient is both well supported and truly immobilized.

Attitude Tip

Proper padding during immobilization is much more than a comfort issue in older patients. Lack of padding under "empty" spaces can lead to unnecessary spinal injuries, and inadequate skin protection at bony contact points can produce pressure sores that occasionally lead to life-threatening infections.

Further Assessment Points

The chest wall becomes stiffer with age, which can make it difficult to identify a flail chest by visualizing paradoxical chest movement. Splinting (taking small breaths to avoid the pain of taking a deep breath) and chest wall pain may be the only clues to significant chest trauma in older patients. Be aware that loss of elasticity of the chest wall means that injury to the underlying lung requires less force in older people. These patients are more likely to develop pulmonary contusions with serious respiratory compromise. They are therefore also more likely to require level-one trauma center support when it is available. Aging blood vessels lose elasticity, so tears of the aorta are more common in older patients who sustain rapid

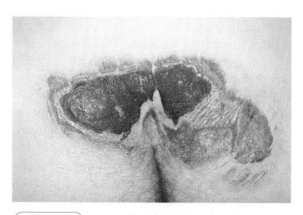

Figure 5-8   This photo shows a sacral pressure ulcer from a backboard. Be sure to pad older patients especially well at the mid-back, shoulders, sacrum, heels, and occiput.

deceleration. Their higher likelihood of needing computed tomography (CT) scans or angiograms for evaluation of a possible aortic injury, or thoracic surgery to repair one, make a trauma center the appropriate destination when available.

In many systems, age alone is a reason to bypass to a level-one trauma center. With identical injuries, the older patient will likely require more interventions than the younger patient. These include emergency department evaluation and treatment, surgical care, intensive care unit services, and rehabilitation. If you are concerned about the level of injury to an older patient, err on the side of early triage to a level-one center trauma center.

Deformity of the extremities may be a result of aging or disease, not injury. You should be familiar with the typical deformities that occur to the fingers in severe arthritis (▼ **Figure 5-10**). Do not confuse this with fractures or dislocations. The **rule of symmetry** is important, especially in the older patient. A physical finding on one side of the body that is present on the other side of the body is more likely to be a normal finding. Bruising found on one arm may be from trauma; if present on both arms, it may be due to age-related thinning of the skin and weakness in the capillary walls that supply the skin (▶ **Figure 5-11**). Be sure to thoroughly question the patient in these cases.

Assessing the Chief Complaint

Determining the chief complaint in the older patient may be difficult due to multiple disease processes and multiple or vague complaints. The

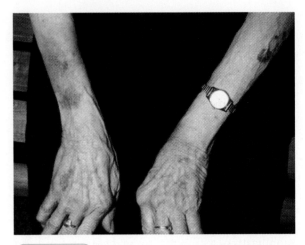

Figure 5-11 Check for symmetrical bruising on both sides of the body. Symmetrical bruising may be a result of age, not trauma.

signs or symptoms the patient presents with on-scene may be present every day. Your job is to get at the root of why they called for your help *today*. In the older patient, you may ask what is *different* about what is bothering them today, what *new* problems they have today, or what is *worse* about their symptoms today.

When patients or caregivers list multiple complaints, it helps to ask them to identify the one thing that is bothering the patient most. If the patient tells you he is weak, having trouble breathing, and has a little discomfort in his chest, ask which one of those is the most bothersome or new today. It may be that the patient has a history of chronic pulmonary problems and is always a little short of breath with some chest discomfort, but the weakness is a new and frightening symptom for this patient. Your assessment would then focus on the weakness. The chest discomfort and difficulty breathing would be considered chronic problems, and the weakness the acute problem that requires your attention.

Remember, though, that the chief complaint may not really be the most life-threatening issue. For instance, if the complaint is inability to ambulate due to swelling in the feet, the patient will probably tell you her chief complaint is that she cannot get around like she used to. However, upon assessment, you may likely determine that her presenting problem is congestive heart failure, which is causing **pedal edema** and thus difficulty in getting around.

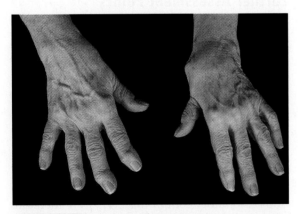

Figure 5-10 Do not confuse typical deformities of the fingers, caused by severe arthritis, with fractures or dislocations. Keep the rule of symmetry in mind.

We often organize our assessment around a set of questions specific to a chief complaint, such as chest pain or back pain. The symptoms described by an older patient may not fit into only one category of complaint or presenting problem. In this case, you should ask questions related to the most prominent or life-threatening complaint or finding first; then, if time permits, move on to other assessment questions (▶ **Figure 5-12**). For example, chest pain is usually a much more serious complaint than nausea. So, if both are offered as complaints, you should ask the questions specific to chest pain assessment first, then move on to the questions specific to nausea as needed.

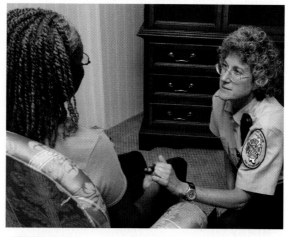

Figure 5-12   To help obtain an accurate history, have only one person interview the patient, asking one question at a time and waiting for a full answer before continuing.

Attitude Tip

Attend to the emotional needs of the patient by asking directly if the patient is frightened, reassuring the patient, asking about previous history of emotional disturbances, and managing any emotional condition as professionally as possible.

CASE STUDY 1 (continued)

In Case Study 1, you encountered a nursing home patient who was confused. As this case continues, you check airway, breathing, and circulation (the ABCs), which are intact; administer oxygen; and take her vital signs, which are within normal limits. You realize that the patient is unable to communicate an accurate past medical history to you, so you enlist the help of the nurse who has arrived with the patient's chart.

The nurse tells you that the patient has a history of heart attack and hepatitis. She has been here at the nursing home for 5 years because she was unable to care for herself. Also, she is a recovering alcoholic. She takes aspirin, atenolol (a beta blocker), and bumetanide (a diuretic). She has adhered to her medications, and did get up to go to breakfast this morning. However, she vomited once after breakfast. It was family members who noticed her change in speech when they came to visit this afternoon.

You have a big advantage in this assessment: there is family present. You turn your attention to the daughter. She states that she comes every Sunday to visit with her mother. Today, as soon as she arrived, she realized that something was wrong. She noticed that her mother had urinated in the bed, and she was unable to get her mother up to go to the bathroom and get changed. Then she noticed the change in her speech and called for a nurse right away. She confirms that her mother is normally able to carry on conversation, aware of her surroundings, and cognitively intact.

What considerations should you keep in mind when transporting this patient?

Identifying Priority Patients

Know how the assessment of the older patient differs from that of the younger adult and apply these principles during your calls. Conclude the initial assessment by identifying priority patients. These are patients who have conditions associated with higher risks of morbidity (illness) or mortality (▼ Table 5-1). If your patient has one or more of these conditions, expedite transport and consider calling ALS if it is available.

TABLE 5-1 Identifying Priority Patients

Priority Patients	Considerations for Older Patients
Poor general impression	Overall less reserves, more likely to deteriorate rapidly
Unresponsive, no gag or cough	Gag response less sensitive
Responsive, not following commands	Determine if this is a change from the baseline mental status
Difficulty breathing	May fatigue earlier (run out of reserves)
Shock (hypoperfusion)	Early shock may be more difficult to identify because the ability to increase heart rate in response to hypoperfusion is compromised
Chest pain with blood pressure of < 100 mm Hg systolic	Baseline systolic blood pressure may be higher; watch for a decrease from baseline blood pressure
Uncontrolled bleeding	Gastrointestinal bleeding more common
Severe pain anywhere	Less pain perception in general; moderate pain may be a priority

Detailed Physical Exam

As previously mentioned, the decision to perform a detailed physical exam is based on the patient's condition. (▶ Table 5-2) lists some of the common physical findings in older patients that may be noted during the detailed physical exam. Keep in mind that these findings will not be present in all your older patients. However, when you do see them, they may be normal changes for this person.

It is not just the history that is complicated with the older patient. The physical exam can be tough, too. Actually gaining access to the body may be more challenging, because the older patient is often very modest and uncomfortable being exposed. Protect privacy by keeping undergarments intact if possible, and covering the patient with a sheet or blanket (▼ Figure 5-13). Additionally, because thermoregulatory function is often impaired in the older patient, they may often feel cold and wear many layers of clothing to keep warm. You will have to remove some of these layers to take lung sounds, apply a heart monitor, or assess skin signs.

A primary aspect of protecting older patients is keeping them warm enough to make them comfortable and prevent shivering. This is a patient comfort measure as well as prevention of a complication that will interfere with your assessment. Maintaining internal body temperature becomes more difficult with age. Fat reserves are

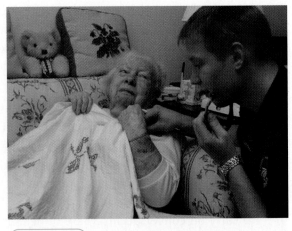

Figure 5-13   The older patient is often very modest and uncomfortable being exposed. Protect privacy by keeping undergarments intact, if possible, and covering the patient with a sheet or blanket.

TABLE 5-2	Physical Changes in Older Patients
Body Part	**Findings**
Head	Thinner scalp; less hair overall Brown spots from sun exposure
Face	Skin wrinkles; nose may enlarge due to cartilage changes Brown spots from sun exposure
Ears	Hearing loss; ears may develop small lumps or contain a hearing aid
Eyes	Decreased visual acuity; pupils smaller; opaque white ring of fatty deposits circling the cornea; eyes can appear more sunken due to loss of **periorbital** fat; cataracts may cloud the lens; prior surgery may result in irregular pupils or a hole in the iris
Mouth	Dentures; teeth less white; varicose veins of the tongue, tooth loss, gum shrinkage
Neck	Decrease in range of motion; increased spinal curvature Stiffness and chronic pain to touch and movement
Chest	Less chest expansion with breathing; bilateral crackles on inspiration that clear with subsequent deep breaths
Abdomen	Decreased muscle tone, loss of ability to become rigid with internal bleeding or infection
Pelvis	Decreased range of motion, frail bones that fracture easily
Extremities	Decrease in range of motion; symmetrically decreased muscle strength; varicose veins; symmetrical bruising; edema, especially in lower legs/feet Decreased capillary refill, loss of muscle mass
Back	Increase in curvature of the spine, frail bones that fracture easily, chronic pain, loss of flexibility (▼ **Figure 5-14**)

lost, skin is thinner, and metabolism slows. Use blankets frequently in older patients where you would just use a sheet in the young. Take care to cover the head of an older patient when it is cold outside. Make sure your ambulance compartment is warm.

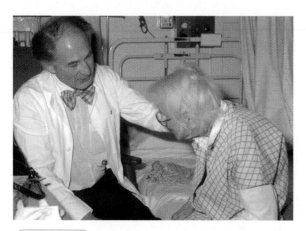

Figure 5-14   Severe kyphosis, or increased curvature of the spine, can occur in older people.

Attitude Tip

Covering the patient with a blanket to protect privacy and keep the patient warm shows respect for the patient and will improve your exam.

Ongoing Assessment

A patient who is initially stable does not always remain stable. Ongoing assessment is more important in older patients than in their younger counterparts. Without careful attention to the appropriate areas of assessment, you could miss a patient's deterioration. There are four elements of the ongoing assessment: repeating the initial assessment, repeating the vital signs, repeating the focused assessment (tailored to the patient's complaint or injuries), and checking the interventions you have implemented.

Repetition of the initial assessment should take place at least every 15 minutes for a stable patient and at least every 5 minutes for an unstable patient. This includes reevaluation of mental status, airway, breathing, circulation, and patient priority. Reassess and record the patient's vital signs, looking for trends toward improvement or deterioration. Repeat the focused assessment. In the medical patient, this means asking the patient how she feels now compared to before. In the trauma patient with a significant mechanism of injury, it will mean repeating the pertinent parts of the detailed physical exam. Last, check the interventions you performed (▶ **Figure 5-15**). Is the patient still receiving oxygen? If you are ventilating, how well is the chest rising? Has any bleeding resumed from a wound you bandaged, or has bleeding started in a new area? How is the neurovascular function of the extremity you splinted? Is your spinal immobilization adequate?

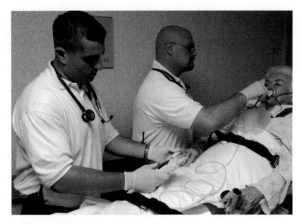

Figure 5-15 Ongoing assessment concludes with checking interventions you have performed. Is the patient still receiving oxygen, for instance, and is it doing what you intended?

Performing the ongoing assessment depends on the patient's condition. You may not have time to perform all of it, or sometimes any of it. Occasionally you will not get past the initial assessment because the patient has life-threatening injuries that demand your constant attention. Fortunately, these patients are uncommon. On most EMS calls, you have the time to reevaluate your patient before you arrive at the hospital.

CASE STUDY 2

You are dispatched to the residence of an older woman with a chief complaint of shortness of breath. On arrival you are met at the door by a neighbor who guides you to the living room of a well-kept older home. Your patient is seated and appears to be in no distress. You introduce yourself, determine the patient's name to be Mrs. Smith, and ask how you can assist her this morning. She states that she called 9-1-1 because when she climbed the stairs today she became breathless. This hasn't happened before, and got better when she sat down. She tried the stairs again and the same thing happened. She is normally very active.

You observe the patient to be alert and oriented. Your partner applies oxygen via nasal cannula at 2 L/min and proceeds to take vital signs. You determine that Mrs. Smith is without chest pain, nausea, fever, or dizziness. Further, she has no allergies, takes one baby aspirin in the morning, and was hospitalized 2 years ago for pneumonia. You also determine that she typically eats breakfast but was "not up to it today."

What is potentially happening with this patient?

PART II: COMMON COMPLAINTS OF THE OLDER PATIENT

This section discusses potential causes and assessment of the top ten chief complaints of older patients, including shortness of breath; chest pain; altered mental status; abdominal pain; dizziness or weakness; fever; trauma; falls; generalized pain; and nausea, vomiting, and diarrhea.

Shortness of Breath

The sensation that one cannot breathe is extremely frightening, and the reality is that it can be life threatening. The older patient is at high risk for respiratory problems due to normal processes of aging. Breathing capacity can decrease by up to 50% during the aging process (▶ **Figure 5-16**). The complaint of shortness of breath (SOB) is common in the older population, and often it is a true medical emergency.

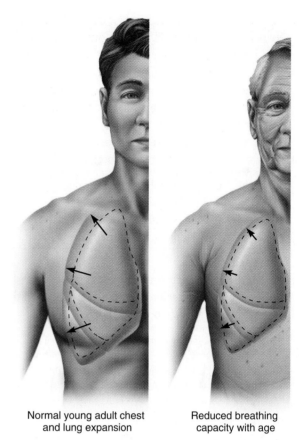

Normal young adult chest and lung expansion

Reduced breathing capacity with age

Figure 5-16   Breathing capacity can decrease by up to 50% during the aging process.

Potential Causes

Shortness of breath is often caused by cardiac problems in the older population. It may be the only symptom of heart attack. Chronic obstructive pulmonary disease (COPD), bronchitis, asthma, emphysema, and congestive heart failure (CHF) can all cause wheezing. A careful history and physical exam may help sort this out. (▶ **Table 5-3**) shows a list of the distinguishing features that will help you separate the classic presentation of the older patient with these diseases.

Remember, too, that shortness of breath can occur for a variety of other medical reasons that are not respiratory or cardiac in nature, such as pain, bleeding, or medication interactions.

Assessment

Remember that the patient may have multiple disease processes or past medical problems. Determine if any of these chronic conditions could be causing the difficulty breathing, or if the patient frequently or always has trouble

breathing (▶ **Figure 5-18**). If so, ask what has made the patient call for help today, or what makes the breathing more difficult today. Attempt to learn which other signs and symptoms are chronic, and which are new or acute. You will likely treat only acute symptoms or chronic symptoms that have worsened. However, never withhold oxygen from any patient complaining of difficulty breathing, regardless of origin or onset.

Medication Tip

The older patient is frequently prescribed many more medications than the younger patient, multiplying the risk of interactions and medication side effects, which can include difficulty breathing.

TABLE 5-3 COPD versus CHF

	COPD	CHF
History	◆ Long-time smoker ◆ Known emphysema or bronchitis ◆ On oxygen, inhalers, steroids ◆ Made worse by upper respiratory infection ◆ Chronic hacking morning cough	◆ Prior heart attacks/angina ◆ Prior coronary artery bypass graft, angioplasty ◆ On nitrates, cardiac meds, furosemide (Lasix) ◆ Orthopnea (▼ Figure 5-17), nocturnal dyspnea ◆ New cough of frothy sputum
Physical	◆ More trouble getting air out ◆ Pink Puffer* or Blue Bloater† ◆ Wide, round, barrel chest ◆ Swelling at the base of the nails (clubbing)	◆ More trouble getting air in ◆ Jugular vein distention (JVD) and pedal/leg edema ◆ Generally normal chest ◆ Point of maximal impulse displaced to right
Treatment	◆ Oxygen ◆ Inhaled beta agonists ◆ No morphine—bad for respiratory rate ◆ Intubation if severe	◆ Oxygen ◆ No beta agonists—bad for heart rate ◆ Furosemide (Lasix), nitrates, possibly morphine ◆ Intubation if severe

*Pink Puffer: Thin, frail, reddened complexion. Breathing fast, using accessory muscles. Has a prolonged expiratory phase with cheeks puffed out to force air out.

†Blue Bloater: Fat, robust, cyanotic complexion. Breathing fast using accessory muscles, but hard to see due to thick short neck. Prolonged expiratory phase, leaning forward.

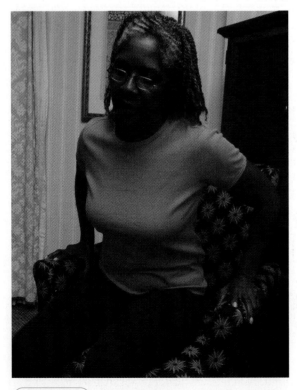

Figure 5-17 Difficulty breathing in the reclined position (orthopnea) is a sign of CHF.

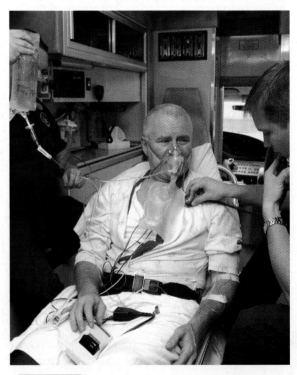

Figure 5-18 Determine if the patient's shortness of breath is caused by a chronic condition, or if the problem is new today.

Chest Pain

Cardiovascular disease is a leading cause of death in the older patient. Chest pain is common in older patients, and often life threatening. A chief complaint of chest pain may have many causes, but should always be taken seriously and treated aggressively because many of the cardiac conditions causing chest pain will be lethal if not treated immediately.

Potential Causes

Cardiac problems can present atypically in older patients, for example, with only a feeling of weakness or SOB. Older people may not have any chest pain, but instead may have shoulder or neck pain, arm pain, back pain, or jaw pain. This type of pain presentation may easily be mistaken for a toothache, pulled muscle, or arthritis. Use the rest of the history and physical exam to rule out or confirm a cardiac condition.

Chest pain is very commonly caused by angina (lack of blood supply to the heart muscle), which causes heart pain. When this is the case, the patient is usually aware of the diagnosis, and probably takes nitroglycerin. Often the patient can tell you if this pain is different in any way from their usual type of pain, and that can be a critical clue to determining the cause. The problem, however, is that chest pain is often attributed to angina when it is really a heart attack in progress. The safest bet for all EMS providers is to treat for the most lethal condition, which would be myocardial infarction.

Another extremely dangerous condition more common in older patients than in younger patients is aortic **aneurysm**, or bulging of the blood vessel. This can lead to blood leakage, or major bleeding if the vessel tears open. A torn aorta will most certainly cause death in minutes if not detected. Classically, these patients report a tearing chest pain that may go to the back.

Pulmonary embolism is also more common in the older patient. This causes pinpoint chest pain with sudden onset, and possibly shortness of breath. Pulmonary emboli have many causes, such as sedentary lifestyle, blood clot in the legs, cancer, vascular injury, and long bone fractures.

Assessment

There are several questions to ask of the chest pain patient that can help you determine the cause of the chest pain. Location of the pain is important. Substernal chest pain (located beneath the sternum) may be a heart attack, while pinpoint chest pain may be a pulled muscle. **Epigastric pain** may be abdominal in nature, and the lack of pain does not rule out a heart attack. Older patients, those who have had open-heart surgery, and patients with diabetes all experience pain differently (or not at all) than younger patients. In your cardiac assessment, it is very important to expose and examine the chest of a patient with chest pain. Inspection of the chest may reveal old scars from previous cardiac surgeries. This would inform you of a history of cardiac problems. A pacemaker or defibrillator may be present under the skin on the upper chest (▼ **Figure 5-19**). Both of these devices are more common in the older patient and give you clues about past arrhythmias. The upper torso may also reveal transdermal medication patches, such as nitroglycerin. It is possible that the patient's complaint is caused by too much or too little of this medication. If your patient is hypotensive and is wearing a nitroglycerin patch, REMOVE the patch! At the very least, the patch will give you a clue about a past medical history of angina, heart attack, or arrhythmia.

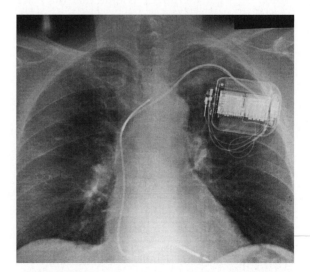

Figure 5-19   Presence of an implanted pacemaker or cardioverter-defibrillator (automated implantable cardio defibrillator [AICD], pictured) beneath the skin gives clues about past arrhythmias.

Medication Tip

If your patient is hypotensive and is wearing a nitroglycerin patch, remove it. It is possible that the patient's complaint is caused by too much or too little of this medication.

Medication Tip

Numerous medications and other ingested substances can lower or raise the heart rate. Ask about beta blockers and calcium channel blockers (lower), as well as respiratory medications, caffeine, tobacco, and other stimulants (raise).

Altered Mental Status

Altered mental status (AMS) is the typical presentation of a large number of underlying problems in the older patient. Frequently, EMS is called because a family member or caregiver notices that a person is "not acting right." Avoid the temptation to assume that because the person is an older patient, he or she is normally altered. Only 2% of persons in their 60s suffer dementia. Therefore, it would be a grave error to assume that the AMS presentation is normal for the patient without first investigating the potentially life-threatening medical or traumatic conditions that may exist.

Attitude Tip

Avoid the temptation to assume that because the patient is older, it is normal for him or her to have an altered mental status.

Potential Causes

Altered mental status is really a presentation, not a chief complaint. However, it is very common for the family or caregivers to notice that someone cannot carry on a conversation, has become forgetful, cannot recognize family members, is lethargic,

sleepy, or even unconscious (▼ Figure 5-20). These noticeable findings are usually a symptom of an underlying condition that has caused the AMS.

A malfunction to nearly any body system can result in AMS. Causes of AMS include seizure, stroke, cardiac dysfunction, respiratory compromise, trauma, hypoglycemia, medication problems (overdoses, underdoses, and interactions), infection, dehydration, hypothermia, hyperthermia, and sometimes dementia. The causes of AMS are not different in the older population than in the younger population, but the frequency of AMS presentation is much higher for older patients. Moreover, AMS can be the only presentation of a life-threatening illness, so it is always important to investigate thoroughly.

Assessment

The altered patient presents a challenge to the EMS provider because a person who is severely altered or unconscious may not be able to protect his or her own airway. Therefore, airway management will need to be started during the initial assessment, and if the cause of the AMS cannot be identified and corrected, then airway management will have to be maintained throughout the call.

In addition to airway management, the altered patient should have vital signs monitored frequently, as changes in the patient's condition are likely. Advanced providers should use routine ALS care, which includes the cardiac monitor and IV placement. The rhythm on a cardiac monitor

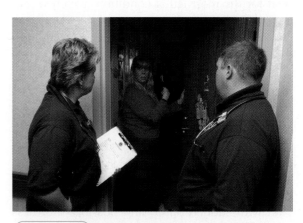

Figure 5-20 It is very common for family or caregivers to call EMS with a concern about altered mental status in an elder.

may provide information about a recent heart attack or arrhythmia that is causing the AMS. Never assume that an existing arrhythmia is old. You must question and establish this accurately because it may be an acute life threat.

Physical Exam

The first step of the physical exam for the AMS patient will be to determine level of consciousness. This process is summarized earlier in this chapter. Check the patient's orientation to person, place, time, and event (▼ **Figure 5-21**).

> ## Communication Tip
>
> **As a matter of respect, always try to interview the patient first rather than assuming an inability to communicate.**

Determination of motor and sensory response is standard in AMS patients. Check grip strength and uniformity, pedal push strength and uniformity, and smile symmetry. An altered gait can indicate a neurological finding. If your patient is ambulatory to the stretcher, observe the gait for coordination and steadiness. Another physical finding important for the altered patient is pupil size and reactivity, which can indicate drug overdoses, head injury, and hypoxia, but recall that patients with prior cataract surgery may always have unequal pupils. Skin temperature can often rule out hypothermia and hyperthermia. When possible, get a blood sugar measurement to rule out the possibility of hyperglycemia or hypoglycemia. The treatment for any of these potential causes for the AMS will be determined by your assessment findings, and will be similar to what you would do for the same condition in a younger patient.

Because 25% of all prescription medications are sold to the older population, medication interactions, overdoses, and underdoses are a very common problem and frequent cause of AMS. Be sure to get a thorough list of all medications, including over-the-counter and herbal medications. Take special note of any new medications, or multiple bottles of the same medication, as you are the only one who will be able to bring this information to the hospital. This is a very critical point that may determine the entire cause of the patient's problem. Older patients can get into trouble with their medications when different physicians prescribe the same medication, or different medications from the same class or family of medications, resulting in an unintentional overdose. Alcohol abuse is not only a problem of youth. Be cautious that reverse prejudice does not make you miss alcohol abuse in the older patient.

> ## Medication Tip
>
> **Multiple medications, prescriptions from more than one doctor, and use of over-the-counter medications and herbal preparations can all cause altered mental status.**

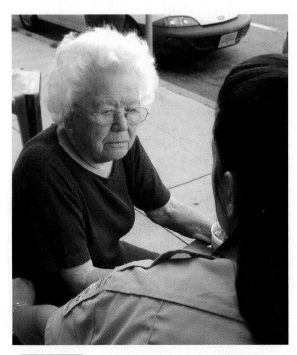

Figure 5-21   In older patients with suspected AMS, determine orientation to person, place, time, and event.

Abdominal Pain

In contrast to the younger patient, the older patient who presents with abdominal pain is more likely to be hospitalized, have surgery, or die from whatever caused the pain (▼ **Figure 5-22**). Early determination of the cause results in a higher chance of successful treatment. The care given by the EMS provider is often the first vital step in that success.

Potential Causes

The potential causes of abdominal pain change as we age. Appendicitis is common at younger ages. It is uncommon in the older patient, but when it does occur, the appendix is more often ruptured and the patient is sicker. We will focus on the causes of abdominal pain that present significant risk to an older person's health.

Older patients suffer from different disease processes than the young. Those illnesses causing abdominal pain in older people that are rare in the young are:

◆ Vascular problems
  ◆ Abdominal aortic aneurysm (AAA)
  ◆ Mesenteric ischemia/infarction

◆ Diverticulitis
◆ Gallstones
◆ Peptic ulcer disease (▼ **Table 5-4**)
◆ Intestinal obstruction from hernia, tumor, or adhesion

Assessment

History

In assessing the older patient with abdominal pain, the patient history is the key to successful care. The expected signs and symptoms associated with a particular abdominal problem may be altered or absent in the older patient. Older patients have a blunted immune response, meaning that they don't develop inflammation and peritonitis (an irritation of the lining of the abdomen from blood, infection, or digestive fluids) like the young. Therefore, they often do not have the symptoms or physical findings typical of younger adults with these diseases.

Older people typically have less abdominal pain perception and fewer associated symptoms. The younger patient with appendicitis classically complains of right lower quadrant abdominal pain, nausea, and vomiting. The older patient may complain of more diffuse pain (scattered rather than localized) without nausea or vomit-

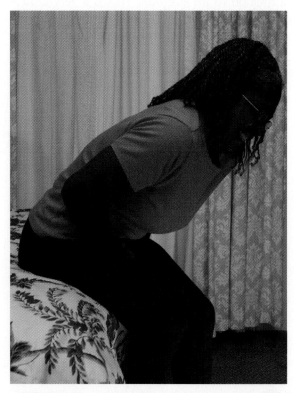

Figure 5-22 Older patients with abdominal pain have higher chances of hospitalization, surgery, and death than younger people.

TABLE 5-4 Arthritis Medicines That Can Contribute to Peptic Ulcer Disease	
Anti-pain and anti-inflammation medications	◆ Aspirin or ASA (acetylsalicylic acid) ◆ Nonsteroidal anti-inflammatory drugs (NSAIDs) Examples: ibuprofen (Motrin); indomethacin (Indocin); ketoprofen (Orudis); meclomenamate (Meclomen); nabumetone (Relafen); piroxicam (Feldene)
Anti-inflammation medication	◆ Steroids (prednisone)

ing, or just not feeling well. However, not every older patient will present differently than expected. The effective EMS provider is familiar with the typical presentation of the patient with abdominal pain, its various causes, and how aging may change the presentation.

It is important to determine the patient's mental status early to gauge the validity of the information provided. Confirm the history or gather additional information from family, caregivers, or bystanders through direct questioning based on your knowledge of abdominal problems in older people. A history of intermittent back pain that preceded the abdominal pain may be due to an aneurysm. Additional history that may increase your suspicion includes tobacco use, medications for high blood pressure or angina, and a previous heart attack. Gallstones typically cause right upper quadrant and epigastric pain after eating greasy food and are often accompanied by nausea, vomiting, and bloating. Although these classic symptoms may not be present with the older patient's current episode, a careful history of any previous bouts may lead to a suspicion of gallstones as the problem. Always inquire about bleeding in vomit or bowels in all older patients.

Diverticulitis generally presents with left lower quadrant pain. The older patient may report the discomfort as pressure or constipation instead of pain. Complaints in the left lower quadrant of the abdomen should cause you to think of diverticulitis (▶ **Figure 5-23**).

Physical Exam

The physical exam begins with observing the patient. Does the patient appear distressed? As with history taking, determine the baseline mental status early to help interpret the patient's response to your exam. The abdominal organs do not necessarily remain in the same location as when young; your knowledge of anatomy will help guide your physical assessment (▶ **Figure 5-24**). The approach is unchanged: observe, auscultate, and palpate.

If you see a distended abdomen, it may be dilated loops of bowel from an obstruction or blood from a ruptured aneurysm. If you hear a whooshing sound (**bruit**) with each heart beat when you listen to the abdomen, it may be from an aneurysm. The absence of bowel sounds could suggest

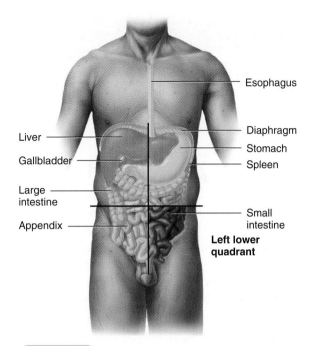

Figure 5-23 Diverticulitis generally presents with left lower quadrant pain.

a serious abdominal problem, should be frequently reassessed during transport, and should be reported to the emergency department. Is the palpated abdomen soft or hard? A hard abdomen is a very serious sign in the older patient. This signals ALS care and rapid transport.

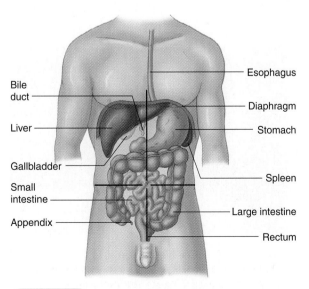

Figure 5-24 The anatomy of the abdomen.

Medication Tip

Medications, including over-the-counter meds, can alter the patient's response to your examination of an abdominal pain complaint. Keep meds in mind as you examine.

Further Assessment Points

The priority older patient with abdominal pain has severe pain or at least one of the following: hypotension, tachycardia, or recent mental status changes. Severe abdominal pain is significant because the older patient has an overall diminished response to pain; severe pain is more likely to be due to a serious illness. Tachycardia or hypotension, even if transient, can indicate the presence of a life-threatening process such as gastrointestinal bleeding, an abdominal aortic aneurysm (AAA), a perforated ulcer, spreading infection from diverticulitis or a non-abdominal process such as a heart attack. Recent mental status changes in the older patient are often the earliest sign of a serious illness.

Management

In your management, remember that ALS is "BLS-plus" not "instead of BLS." BLS care includes appropriate transport in the position of comfort in a warm environment (▼ **Figure 5-25**). Collect and transport all prescription medication and any re-

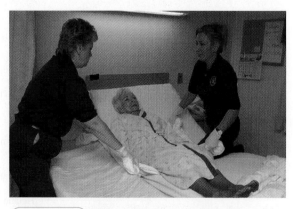

Figure 5-25　The biggest threat to the older patient with abdominal pain is a delay in identifying the underlying cause. Timely EMS care and transport will lead to a better patient outcome.

cently used over-the-counter medications. For the priority patient, apply oxygen and expedite transport. Keep the patient from eating or drinking; this complicates the administration of anesthesia should the patient require surgery.

ALS treatment adds venous access, cardiac monitoring, and the potential for pain control. Fluid administration should align with the patient's condition. Treat tachycardia and/or hypotension with bolus therapy, constantly reassessing the patient's response. It is important to keep in mind the potential for fluid overload that can result in pulmonary edema. However, it is even more important to recognize inadequately treated shock. Also, be sure to consult with the receiving physician before administering pain medication in older patients with severe abdominal pain.

Dizziness or Weakness

Dizziness is a common complaint among older people. A patient who experiences dizziness is more likely to experience a fall, fracture a hip, and end up in a long-term care facility—or die as a result of the fall. Dizziness that does not have a diagnosable cause, such as orthostatic hypotension, is primarily a sign of depression or anxiety or the presence of a chronic illness. Patients may also report "weakness" with similar signs and symptoms as dizziness.

Potential Causes

Your patient's complaint of dizziness can be caused by a single factor or a combination of factors. These factors can be divided into balance, injury, oxygen, energy, or psychological factors. Damage to the body's balance mechanism in the inner ear by inflammation, infection, or injury can cause dizziness. Direct brain injury from a stroke or from trauma can also result in dizziness. A low oxygen supply to the brain can be caused by a blood pressure that is too low (hypotension or arrhythmia) or too high (hypertension), or from too few red blood cells (**anemia**). Low blood pressure can be constant or transient. Constant low blood pressure can be due to shock of any cause, or a heart beat that is irregular, too fast, or too slow. Transient hypotension may be due to mild dehydration, intermittent heart rhythm irregularities, or medication effects. Glucose is the only energy source for the brain; if it is too low, dizziness can be one of the symptoms (▼ Figure 5-26). Dizziness may also be one of the many symptoms associated with depression and anxiety.

Assessment

History

Dizziness means different things to different people. Your patient may describe the dizziness as spinning (**vertigo**), lightheadedness, weakness, being unsteady, wooziness, or having a loss of balance. You can separate your patients into two categories by asking whether the patient experiences vertigo. The patient may feel that he himself is spinning, that the surroundings are spinning, or both. Patients with vertigo are more likely to have a balance problem from the inner ear than from any other cause. They often report spinning when they move their heads in a certain manner. Lying quietly often makes the vertigo better. Brain injury patients can also develop vertigo. Vertigo patients often also have vomiting. Make sure you assess for this, because it is a very helpful tool.

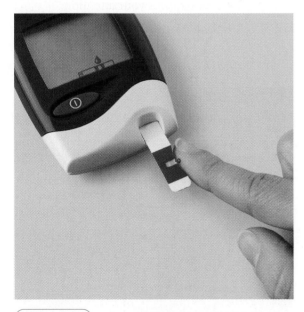

Figure 5-26 If a patient's glucose level is too low, dizziness can be one of the symptoms. A glucometer can be used to test blood glucose levels.

> **Communication Tip**
>
> **Dizziness means different things to different people. You can separate these patients into two categories by asking whether the patient experiences vertigo.**

Patients with dizziness but no vertigo can be further divided into patients with dizziness at rest and those with dizziness when active. Possible reasons for dizziness at rest include an irregular heart rate and severe hypotension. Determine if the patient has heart problems, or a pacemaker, and what medications he or she takes. Certain heart medications can make the heart beat too slowly, and some over-the-counter medications, such as certain cold compounds and herbals, can cause the blood pressure to increase.

Assess if the dizziness occurs with a simple activity such as sitting up from bed or getting out of a chair. If these occur, consider low blood pressure, dehydration, or anemia. Determine if the patient has been eating and drinking fluids on a regular schedule. Ask the patient if they took any medication before the onset of dizziness. Medicines that are used to treat high blood pressure (antihypertensives) can be the culprit. Determine if your patient has diabetes and whether there are additional signs of low blood sugar, such as tremors or sweating.

> **Medication Tip**
>
> **Certain heart medications can make the heart beat too slowly and some over-the-counter medications can cause the blood pressure to increase. Either of these effects can cause dizziness.**

Physical Exam

Normal vital signs, oxygen saturation, and blood sugar should help rule out most potentially life-threatening causes of dizziness such as hypotension, heart rhythm problems, or hypoglycemia. Orthostatic (postural) vital signs may identify a low circulating volume that causes the dizziness when the patient is erect. To do this, take the blood pressure and heart rate when the patient is lying quietly. Then, have the patient stand, observe for unsteadiness, and ask if the patient feels unsteady. Recheck after approximately 1 minute of standing (▼ Figure 5-27). If the systolic blood pressure decreases by 20 mm Hg or more or the diastolic blood pressure decreases 10 mm Hg or more from the first reading, or if the pulse increases by 20 beats/min or more, the patient is said to have orthostatic hypotension.

Is **nystagmus** present? These jerky eye movements can be seen with dizziness caused by problems in the balance mechanism of the inner ear or in the brain. Auscultate for bruits (whooshing) over the carotid arteries and gently palpate for any decrease in pulsatile force. These may be signs of decreased blood flow to the brain. Is there evidence of a previous stroke, such as a facial droop, arm drift, or slurred speech? Check for scalp tenderness, bruising, or swelling from a recent trauma. Note any difficulties with standing or walking.

Further Assessment Points

Patients with dizziness due to hypotension, abnormal heart rhythm, evolving stroke, or a history of a recent head injury are priority patients. Hypotension may be simple dehydration or significant shock. The abnormal heart rhythm can be a simple decrease in rate or an unstable rhythm like ventricular tachycardia. Patients with an evolving stroke are a priority because of the potential for treatment with clot-busting drugs. Changes in assessment after any head injury may indicate a worsening condition. These patients require priority transport and treatment. Nonpriority patients with dizziness are at risk for becoming priority patients from falls due to their dizziness.

Fever

Fever is part of the body's response to infection. It is defined as an oral temperature of 100°F or higher (▼ Figure 5-28). In older people, fever can be defined as a rise of 2°F from the person's baseline temperature. Because older individuals can have a lower baseline body temperature and are less able to develop a fever when infected, the presence of a fever in an older person is a significant finding that requires your attention.

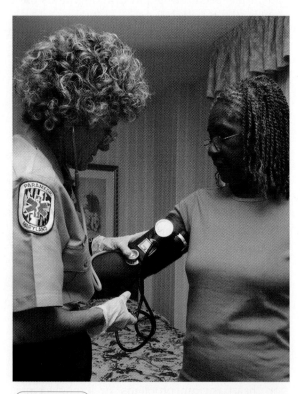

Figure 5-27 Orthostatic (postural) vital signs may identify a low circulating volume that causes the dizziness when the patient is erect. Recheck blood pressure after the patient has been standing for about 1 minute.

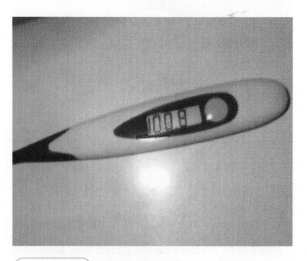

Figure 5-28 Fever is defined as an oral temperature of 100°F or higher.

Potential Causes

Before the development of antibiotics, dying from "old age" often meant death from pneumonia. This is still a very common cause of fever in older people, and despite antibiotics, pneumonia is a common cause of death. Infections of the urinary tract are also common. Other causes include infection in the blood, gastroenteritis, and soft-tissue infections, especially from pressure ulcers. Temperature elevation is much less frequently caused by non-infectious problems, which include heat stroke, malignancy (cancer), **thyroid storm**, and aspirin overdose, to name a few.

Assessment

History

Begin by asking about the patient's baseline temperature. In a nursing home environment, documentation of the patient's baseline temperature should be available. In an older patient with a temperature and a recent change in mental status, suspect a serious infection. Even if the temperature is normal or only slightly elevated, recent mental status changes could suggest infection. Commonly associated symptoms may be diminished or absent. The older patient with pneumonia may not have a cough. Burning on urination may be absent in the older patient with a urinary tract infection. What may be present instead is a change in daily living. The patient's eating habits may be altered. The person may be less active or more fatigued. Ask the patient or caregiver if daily activities have recently changed. Is the patient on medication that alters the fever response (acetaminophen [Tylenol], aspirin, or NSAIDs) or alters the ability to fight infection, such as steroids (prednisone)? How about over-the-counter medications? The patient may admit to using cough syrup, but forget to tell you about the cough.

Medication Tip

Medications that alter fever response (acetaminophen [Tylenol], aspirin, or NSAIDs), alter the ability to fight infection, such as steroids (prednisone), or are used to treat a possible infection (cough syrup) can all be tips to infection when a patient has little or no fever.

Ask about the patient's immunization status. Viral infections such as the common cold do occur in older people. Most devastating can be influenza, thus the importance of a yearly flu vaccination in the fall (▼ **Figure 5-29**). Pneumovax, the pneumonia vaccine, is generally administered only once. It provides protection from the bacteria *Pneumococcus*, one of the most common causes of bacterial pneumonia. Determine the presence of any other diseases that may elevate infection risk. Diabetes increases the overall chance of infection; pneumonia and bronchitis are frequently seen in patients with COPD; kidney stones and gallstones can cause infection; and pressure ulcers often grow a variety of bacteria that can result in local infection or blood-borne (system-wide) infection.

Physical Exam

The focus of your exam of the febrile older patient is to find any immediate life threats and to help determine the source of infection. The patient may be sicker than he or she appears on initial contact. Heart rate may not increase with temperature as expected. Respiratory rate normally stays in the higher range of normal. Low oxygen saturation may be the first indication of a pulmonary infection. Are there any signs of increased work of breathing? As you perform a head-to-toe exam, note any skin areas that are red, warm, tender, or swollen, indicating possible infection. Look for pressure ulcers that may develop over high-pressure areas such as the heels, sacrum, and buttocks. Do these wounds look

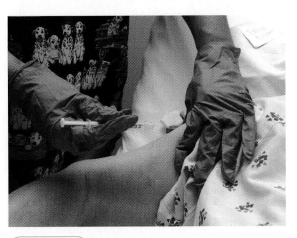

Figure 5-29 Getting your patient's vaccination history may help you assess the likelihood of infection.

clean or dirty? Are they red, swollen, and draining? What is the color of the drainage?

Check for neck flexion—is it stiffer than normal? This could indicate meningitis. Listen for diminished breath sounds or crackles on one side or the other that do not clear after several inspirations. This may indicate a pulmonary source for the fever. Local or generalized abdominal tenderness to palpation may be the result of infection. Tenderness to percussion (tapping) of the back over the kidneys in the patient with a fever is consistent with a urinary tract infection involving the kidney. In the physical exam of the older patient with a fever, there is often a lack of the typical signs of infectious disease as seen in the younger adult.

Further Assessment Points

Fever in the older patient means serious infection until proven otherwise. *You must assess these patients for the existence of sepsis and septic shock.* If found, then they must have priority ALS care. Give fluids for the hypotension. Remember, more older people die from their infections than younger adults, even though they may appear less ill than the younger adult with the same infection. The older febrile patient has fewer associated signs and symptoms when compared to the younger adult. In addition, the presence of chronic disease and use of routine medications may increase the potential for infection while confusing the assessment process.

Infections are common in older people, with or without generating a fever. Presenting signs and symptoms may be minimal. Any increase in body temperature should lead you to suspect infection. The course of infectious disease in the older patient is typically longer and more severe. Early detection allows for early treatment and a better outcome. The assessment and treatment you provide in the field may be the key to effective, timely treatment.

Trauma

In cases of trauma, it is important to keep in mind the differences between older and younger patients. Rapid initial evaluation of ABCs must be accomplished, followed by a detailed history and physical exam as appropriate (▶ **Figure 5-30**).

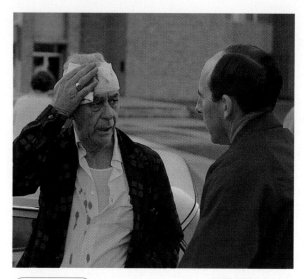

Figure 5-30 In assessing the older trauma patient, the goal is to gather the most information possible while minimizing the time required for transfer to definitive care.

Because older patients are more complex, the goal of assessment is to gather as much information about the patient as possible while minimizing the time necessary for transfer to definitive care.

Potential Causes

Although older patients may experience trauma in the traditional sense, there are two special concerns that you should keep in mind when assessing older trauma patients: elder abuse and underlying medical causes.

When the trauma occurred at the older patient's residence, be sure to screen carefully for signs of elder abuse or an unsafe living environment that could have contributed to the trauma. Elder abuse is discussed at length in Chapter 14.

Older patients may have several medical conditions that could lead to trauma. For example, a patient who undergoes a stroke while driving a vehicle could crash as a result. Older patients may also be on several medications for these medical conditions. Medication problems can lead to a change in mental status that results in trauma. Because of the complexity of the older patient, taking a thorough history is crucial. Collect information from the patient and from bystanders if possible. Obtain as much information as you can, in the time you have.

Assessment

History

Once the scene is safe, begin to gather information regarding the incident. As previously mentioned in this chapter, past medical history plays a critical role in the older patient's response to trauma. It is essential to gather as much information as possible about the patient's medical history from the patient and those familiar with the patient when possible. Certain medical conditions and medications may influence treatment decisions, as well as decisions about whether or not to transfer the patient to a trauma center. Medical conditions such as heart disease and COPD can greatly reduce the body's ability to respond to trauma, and baseline hypertension can cause misleading findings about the patient's perfusion status. The use of an anticoagulant, such as Coumadin (warfarin) or dicumarol, is of particular concern in the older trauma patient because it can cause prolonged bleeding from a relatively minor injury. Over-the-counter remedies such as aspirin, garlic, and ginkgo can also act as anticoagulants.

Physical Exam

As with any trauma patient, the physical exam should be conducted in the most efficient manner to minimize on-scene time. Keep in mind that the physical exam should be performed systematically to ensure completeness, yet should be dynamic so that it may address the needs of individual patients.

During this part of the assessment, assign a Glasgow Coma Scale (GCS) score to the patient by asking simple questions and having the patient follow simple commands (▶ **Figure 5-31**). In older patients, the GCS is one of the best measures of the chance for a positive outcome.[1] Any older patient with a head injury and a score of less than 15 who normally has a score of 15 should be transferred to a trauma center. Many older patients have a pre-existing decrease in cognitive function, diminished affect, and memory loss, making it difficult to determine the presence or extent of a head injury.[2] However, it is important not to assume that a decreased level of consciousness is the baseline mental status of an older patient. If people familiar with the patient are available, ask them questions such as, "What

GLASGOW COMA SCALE

Eye Opening	
Spontaneous	4
To Voice	3
To Pain	2
None	1

Verbal Response	
Oriented	5
Confused	4
Inappropriate Words	3
Incomprehensible Words	2
None	1

Motor Response	
Obeys Command	6
Localizes Pain	5
Withdraws (pain)	4
Flexion (pain)	3
Extension (pain)	2
None	1

Glasgow Coma Score Total	15

Figure 5-31   Transport any older patient with a head injury and a Glasgow Coma Scale score lower than what is normal for the patient to a trauma center.

was he like an hour ago? What was he like yesterday? Does he usually talk like this? Can he usually move his arms and legs?" in order to have a point of reference for evaluation. When uncertain, triage an older trauma patient to a trauma center.

When assessing the abdomen of an older patient, it may feel tense and distended, but the abdominal wall of an older person has less musculature, which makes a negative finding less reliable. Any older trauma patient who complains of abdominal pain should be suspected to have an internal organ injury, even if the abdominal examination is entirely normal.

Before evaluating a patient's range of motion for a specific limb complaint, find out if the patient has a history of arthritis or previous joint replacements, and be sure to ask about the patient's normal range of motion. Excessive flexion or extension of replaced or arthritic joints may lead to injury or damage to the limb and should therefore be avoided.

> ### Attitude Tip
>
> Arthritis and other joint problems may limit an older patient's normal range of motion. When possible, get a history before moving a limb or joint, and always examine gently.

Remember that hip fractures are serious injuries. A patient may lose a liter of blood or more with a hip or femur fracture. Be sure that you assess the hip or femur for an expanding hematoma. Ice and immobilize this serious fracture as you would a wrist or ankle fracture. This is accomplished by taping a covered ice pack over the site of the fracture. The hip can be supported by taping the patient's knees together with a pillow or blanket between the thighs. Support the fractured leg in a position of comfort with other pillows or blankets. Management of the older trauma patient is covered in Chapter 7.

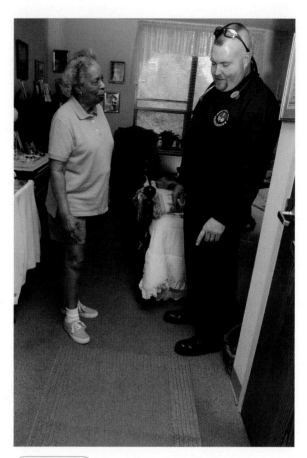

Figure 5-32   You can impact an older patient's health by reporting fall risks noted at the scene, and by injury prevention through fall-risk assessments.

Falls

Falls are the number one cause of injuries in older people. They are the reason for the majority of hospital trauma admissions, and a leading cause of death from injury (▶ **Figure 5-32**). Falls are discussed in detail in Chapter 6.

Generalized Pain

Pain is whatever, wherever, and whenever the individual in pain determines it to be. On any given day, older people experience pain about twice as often as younger adults. Surveys indicate that pain occurs in 25% to 50% of older people who live in the community and 45% to 85% of older people who live in nursing homes. This pain can be long-standing (chronic) or of recent onset

(acute). The cause of the pain may be obvious, as in a deformed extremity after a fall—or a bit cloudy, as in, "I hurt all over." In either event, your intervention can help decrease the patient's pain or the response to pain.

Potential Causes

The causes of acute pain in older people are the same as in younger people, and generally are the result of acute illness or injury. On the other hand, chronic pain in older people tends to be the result of the normal aging wear and tear, and often the effects of chronic disease. Some of the more common causes are musculoskeletal and neurologic disorders, cancer, and depression. Musculoskeletal examples include arthritis, bone disorders such as brittle bones (osteoporosis) and soft bones, soft-tissue pain and back pain from arthritis, compression fractures, and narrowing of the spinal canal. Neurologic examples include a persistent pain that occurs after shingles (herpes zoster infection) and the pain associated with nerve damage from diabetes (<u>**diabetic neuropathy**</u>). Cancers occur more frequently in older people; pain can arise from the tumor or its spread, or from the various cancer treatments. Psychiatric problems such as depression can cause pain or worsen a patient's existing pain. The pain experience can also cause a patient to feel depressed, which may make the pain worse. It is important to remember that pain is an emotional experience.

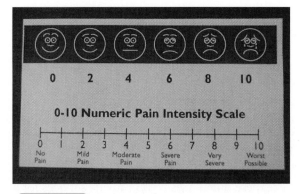

Figure 5-33   Visual scales use numbers, faces, or both to document the pain experience.

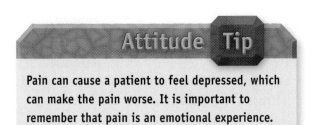

Attitude Tip

Pain can cause a patient to feel depressed, which can make the pain worse. It is important to remember that pain is an emotional experience.

Assessment

History

The history is key to evaluating the patient's pain. Use open-ended questions to hear about the pain in the patient's own words. Follow up with appropriate direct questions to complete the familiar mnemonic, OPQRST (onset, provocation/palliation, quality, radiation, severity, and time).

Use a pain scale to be consistent and accurate. Visual scales use numbers, faces, or both to document the pain experience (▶ **Figure 5-33**). Simple verbal pain scales can be used when the patient is visually impaired. This includes verbalizing the numeric pain scale or using simple descriptive terms for the intensity of pain: none, mild, moderate, severe, very severe, worst possible.

An accurate history will reveal the most information concerning the patient's pain. If the patient cannot provide a history, it is important to enlist the assistance of family, friends, or caregivers. If minimal history is available, assume pain is present and manage accordingly.

Physical Exam

The initial assessment should determine if the pain complaint is the result of an immediate threat to life. The outward expressions of pain, such as grimacing or groaning, may be diminished or absent in the older patient despite significant pain. Vital signs may or may not be altered by the pain experience. Interpret altered vital signs as secondary to an illness or injury, and not pain, until proven otherwise. For example, the tachycardic older person with gastric ulcer pain has tachycardia due to blood loss, not pain, until proven otherwise. If the patient is stable and the pain is acute and localized, a focused exam is indicated (▼ **Figure 5-34**). For more generalized or chronic pain complaints, the head-to-toe or detailed physical exam is performed but may not provide an abundance of information.

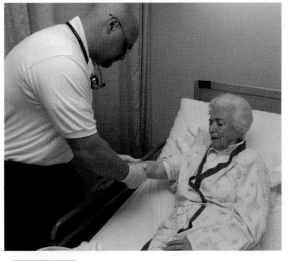

Figure 5-34   If the patient is stable and the pain is acute and localized, a focused exam is indicated.

Further Assessment Points

Older patients may hesitate to complain of pain for several reasons. They may believe that pain is a normal part of aging, fear they will not be believed, worry about lengthy hospitalization, or fear that the pain is due to a serious illness such as cancer. Older people often live with daily pain and their outward expression may be muted. Cultural differences may also alter an older person's response to pain. It is important to recognize these differences if you provide services for a diverse population. The foundation for pain assessment and management is to believe the older patient's complaint of pain.

Management

Pain is a very personal experience. To be successful in the management of the older patient with pain, you must demonstrate empathy and interest in the patient's problem. Empathy, interest, and a gentle touch may be the only treatment you can offer. *They are effective.* Prevent additional discomfort through careful and gentle transfer of the patient. Considerations such as padding the backboard, if one is needed, or assuring that the patient is in the position of comfort during transport are the signs of an effective and knowledgeable provider.

The ALS provider may additionally provide pain medication, depending on local protocol and patient condition.

> ### Attitude Tip
>
> To be successful in the management of the older pain patient, the EMS provider must demonstrate empathy and interest in the patient's problem.

Nausea, Vomiting, and Diarrhea

Potential Causes

The causes for nausea, vomiting, and diarrhea can originate inside or outside of the gastrointestinal tract. They often share the same general causes, such as infection, medication side effects, or psychological origin. Viral infections frequently cause gastroenteritis at all ages, with resultant nausea, vomiting, and diarrhea. Another important cause of infection is food poisoning, most commonly caused by bacteria. *Campylobacter*, *Salmonella*, *Shigella*, and *E. coli* are frequent or well-publicized bacterial causes of food poisoning. Medications can also result in these gastrointestinal side effects. Because older people take more medication than younger people, you can expect more medication-induced nausea, vomiting, and diarrhea. Frequent offenders are antibiotics and anti-cancer medications.

> ### Medication Tip
>
> Antibiotics and cancer medications are frequent offenders among the causes of nausea, vomiting, and diarrhea.

Everyone reacts to stress differently and with many individuals, the gastrointestinal tract is sensitive to the individual's emotions. Thus, any of these three gastrointestinal problems can be the result of the body's response to stress or extreme emotional experience. There are many additional causes for nausea and vomiting, such as an obstructed, distended, or twisted bowel; motion sickness; inner ear infection; poisoning or overdose; diabetes; previous surgery; cardiac ischemia or brain irritation from increased intracranial pressure; infection of the brain itself (encephalitis), or the brain coverings (meningitis). Additional causes of diarrhea include inflammatory bowel disease, traveler's diarrhea, and constipation. Constipation is a common problem in older people and can result in diarrhea when liquid stool moves past the fecal obstruction. Another cause with an increased incidence in older people is lactose intolerance. The decreased ability to digest milk sugar, or lactose, can produce diarrhea when milk products are ingested.

Assessment

History

Initially determine if the nausea, vomiting, or diarrhea is acute or chronic. If acute, has there been any recent change in diet or medication? Has the patient traveled to a foreign country prior to onset of symptoms? Determine the onset, frequency, appearance, color, and odor of the vomit or stool. Ask if anyone in the home or long-term care facility has experienced onset of the same complaints. If chronic, has there been any change in the usual pattern of symptoms? Are there any new symptoms such as bleeding, abdominal pain, dizziness, or chest pain?

Physical Exam

First, look for any life-threat indicators such as a poor general impression, change in mental status, or altered vital signs. Determine the presence of dehydration through vital signs and other signs such as dry mucous membranes or low blood pressure. Use the detailed physical exam to determine the need for further field treatment and to provide clues as to the cause of the problem. If the patient has been vomiting, listen closely to the breath sounds for any evidence of aspiration, such as fine or coarse crackles. Note the characteristics of any observed vomitus or stool such as consistency, color, odor, or presence of blood.

Further Assessment Points

Recall that nausea, vomiting, and diarrhea can be the result of a problem inside or outside of the gastrointestinal system. Either can result in signif-

icant fluid loss, alterations in the acid-base balance or abnormal levels of body sodium, potassium, chloride, and bicarbonate (electrolytes). Determine the presence of signs or symptoms of gastrointestinal bleeding: bright red blood in the vomit (hematemesis) or stool indicates active bleeding; digested blood in the vomit (coffee-ground emesis) or dark, tar-like stools indicate previous bleeding in the stomach or small intestine. The importance of being familiar with non-gastrointestinal causes for nausea, vomiting, and diarrhea is in recognizing any serious underlying problem such as cardiac ischemia that would merit immediate EMS treatment.

Summary

The assessment of the older patient is more complicated and requires a greater level of knowledge from the EMS provider. This knowledge leads to a more comprehensive history and physical exam, which in turn lead to a better assessment, which can save lives. Your hard work to master these skills will pay off in the improved care you can now offer to this large segment of your patient population.

Case Study Summaries

CASE STUDY **1** SUMMARY

As with any patient, ensure that ABCs are intact and that no life-saving measures are needed immediately.

This patient's ABCs were intact. The patient had no chief complaint when asked. Oxygen was applied due to her altered mental status, and her vital signs were found to be a heart rate of 58 beats/min, weak and regular; a respiratory rate of 14 breaths/min with normal tidal volume; a blood pressure of 106/66 mm Hg; lung sounds were clear bilaterally; and skin was cool, pale, and dry.

The physical exam was within normal limits except the altered mental status, aphasia, vomit-ing one time that morning, weak grips, distended abdomen, incontinence of urine, and inability to ambulate.

 When assessing an older patient, keep the GEMS diamond in mind. Older patients are more susceptible to changes in temperature. This patient's cool environment could be contributing to her problem. Aspects of the environment such as the loud TV and the smell of urine are also red flags that something is wrong.

CASE STUDY **1** SUMMARY *(continued)*

When transporting an older patient, take into account the patient's fragile skin and potential curvature of the spine. Ensure that the patient does not stay in the same position for more than 2 hours. In this case, the patient was prepared for transport to the emergency department by placing her on the stretcher on her left side in case she vomited again.

She was covered with several blankets to warm her. A heart monitor was attached and an IV of normal saline at a TKO ("to keep open") rate was started. The blood glucose level was checked and found to be 82 mg/dL. The mental status assessment and vital signs were repeated twice en route to the hospital. Findings were reported to the emergency department staff.

Later, it was found that the patient had suffered a transient ischemic attack (TIA), and was doing much better. Her symptoms were worsened by mild hypothermia and an alcohol level of 0.12. The daughter found a small flask of vodka in her purse when she retrieved her insurance cards from it.

Several factors contributed to the assessment findings in this case. The low heart rate could be normal for this patient, as a result of the atenolol (a beta-blocking agent), caused by the alcohol, or the TIA itself. Her confusion, weakness, and incontinence could also have been caused by any of the above. Despite her many symptoms, there was little prehospital treatment indicated, although identifying a cerebrovascular accident (CVA) as a likely cause may have made her a candidate for clot-dissolving medication in the hospital if timing and severity of symptoms were right. The most important thing EMS did for this patient was to gather important history information and conduct a thorough physical exam. This narrowed the list of possibilities from dozens to a likely two or three.

Because of your understanding of the decreased pain sensation in the older patient, you should suspect a possible cardiac problem even with the absence of chest pain.

This patient's vital signs were found to be a blood pressure of 160/84 mm Hg, a pulse of 90 beats/min, respirations of 20 breaths/min, and an oxygen saturation of 94%. The focused exam revealed no jugular vein distention, a regular heart rate, lung crackles in the bases of both lungs that did not clear with deep inspiration, and the absence of swelling in the legs. The fluid in the lung should further add to your suspicion of a heart condition, most likely a heart attack. Although there is no pain, you should be familiar with the lack of system reserves in the older patient and be aware that the damaged heart may be less able to pump the blood out of the lungs well enough to prevent shortness of breath with exertion. Based on this information, you should determine the patient to have a priority condition and explain to your patient the need for further evaluation at the hospital. Expedite transport and request an ALS intercept if available.

This patient was diagnosed at the receiving facility with a limited myocardial infarction and discharged to home after a brief hospital stay. Knowledge of older patients led to the correct field assessment and treatment, and resulted in returning Mrs. Smith to her active life.

Endnotes

1. Osler T, et al. Trauma in the geriatric. *The American Journal of Surgery.* 1988;156:539.

2. Coodley EL, Carston D. Trauma in the geriatric patient. *Trauma.* 1985;5:8, 14.

Suggested Educational Resources

1994 Emergency Medical Technician-Basic: National Standard Curriculum. Available at http://www.nhtsa.dot.gov/people/injury/ems/nsc.htm#emt.

Andresen GP. *As America Ages: Assessing the Older Patient.* Available at http://wwwqa.medec.com/rnweb/ce/misc/ages.html.

Clinical Geriatrics. Journal online. Available at http://www.mmhc.com/cg/.

The Merck Manual of Geriatrics. Text online. Available at http://www.merck.com/pubs/mm_geriatrics.

Chapter Resources

Falls

1 Discuss problems with mobility in older people.

2 Discuss medical risk factors, medications as risk factors, and environmental risk factors that make older people prone to falls.

3 Discuss the relationship between medical conditions in the older patient and trauma in the older patient.

4 Discuss strategies for prevention of falls in older people.

CHAPTER 6

Colleen Christmas, MD

Ann Marie Spellbring, PhD, RN

CASE STUDY 1

You are dispatched for an 83-year-old man with Parkinson's disease and mild left-sided weakness. He has recently experienced two falls in the kitchen that were related to rising from his chair at the table. These did not result in serious injury. He is receiving medications for Parkinson's disease and several other conditions. This call is for another fall in his home.

What factors do you need to consider?

What are his key risk areas?

Falls

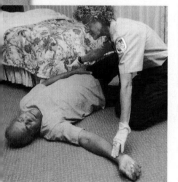

Occurrence Patterns and Outcomes Associated with Falls

Falls are a common reason for calls to 9-1-1, although the actual number of falls far exceeds the number of times a patient is examined by a medical provider. Because many older patients are reluctant to report falls and often simply don't recall having fallen, the true prevalence of falls in the community (as opposed to institutions) is difficult to determine accurately. It is estimated that about 30% of people over the age of 65 and living in the community fall each year, and about half of these will have multiple falls.[1] The rate of falls increases with age. The prevalence is even higher in institutionalized patients; about 50% of ambulatory nursing home residents fall per year, though it is not clear whether nursing home residents truly fall more frequently, or falls are simply documented more often in a supervised setting.[2]

Attitude Tip

A fractured hip can lead to a rapid decline in the patient's quality of life and/or death within the coming year or less. Don't treat these patients as "just another fractured hip."

Though most people consider the physical injuries that may result from falls, it is important to keep in mind that falls have profound effects on many aspects of an older patient's quality of life. For instance, not only are falls a leading cause of death in the older age group, but about 50% of falls result in lesser injuries (such as soft-tissue trauma and lacerations) requiring treatment. Fortunately, hip fractures occur in only 1% of falls, but 5% of falls result in other types of fractures.[3] Head trauma (including concussion and subdural hematomas) is also an uncommon but serious consequence of falls.

Perhaps most devastating of all are the psychological and social impacts of falls. About half of people report they have been unable to get up after falling (▶ **Figure 6-1**). Ten percent may

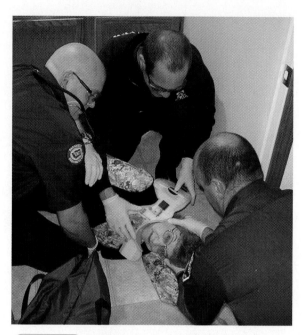

Figure 6-1   About half of older adults who have fallen report not being able to get up afterward. Ten percent may be "down" for more than 24 hours.

remain on the ground for over 24 hours, with resultant risk of pressure ulcers, pneumonia, deep venous thrombosis, **rhabdomyolysis** (disintegration of muscle fibers), and fluid and electrolyte abnormalities. The possibility of not being found certainly contributes to the fear of falling. Interestingly, 40% to 73% of older people who have fallen report that they restrict their daily activities because of a fear of falling, but a striking 20% to 46% of people *who have never fallen* also report that they do so because this fear is so intense.[3] In addition, older patients who fall tend to use health care resources more often. Falling is a very common reason that older individuals must give up their homes and move into a more supervised setting.

Risk Factors for Falls

Though it is clear that many falls are related to mobility problems in older individuals, it is often a useful exercise to ask the patient, "But why did you fall *today*?" Indeed, the causes of a fall are often multiple—resulting from a combination of age-related changes in balance and strength, diseases that affect balance (such as cataracts or strokes), environmental factors (a loose rug or wet floor), and often an acute medical problem such as a urinary tract infection (UTI) or hypoglycemia. It is particularly important to seek the medical causes, since falling is frequently a nonspecific presentation of an acute medical disease and it can be the only symptom of a serious illness.

It is also important to evaluate the patient for the presence of risk factors for falls and injuries and to determine the contributing factors to each fall, since many such risk factors and contributors are subject to interventions that could reduce the chance of a subsequent fall. In fact, a study of falls in community-dwelling older individuals showed that, for each risk factor for falling that was identified and modified, the chances of falling in the next year were reduced by 11%.[4] Thus, EMS providers are in a unique position to make an enormous impact on the quality of life of the older patients they serve.

There are many known intrinsic risk factors for falls and injuries. They can be grouped into major categories (▼ **Table 6-1**).

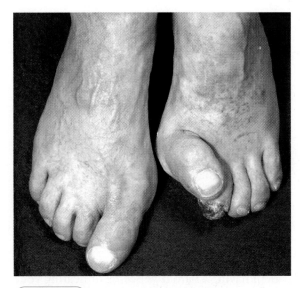

Figure 6-2   Musculoskeletal disorders that cause bony deformity or leg or foot weakness are a risk factor for falls in older adults.

TABLE 6-1   Intrinsic Risk Factors for Falls and Injuries in Older Adults

◆ **Sensory impairment** particularly vision, hearing, and **proprioception** (perception of movement and body's position).

◆ **Brain diseases** that affect balance. Stroke and Parkinson's disease are the classic ones.

◆ **Dementia**, which influences balance, judgment, and problem-solving ability.

◆ **Musculoskeletal disorders**, especially those that cause leg or foot weakness or bony deformity (▶ **Figure 6-2**).

◆ **Medications**, particularly those with sedative effects such as sleep aids and anxiety medications; also, simultaneous use of many medications (polypharmacy).

◆ **Depression** and the use of antidepressant medications.

◆ Use of **alcohol**.

◆ Advanced **age**: the older the patient, the more likely are falls and injuries.

◆ **Poor energy-absorbing capacity** of tissues ("onion skin") or bone (osteoporosis).

Assessing a Patient Who Has Fallen

Investigating the cause of a fall is at least as important as treatment of the injury sustained, yet this process is often overlooked. Determining the cause or causes of a fall requires only a few brief questions of the patient or witnesses to the event. The key components of a fall history can be remembered by the acronym SPLATT (▼ **Table 6-2**). Environmental factors frequently contribute to the cause of a fall as well.

Inquire what exactly the patient was doing and feeling at the time of the fall. Does he or she

TABLE 6-2   Essential Components of a Fall Assessment: SPLATT

Symptoms
Previous falls
Location of fall
Activity at time of fall
Time of fall
Trauma, both physical and psychological

Adapted from: Tideiksaar R. Preventing falls: How to identify risk factors and reduce complications. *Geriatrics* 1996; 51: 43–53.

know what caused the fall? Did he or she have any warning symptoms? It is important to ask specifically if the patient "passed out" or lost consciousness, causing the fall, or if he or she struck their head or lost consciousness when hitting the ground. Ask if the patient has any of the risk factors listed in Table 6-1 above.

Next, ask about and examine the patient for any injuries requiring treatment. While examining the patient in search of injuries, also look for clues that would indicate the patient has any of the risk factors for falls ▼ Figure 6-3 . For example, does the patient smell of alcohol? Are there pill bottles nearby? Are there signs of mobility problems, such as a walker? Is the patient having a hard time seeing or hearing you? Is the environment well lighted?

The exam focuses on evaluation of the patient's complaint, such as examining a painful ex-

tremity to determine if a fracture may be present, but remember that older patients are very prone to injury even from minor trauma. A thorough exam may be required to determine the full extent of injuries. One study demonstrated that, in older patients presenting to an emergency department with one complaint from a trauma, nearly one quarter were found to have a second injury they were not aware of.[5] The management of the older patient who has fallen begins with investigating the cause of the fall. If there is a medical condition that caused the fall, treat as appropriate. A full discussion of the treatment of traumatic injuries in older patients is covered in Chapter 7.

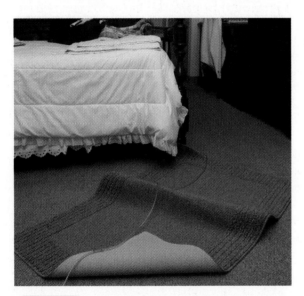

Figure 6-3 Environmental hazards are among the risk factors for falls.

Preventing Falls and Injuries in Older Patients

Role of the EMS Provider

The EMS provider is in a strategic position to be proactive in the prevention of falls and injuries in the older adult population. Research has demonstrated that an older person has an increased risk of falling when the number of risk factors increases. In addition, many older adults who fall do so repeatedly. One of the best predictors of falls among older persons is having a history of a previous fall; therefore, it is important to identify such a history. The identification of risk factors and the prevention of subsequent falls should include a review of medications, improvement of sensory function, elimination of environmental obstacles, and promotion of an exercise program that can help an older adult regain strength and balance. The EMS provider should also be knowledgeable about community resources and appropriate rec-

CASE STUDY 2

You are dispatched to the home of an 84-year-old woman by a neighbor who has not seen the patient in two days but could hear the television blaring all day and night. When you arrive on the scene, the woman is on the floor, awake but very confused and unable to tell you what happened.

What can you do to help determine the contributing factors to her fall?

What adverse effects can be caused by lying on the floor for up to two days?

| Agency | AERS
Adult Evaluation &
Review Services | DSS/APS
Department of Social
Services/Adult Services | Department of Aging | Bureau of Long-Term
Care and Bureau of
Mental Health |
|---|---|---|---|---|
| Contact Numbers | 410-555-2740
M-F 8:30-4pm | 410-555-3000 Press 2 | 410-555-2594 | 4 Centers (See below) |
| Type of Referral | Medical Problems | At Risk/Abuse | General Assistance | Mental Health |
| Age/Requirements | Adult
Baltimore County resident | Adult 18+
Baltimore County resident | 60+
Baltimore County resident | 60+
Baltimore County resident |
| Referral Issues | • Coordination of medical care
• Coordination of medications
• Access to home health care
• Access to meals on wheels
• Access to medical equipment
• Evaluation for alternative living/nursing home entry
• Access concrete services
• Provide nursing assistance | • Maltreated/neglected
• Inadequate food
• Inadequate clothing
• Inadequate shelter
• Lack of essential medical care
• Adult foster care/Project HOME
• Homeless services
• Food stamps/Medical assistance
• Housing services | • Assistance with application for financial assistance
• Accessing funds for one-time emergencies
• Accessing concrete services
• General information
• Transportation
• Caregiver issues | • Assessment and evaluation of mental health problem
• One-to-one counseling
• Psychiatric evaluation and prescription of meds

Southwest 410-555-7240
Northwest 410-555-9553
North & East 443-555-2221
Southeastern 410-555-7167 |

Figure 6-4   EMS providers can provide a valuable service to older patients at risk of falls by being prepared to recommend community resources related to falls and fall prevention.

ommendations to make to older adults and families about fall prevention (▲ Figure 6-4).

Reducing Medications

Persons who have fallen should have their medications reviewed and perhaps changed or discontinued. Medical research consistently demonstrates a strong relationship between falls and the use of **psychotropic** and **psychoactive** medications that cause sedation, dizziness, or loss of balance. Examples of these types of medications include benzodiazepines, sedative-hypnotics, antidepressants, and antipsychotics.

Cardiovascular drugs and antihypertensives can place an older adult at risk for falls by causing low blood pressure. Orthostatic hypotension can be triggered by certain types of cardiac drugs such as digoxin, antiarrhythmics, and diuretics. Also, alcohol—even in very small doses—can affect gait and balance and place an older adult at risk for falls. Several studies have suggested that not just certain types of medications, but also the number of medications can contribute to a fall. The American Geriatrics Society's "Guideline for the Prevention of Falls in Older Persons" recommends medication reduction in older persons taking four or more medications.[6]

Improving Sensory Function

Poor visual acuity has been identified as a contributor to falls. Lighting is the environmental factor most easily adapted in order to improve vision and reduce the risk of falling.

> **Medication Tip**
>
> The American Geriatrics Society recommends paying particular attention to medication reduction in older persons taking multiple medications.

Lighting should be bright and at consistent levels throughout the home, with glare and reflection minimized. A 100- to 200-watt bulb should be used for close work and a 75-watt bulb for watching TV. When possible, a nightlight in the bedroom, bathroom, hallways, and kitchen will ease the transition from darkness to brighter light. Motion-sensor-operated nightlights that turn on when an older person enters the room and turn off when the room is unoccupied are inexpensive and easily obtained at local hardware stores. Further, it is recommended that an older person have a yearly eye exam. After older persons fall or if an older person has risk factors for falling, he or she should be asked if they are experiencing any difficulties related to vision and should visit a physician promptly to have visual testing and correction of any problems identified.

Exercise and Balance Training

Difficulty with balance, mobility, and performing activities of daily living (ADLs) are possibly the most important indicators of fall risk. Lower extremity weakness is also a major risk factor. An easy test to evaluate gait, balance, and strength is the "get

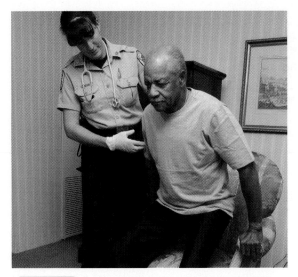

Figure 6-5   The "get up and go" test is an easy way to evaluate gait, balance, and strength, and thus the overall risk of falling.

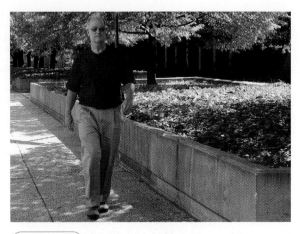

Figure 6-6   Moderate, weight-bearing exercise improves balance and bone density. Walking and dancing are inexpensive examples.

up and go" test (▲ Figure 6-5). This test can be performed in the home setting by asking the older person to rise from a chair that has been placed 10 feet from the wall, stand in place for a few seconds, walk to the wall, turn around and walk back to the chair, and sit down. Observe whether or not the patient needs to use his or her hands to rise from the chair and how steady he or she is while walking and turning. This test requires little time and provides an excellent assessment of the older person's overall mobility and risk of falling.

One of the major contributions to muscle weakness, as well as gait and balance instability, is the lack of physical activity among older adults. Although muscle bulk and strength decrease with age, this can be partially offset with exercise. In addition, exercise improves bone strength and balance, and reduces falls. A reasonable goal is to get the patient to increase activity levels with an eventual target of exercising a total of 30 minutes, either in one session or divided into multiple small sessions throughout the day, on most days of the week (▶ Figure 6-6).

Attitude Tip

More aggressive assessment, field management, and communication of important observations made at the home can result in decreased morbidity and mortality, and in improved outcomes for injured patients.

Walking and dancing are weight-bearing exercises that may improve balance and bone density and are very inexpensive. Balance training, particularly T'ai Chi, has proven to reduce falls in frail older individuals. Most importantly, the patient should pick exercises that he or she is likely to continue to perform life-long and in a setting that encourages adherence to the program. Preferences will differ regarding structured classes, exercising with a spouse, or exercising alone. The EMS provider's familiarity with local resources available through senior centers and community colleges can be helpful to the patient. Often the local chapter of the Arthritis Association can provide a list of exercise facilities for seniors. Some patients may need an evaluation by a physician or physical therapist to help them determine a safe and optimal exercise regime for their individual needs.

Use of Assistive Devices

An older person's gait and balance may improve with the use of an assistive device (▶ Figure 6-7). Canes and walkers increase the base of support, but an older person needs instruction on how to use them, for they can be a hazard if used improperly. A knowledgeable health care provider may do this. The ambulation device should be assessed regularly for problems such as loose hardware on walkers or a worn rubber tip on a cane. When these types of problems are present, the assistive device will not give adequate support. In the home setting, it is important to evaluate the older adult's use of the device. A cane is properly held on the side opposite the affected extremity,

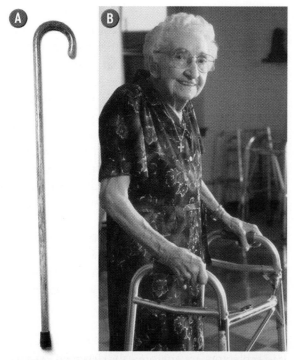

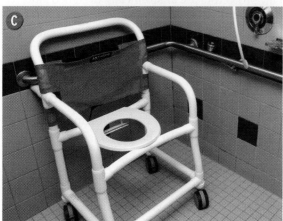

Figure 6-7   Types of assistive devices. **A.** Canes. **B.** Walkers. **C.** Shower chairs.

advancing the cane and affected extremity together. For a walker, it is important to evaluate its use in relation to narrow hallway passages and doorways, space availability in the bathroom and other rooms of the house, and type of flooring. Even standard walkers can tip over, so advise the patient to keep the walker ahead and step into it. The bathtub tends to be a particularly hazardous area of the home. To reduce the risk of falling in the bathtub, many people will use a tub bench, a secure seat that allows them to sit rather than stand in the shower. Proper use of an assistive device will decrease the risk of falling and serve as an aid to impaired gait and balance.

Making the Home Safe

Approximately 70% of falls occur at home, and a clear environmental factor is involved in about half of all falls.[1] This is important to keep in mind because it suggests that a careful assessment of the safety of the home may yield dramatic reductions in fall risk. Again, this is a golden opportunity for the EMS provider to effect a change that results in dramatic improvements in quality of life for an older individual, an opportunity not available to all health care providers. A checklist of common hazards associated with falls in the home, such as that proposed by the U.S. Consumer Product Safety Commission, can be given to the patient and family. This Home Safety Checklist is found in Appendix C.[7]

Modifications can then be made in the home to improve its safety, such as removal of loose throw rugs, moving most frequently used items to easy-to-reach shelves, and installing necessary durable equipment (eg, toilet risers and grab bars, bathtub/shower chairs or benches and grab

CASE STUDY 3

A 74-year-old woman with diabetes and congestive heart failure falls in her apartment at an assisted-living facility. She is not apparently injured, and just wants the EMS provider to reassure her she is well enough not to go to the hospital. She walks with a walker and has had one prior fall. She takes a total of seven medications. You have interviewed and examined her, and find no acute medical causes of the fall and no injury. She declines to go to the hospital for any further evaluation.

What can you advise to reduce her chances of calling you next week with another fall?

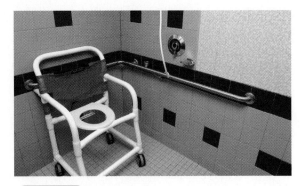

Figure 6-8 Installing equipment such as grab bars and shower chairs helps maintain safe activities of daily living for older adults at risk of falls.

bars) to maintain safe activities of daily living (▲ **Figure 6-8**). Medical device catalogues that can be obtained from local pharmacy stores or mail order companies provide the necessary supportive equipment to improve safety, though for some patients cost may be a concern.

> ## Attitude Tip
>
> Identifying home hazards that may cause falls is an opportunity for the EMS provider to improve quality of life dramatically for older patients, an opportunity not available to all health care providers.

Stairs in particular can be hazardous to an older person. It has been estimated that 10% of falls occur on stairs, usually while descending the stairs[1]; this may be due to misjudgment about the next or the last step. Recommendations to correct this problem include placing a contrasting marker such as tape at the end of each step, and securely installing hand rails on each side. For patients who are unable to use the home safety checklist themselves, a social worker or health care provider such as an occupational therapist may assist in evaluating home safety and making recommendations for improvement. The EMS provider is often in an ideal position to refer the patient for this help.

Proper Footwear

If an older person has any foot problems, this can increase fall risk. Abnormalities of the feet, such as corns, bunions, and hammertoes, can affect safe mobility. Unusually long toenails or painful bunions should be corrected, which may mean a visit to the podiatrist. In addition to problems

with the feet themselves, improperly fitting shoes can lead to walking difficulties that place older adults at risk of falling. When they have foot problems or swelling, they often deal with these problems by wearing larger shoes or slippers that they can simply slip into. This does not provide for proper fit and support, and so can lead to further problems related to falls. In order to keep a larger shoe on the foot, an older person may develop a shuffling walk that can lead to tripping. Shoes that are narrow and squeeze the foot can contribute to foot pain when walking. The best recommendation is a shoe that fits the entire foot, such as a walking shoe with a low heel and nonskid bottom. Rubber- or crepe-soled footwear is also recommended. Instruct older adults to avoid walking in stocking feet and to eliminate loose slippers.

Hip Protectors

Hip protectors are anatomically designed external hip pads that fit over the side of each hip in the pockets of a stretchy undergarment (▼ **Figure 6-9**). They can be worn under a skirt or pants. There are currently about 10 different hip protectors on the market. The majority of hip fractures result from a sideward fall in which there is impact to the **greater trochanter** of the proximal femur (the bony prominence on the proximal lateral side of the thigh, just below the hip joint). Padding this area cushions the force of the fall, and therefore may prevent a fracture. Any older adult who is at high risk of falling, who may have osteoporosis, muscle weakness, or difficulty with gait and balance, could consider wearing these to reduce the chance of a hip fracture. In one recent study of

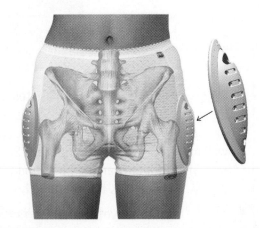

Figure 6-9 By cushioning the force of a fall, hip protectors may prevent a hip fracture.

ambulatory older adults who were at increased risk for hip fracture, the risk of a fracture was reduced by 60% if they were wearing a hip protector at the time of the fall.[8, 9] Some older persons find wearing the hip pads uncomfortable, or are unwilling to wear them as a part of daily clothing, so they may not be suitable for everyone.

Personal Alarms

A personal emergency response system (PERS) consists of a small battery-powered transmitter or portable help button carried by the user and usually worn on a wristband or a chain around the neck (**▼ Figure 6-10**). It also can be carried on a belt or in a pocket. The batteries need to be checked periodically to be sure they work. The receiving unit is connected to the person's telephone, and acts as an automatic dialing machine that contacts an emergency response center for assistance. For this type of system to work well, an older adult needs to accept the concept and be compliant in wearing the transmitter.

There are several psychological benefits to an older adult participating in the PERS. These include an increased sense of security, reduced fear of falling, and increased sense of autonomy and independence. A PERS can be purchased, rented, or leased, but Medicare, Medicaid, and other insurance companies do not pay for purchase of the equipment. Rental may be available through national manufacturers, local distributors, hospitals, and social service agencies. The installation fee and subsequent monthly fees are relatively inexpensive.[10] The Fed-eral Trade Commission provides information on personal emergency response systems.

Teaching the Older Adult to Get Up Safely After a Fall

In order to prevent a long time "down" after a fall, and to build the confidence of a person who has fallen already, the older adult needs to be taught what to do if a fall occurs. The first lesson is, "Don't panic!" If there is some way that an alert can be given, the patient should not get up until checked. If injury makes it impossible to get up, the patient should keep warm by using anything available such as a coat, rug, or blanket. Instructions for ways to get up safely include:

- ◆ Roll onto the stomach, get up on all fours, and crawl to a nearby piece of sturdy furniture.
- ◆ Shuffle on the bottom or side of the body to a telephone or piece of sturdy furniture.
- ◆ Scoot up the stairs and stand when able to.

For patients with mobility problems, it is wise to keep a cordless telephone at hand at all times.

Summary

Falls in the older population are associated with very high **morbidity** and mortality. Mobility problems significantly contribute to the risk of falling in older people, but it is important to keep in mind that most falls have multiple causes; they result from intrinsic age-related changes and disease effects on many systems, often combined with acute medical problems and environmental factors. Carefully assessing the situation surrounding a fall can provide important clues to the causes of the fall and also to factors that can be modified to reduce the chance of subsequent falls. An EMS provider can play a pivotal role in the prevention of falls in the older population.

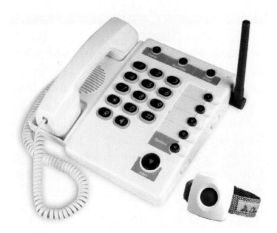

Figure 6-10 A personal emergency response system (PERS) can be worn on the wrist, at the belt, or around the neck. For it to be effective, the patient must check batteries regularly and wear the device consistently.

Case Study Summaries

CASE STUDY 1 SUMMARY

You will want to review the circumstances of the fall, identify risk factors for subsequent falls, and identify injuries. Keep in mind the GEMS diamond during his assessment. His initial key risk factors for falls are muscular weakness, gait instability from his Parkinson's disease, use of medications that may affect balance, and his history of prior falls, though he will need a more thorough evaluation to identify other risk factors.

CASE STUDY 2 SUMMARY

After completing an examination to determine the extent of injury to the patient, assess the environment to look for clues to the contributors to her fall. Do you smell or see alcohol? Are there loose rugs or cords nearby? Is the room well lighted? Do you see assistive devices in the home that could suggest she has balance problems? Find her pill bottles and document her medications. Is she taking medications that may have contributed to her fall, or taking a high number of medications? Does she have any evidence of an acute medical illness on examination (such as labored breathing and rales on lung examination, suggestive of pneumonia)?

Adverse effects from long "down-time" include pressure ulcers on the skin, deep venous thrombosis, pneumonia, dehydration, hypoglycemia, rhabdomyolysis, and fear of falling.

CASE STUDY 3 SUMMARY

There are often many risk factors for falling that can be identified and altered to reduce the chances of a subsequent fall. Because of her diabetes, she should be sure to have her eyes examined and have a physician assess her proprioception. If either of these senses is awry, treatment should be instituted. She should discuss her medications with her physicians in an attempt to reduce the total number of medications, and eliminate any that may be contributing to falls. You could provide her with a home safety checklist to review in her home, with the plan to alter any unsafe environmental factors found. You could also watch her stand and walk with her walker; if she is unsteady in doing so, she should see her physician or physical therapist. She could also start an exercise program to improve her strength and balance. There is actually quite a lot you can do for her!

Suggested Reading

The American Academy of Orthopaedic Surgeons website, http://www.aaos.org.

A nice review article is Tideiksaar R. Preventing falls: How to identify risk factors and reduce complications. *Geriatrics*. 1996; 51: 43–53.

A helpful text on the subject is Tideiksaar R. *Falling in Old Age*. New York: Springer; 1997.

Endnotes

1. Tinetti ME, Speechley M., Ginter SF. Risk factors for falls among elderly persons living in the community. *N Engl J Med*. 1988; 319: 1701–1707.

2. Rubenstein LZ, Robbins AS, Schulman BL, Rosado J, Osterweil D, Josephson KR. Falls and instability in the elderly. *J Am Geriatr Soc*. 1988; 36:266–278.

3. King MB, Tinetti ME. Falls in community-dwelling older persons. *J Am Geriatr Soc*. 1995; 43:1146–1154.

4. Tinetti ME, Baker DI, McAvay G, et al. A multifactorial intervention to reduce the risk of falling among elderly people living in the community. *N Engl J Med*. 1994; 331: 821–827.

5. Levy DB, Hanlon DP, Townsend RN. Geriatric trauma. *Clin Geriatr Med*. 1993; 9:601–620.

6. American Geriatrics Society. Guideline for the prevention of falls in older persons. *J Am Geriatr Soc*. 2001; 49: 664–672.

7. U.S. Consumer Product Safety Commission. Safety for older consumers home safety checklist: CPSC Document 701. Washington, DC: Author. Available at: http://www.cpsc.gov/cpscpub/pubs/701.html.

8. Kannus P, Parkkari J, Niemi S, et al. Prevention of hip fracture in elderly people with use of a hip protector. *N Engl J Med*. 2000; 343: 1506–1513.

9. Lauritzen JB, Petersen MM, Lund B. Effect of external hip protectors on hip fractures. *Lancet*. 1993; 341:11–13.

10. Federal Trade Commission. Information on personal emergency response systems. Available at: http://www.ftc.gov/bcp/conline/pubs/services/pers.htm.

Trauma and Musculoskeletal Disorders

1 Discuss the epidemiology of trauma in the older population, including the risk factors for motor vehicle crashes, pedestrian accidents, falls, burns, penetrating trauma, and elder abuse.

2 Discuss the assessment findings common in older patients with traumatic injuries, including orthopaedic injuries.

3 Discuss assessment of the older patient with complaints related to the musculoskeletal system.

4 Discuss intervention, management, and transport considerations in the older patient with traumatic injuries.

5 Describe management, intervention, and transport of the older patient with complaints related to the musculoskeletal system.

6 Review splinting, immobilization, and packaging considerations in treating older patients, including those with physical deformities.

7 Describe the incidence, morbidity/mortality, risk factors, and preventive strategies for osteoporosis, osteoarthritis, and rheumatoid arthritis.

CHAPTER 7

Matthew J. Belan

Andrew N. Pollak, MD, EMT-P, FAAOS

CASE STUDY 1

You are dispatched to the scene of a single-car motor vehicle crash into a tree with mild to moderate damage done to the vehicle. On your arrival, the driver of the vehicle, a 72-year-old man, is still seated in the vehicle, appears to be confused and unaware of what happened, and has left facial droop. Numerous bystanders report that nothing was seen in the roadway that would have caused the driver to swerve, and that the vehicle did not appear to brake prior to the crash. While evaluating the patient, a medical information wristband indicates that the patient has hypertension, a cardiac condition, and takes Coumadin.

What is the likely reason why the driver crashed the vehicle?

How should this patient be treated?

Trauma and Musculoskeletal Disorders

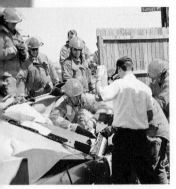

Introduction

In general, older individuals tend to be less active than younger people. Despite suffering from injuries less frequently, older patients tend to be more seriously injured and have a higher incidence of complications. The older patient's body does not respond to injury in the same manner as that of a younger individual, and treatment should reflect this. The purpose of this chapter is to identify the changes associated with aging with regard to how they affect the decisions made by EMS providers who treat older trauma patients. Strategies for treating older patients with a variety of injuries are provided, as well as tips on how to prevent injuries from occurring.

Attitude Tip

Remember that older trauma patients *do* benefit from the aggressive prehospital and in-hospital care they receive! In related studies of patients older than 70 with multiple injuries, it was found that 89% returned home after the trauma, rather than to long-term care facilities.

Epidemiology of Injury in the Older Population

Traumatic injury is the seventh leading cause of death in the United States for people age 65 or greater.[1] As the number of older people rises, the number of older patients suffering from traumatic injuries will also rise.

Motor Vehicle Crashes

Older people tend to be involved in fewer motor vehicle crashes than younger people. In 1998, 14% of all licensed drivers were over the age of 65; however, drivers in this age group accounted for only 8% of all vehicle crashes. As a comparison, 5.4% of licensed drivers were under the age of 19, yet accounted for 13.8% of all crashes during the same period.[1] Most accidents involving older patients occur at intersections, including those with traffic signs, suggesting that older persons may be less able to make quick decisions while operating a vehicle.[2] Older patients who are involved in a motor vehicle incident are nearly twice as likely to be admitted to the hospital after the incident, and are twice as likely to die from their injuries when compared to individuals in younger age groups.[3]

Pedestrian Accidents

Only 11% of all pedestrians who are struck by a vehicle in the United States are older than 65 years of age. Despite this low incidence of injury, nearly 25% of all pedestrian fatalities occur in older patients. This patient population has the highest rate of death of any age group from being struck by a vehicle.[1,4] Changes in vision, hearing, posture, and motor ability predispose older people to a greater risk of pedestrian accidents due to a decreased ability to see traffic signals and detect oncoming traffic (▼ Figure 7-1). Additionally, older people tend to walk at a rate slower than the 4 feet per second for which most traffic signals are designed. Other factors that place the older population at risk for being struck by a vehicle include changes in cognitive function, memory, and decision-making.[4]

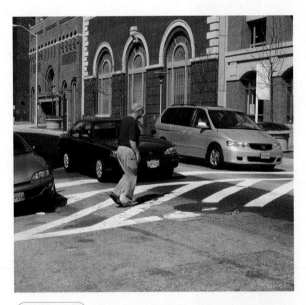

Figure 7-1 Changes in vision, hearing, posture, and motor ability predispose older people to a greater risk of being struck by a vehicle.

Falls

Falling is the leading cause of injury for people over 65 in the United States. [5,6] As a result, it is essential for EMS providers to understand the factors that predispose older people to falling as well as the risks associated with falls. Detailed information related to falls may be found in Chapter 6.

Burns

Burns are a common source of injury for patients of all ages and are often associated with activities of daily living and employment, such as cooking and working with chemicals. The age group at greatest risk for experiencing a burn injury is the over-75 population.[7] Unlike other age groups, this population most commonly is burned by space heaters, cookers, and flammable liquids.[7] This fact likely reflects their decreased mobility and impaired cognitive ability and slowing of peripheral sensory nerves, which can lead them to become trapped in a burning structure, fall into a free-standing space heater or stove, or react more slowly to the sensation of being burned.[7]

As with other forms of injury, older patients have a higher rate of morbidity and mortality associated with burn injuries compared to younger patients. In 1998, a total of 3,300 people died in the United States as the result of burns and fires, with people older than 65 years of age accounting for 1,300 deaths.[1] This is probably because the older patient is less likely than a younger patient to meet the immense physical demand that is placed on the body after suffering a burn. Two types of mortality are associated with burn injuries in the older patient: early death from hypovolemia and/or cardiovascular collapse, and late death associated with infection.[2]

Penetrating Trauma

Older men are much more likely to suffer death from a firearm than are older women. In the United States in 1996, nearly 5,000 older patients died as the result of gunshot wounds, with suicide committed by males accounting for over 4,000 of those deaths.[1] Studies indicate that older patients who suffer from a gunshot wound are 2.5 times more likely to die from the injury than a younger patient, and that those who are victims of a stabbing are 4 times more likely to be mortally wounded.[2]

Elder Abuse

Unfortunately, many older people are subjected to physical, financial, and mental abuse by caregivers, neighbors, family members, and other individuals who may even target the older population as "easy prey." The injuries resulting from physical abuse may seem similar to those that result from other mechanisms of injury. Assaults account for 4% to 14% of all trauma admissions in the United States for older patients and most commonly are committed with blunt objects.[4] Abuse should be considered in any older patient with a traumatic injury. Elder abuse and neglect are discussed in detail in Chapter 14.

Physiological Changes Associated with Aging That Impact Trauma

Nearly every part of the body undergoes some type of change during the aging process. (These changes are reviewed in detail in Chapter 2.) Changes in the pulmonary, cardiovascular, neurologic, and musculoskeletal systems in particular all significantly affect an older person's susceptibility to injury and response to trauma.

Changes in the pulmonary system commonly contribute to the cause of death in the older trauma victim. The primary cause of decreased pulmonary function is from the loss of lung and chest wall elasticity. These changes contribute to higher rates of broken ribs with trauma and higher risks of developing **atelectasis** (partial lung collapse) and pneumonia.[4]

Changes in the heart and blood vessels predispose older trauma victims to a reduced ability to maintain adequate circulation. They are less able to increase their cardiac output, heart rate, and blood pressure in response to blood loss or increased demand for improved circulation, and similarly do not adapt to increases in volume in the circulatory system. Cardiovascular collapse is often a reason for death in the acutely injured older patient. This is particularly important to consider in the older patient with burns, because burns can be associated with marked fluid shifts within the body, which may be very poorly tolerated in the older person. As a result of the normal and pathological changes in the cardiovascular system associated with aging, the usual indicators of volume status, such as heart rate and blood pressure, may be unreliable in this population.

Changes in the brain and surrounding structures make head injury in the older patient population second only to profound shock as the leading cause of traumatic death.[4] As a person ages, the brain shrinks resulting in a higher risk of developing bleeding within the skull, known as a subdural hematoma. Older patients often do not show signs or symptoms of a head injury immediately following injury because there is more space for blood to collect. Thus, examination of the neurologic system in an older trauma patient must be repeated frequently.

Numerous changes occur in the musculoskeletal system with aging that affect trauma and injury. Most notable are the loss of bone and muscle mass and strength. Other changes that occur frequently in the older population include the development of **kyphosis**, a condition in which the back becomes hunched over (▼ **Figure 7-2**); arthritis, which reduces the flexibility of joints, decreases range of motion, and causes pain; and diminished strength, which re-

sults from changes in the composition of muscle fibers. All of these contribute to an increased propensity toward trauma and injury. Older people also tend to become progressively less active. This occurs for many reasons, including prior injury, medications, illnesses, and a decreased level of energy. In response to being less active, conditions such as arthritis and muscle weakness can be aggravated, leading to further reduction in activity.

With aging, the size, number, and functioning of muscle cells in the body decrease, resulting in a progressive loss of strength at the rate of approximately 10% per decade after age 40. The greatest loss of muscle mass occurs in the fatigue-resistant fast twitch muscle fibers, such as those found in the calf, that are used for postural stability. Additionally, muscle fibers contract less forcefully in the older patient.[8,9] The end result of these changes is that older people have a loss of strength and power. Exercise and strength training restore a significant amount of an older person's strength power (▼ **Figure 7-3**).

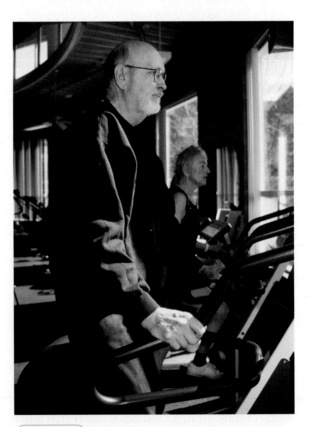

Figure 7-3 Exercising and strength training will restore a significant amount of an older person's strength.

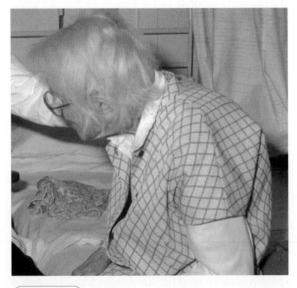

Figure 7-2 Older people often develop kyphosis, in which the back becomes hunched.

Particular Musculoskeletal Injuries

Spine Injuries

Injuries to the spine are a frequent problem in older people. Spinal injuries may be broadly classified as stable or unstable. A **stable spinal injury** is one that has a low risk for leading to permanent neurological deficit or structural deformity; an **unstable spinal injury** is one that has a high risk of permanent neurological deficit or structural deformity. The injuries that older patients incur while performing normal daily activities are most commonly stable ones, whereas unstable injuries tend to result from a significant trauma, such as falls from a substantial height or motor vehicle crashes.

Injuries to the upper cervical spine are potentially lethal because the nerves that stimulate the diaphragm originate from here. An injury at this level or higher may lead to death secondary to an inability to breathe. Many cervical spine injuries in older patients result from hyperextension of the neck as the result of a fall or striking the head on the windshield during a motor vehicle crash. Because of coexisting arthritis, relatively small hyperextension injuries can cause the spinal cord to be squeezed, leading to dysfunction known as **central cord syndrome**. Central cord syndrome results in weak or absent motor function that is more pronounced in the upper extremities than the lower extremities. Although this type of spinal cord injury is usually not permanent, recovery may often take several months or even years.[10]

Osteoporosis in the thoracic and lumbar spine contributes to a high rate of injury in this area in the older population. Three types of fractures are common in the thoracolumbar region: compression fractures, burst fractures, and seatbelt-type injuries. **Compression fractures** are stable injuries in which often only the anterior third of the vertebrae is collapsed. This type of fracture often results from minimal trauma, from simply bending over, rising from a chair, or sitting down forcefully.[11] This is by far the most common type of spine fracture seen in the older patient population. **Burst fractures** typically result from a high-energy mechanism of injury, such as a motor vehicle crash or a fall from substantial height. These fractures are unstable and may lead to neurological injury secondary to shifting of the vertebrae with damage to the spinal cord. **Seatbelt-type fractures** involve flexion, and there is a distraction component (energy being dispersed in two opposite directions) that causes a fracture through the entire vertebral body and bony arch. This type of injury typically results from an ejection or in those wearing only a lap belt without a shoulder harness.[11]

Injuries to the spinal cord are usually associated with neurological deficits, which may be complete or incomplete. An example of an incomplete injury is the previously described central cord syndrome. Patients with an incomplete spinal cord injury may recover function over time, but those with a complete spinal cord injury are not likely to regain function.

Upper Extremities

Injuries to the upper extremities typically pose a minimal risk of death, but loss of function of the extremity can greatly reduce the older person's independence and will often lead to a permanent reduction in function, even after healing. The effective use of the upper extremities depends upon an intact shoulder, elbow, and wrist—sites that are often injured by the older patient.

The **rotator cuff** is composed of four muscles that attach to the humerus to allow motion and provide stability to the arm and shoulder. With time, the rotator cuff undergoes progressive degeneration, making it highly susceptible to injury. Many older people will often have pre-existing tears within the cuff from this degeneration. Older patients who sustain a traumatic injury to the shoulder region are at a higher risk for further damage to the rotator cuff leading to instability about the shoulder, pain, and decreased upper extremity function.

Fractures, dislocations, sprains, and strains are all injuries that can occur about the shoulder in older patients. Osteoporosis predisposes many older people to fracture of the proximal humerus. Falling onto an outstretched arm or falling onto the arm while carrying something in it is a common mechanism of such injury.[12]

Distal forearm and wrist fractures are other common injuries that occur in older patients because of osteoporosis. Falls are a frequent cause of this type of injury, with fractures occurring as the patient extends the arm and lands on an outstretched wrist.

Pelvis

Fractures of the pelvis in older patients often occur as the result of a combination of decreased bone strength due to osteoporosis and a low-energy mechanism of injury, such as a fall from standing position. More serious high-energy fractures can pose a significant threat to life. Injuries of this type can be encountered in a person who has fallen from a significant height, been involved in a high-speed motor vehicle crash, or been struck by a car. High-energy injuries may result in fracture in two places in the pelvis with displacement of a segment of the pelvic ring (pelvic ring disruption). Pelvic ring disruption can lead to hemorrhage from the blood vessels that pass through the pelvis, or injury to the bladder, intestines, or lumbosacral nerve plexus. Older patients are less able than younger patients to tolerate the blood loss and other organ system injuries that are commonly associated with high-energy pelvic ring disruptions.

The **acetabulum** (hip socket) is another site in the pelvis that may be injured as the result of high-energy trauma in older people. Injuries to the acetabulum can occur as the result of an injury in which the knee is driven into the dashboard or ground, with the head of the femur driven through the acetabulum. Owing to the diminished strength of bone, older patients are at a higher risk for this type of injury from lower energy insults than would be required in younger patients.

Hip Fractures

One common debilitating musculoskeletal injury that occurs in older patients is a hip fracture. A hip fracture is a fracture of the head, neck, or proximal portion of the femur. Following a hip fracture, patients often have decreased mobility and independence and can require prolonged rehabilitation. This can be physically and emotionally challenging for both the patient and his or her family. Despite advances in treatment, many older people will be permanently impaired, and nearly 20% will die within the first 12 months following injury.[13]

Treatment of hip fractures depends upon the type of injury sustained as well as the condition of the bone in the hip.

Injuries to the Lower Extremities

Distal femoral fractures are more common in older patients, whereas femoral shaft fractures typically occur in younger patients. Knee joint arthritis with associated stiffness may predispose the older patient to fractures in the distal femur near the knee, while increased mobility in younger patients may result in stresses being concentrated farther up the shaft of the femur. Because of osteoporosis, however, femoral shaft fractures can occur in older patients from a low-energy twisting motion, for example, during a low-level fall such as from missing a step.

Proximal fractures of the tibia may occur from a direct impact to the bone, or by a medial or lateral rocking motion. A fracture may occur to the shaft of the tibia through a direct force, such as that from a motor vehicle striking the leg, or by a twisting force that leads to a stress fracture.

Injuries about the ankle in older patients often result from an injury in which the foot rolls under the leg, causing a fracture of the bone. This type of injury is commonly seen as an older person attempts to step down from a curb or step and misjudges the height. Another common cause for this pattern of injury is depressing the brake pedal with great force in anticipation of and during a collision.

Injuries Associated with Prosthetic Joint Replacement

Prosthetic joint replacements are used commonly in the hip, knee, shoulder, and other regions of the body (▶ **Figure 7-4**). The primary reason for the use of prosthetic joints in the older patient is

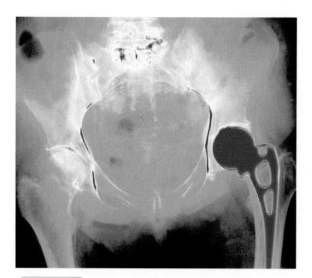

Figure 7-4 Prosthetic joints replace joints, but depend on the remaining bone for support and stabilization.

arthritis. The devices are implanted to replace joints; however, they rely on the remaining bone for support and stabilization. Fractures that occur in close proximity to implanted devices may compromise stability of the prosthesis. Common reasons for fractures of this type are reduced bone strength from osteoporosis, or stressful movement because of poor prosthesis fit, or loosening of the prosthesis from infection or injury.[10] Dislocation of hip replacements can occur if there is excessive motion of the hip joint, especially within the first 6 weeks after prosthesis implantation.

Assessment of the Older Patient

As discussed in Chapter 5, in assessment of the older trauma patient, it is important to keep in mind the differences between a younger patient and an older patient.

One challenge while assessing older patients is determining whether pain being experienced following a traumatic event is acute or chronic. <u>Acute pain</u> represents the body's means of indicating the presence of a new injury; <u>chronic pain</u> is experienced repeatedly and includes behavioral as well as physical factors.[14] It is important always to question patients in detail about the nature of the pain that is being felt and how it compares to the level of discomfort normally experienced. You should always assume that pain is real. The goal of evaluating a patient's complaint of pain is to determine whether the pain being experienced indicates a new injury or represents an aggravation of a pre-existing condition ▶ **Figure 7-5** .

Scene Size-Up

After establishing that the scene is safe, begin to gather information regarding the incident. First, determine the nature of the emergency. Although it may be easy to assume that an older patient found in a damaged vehicle was in a car crash and

CASE STUDY 2

You are dispatched for a 68-year-old woman with back pain. When you arrive, the patient tells you that she has had the pain for several days and it led to severe discomfort, inability to sleep, and trouble moving about the house. When you question her about when the pain began, she reports that it started when she was getting up from her chair after reading the paper. She also advises you that she has been less active over the past year because of joint pain, has not been eating as well as she used to, and that her doctor wants her to take a calcium supplement.

> **How is this patient likely to have injured her back?**

> **What risk factors are present in this patient for the development of osteoporosis?**

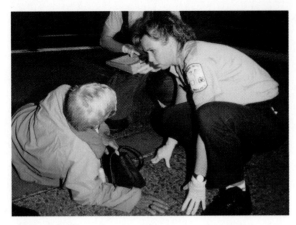

Figure 7-5   It is important to assess whether pain following a traumatic event is acute or chronic.

is therefore purely a trauma patient, medical conditions such as syncope secondary to cardiac arrhythmia need to be ruled out as a potential cause of the crash. Information from bystanders, such as the patient's level of consciousness before the crash, is useful in making a determination about the entire scope of the emergency.

Attitude Tip

Do not assume that you know the nature of the injury. You need to gather complete information, such as prior medical conditions, to make an assessment.

It is easy to make assumptions about falls as well, but recall that there are numerous medical reasons for falls occurring in the older population. Therefore, evaluate the scene for trip hazards, walkers, and canes to determine the nature of the fall, and ask bystanders and the patient about the fall and the events immediately preceding it.

You also need to gather information about the environment in which the incident occurred. The older patient who has fallen may not recall when the fall occurred. You should inspect the scene for indications as to when the patient may have fallen, so that a time down may be estimated. Clues as to when the patient fell include newspapers, meals found sitting out, appliances left on, and the patient's attire. It is also important

once again to interview bystanders and neighbors who may watch for the well-being of the patient to find out when they were last contacted or seen.

Mechanism of Injury

Mechanism of injury is an important factor in establishing an index of suspicion and developing a treatment plan. Any patient who has a penetrating injury proximal to the knees or elbows should be transported to an appropriate trauma center for evaluation based on the high probability of internal injury to major structures. Evaluation of the blunt trauma patient is not as clear cut. You need to carefully integrate the physical findings with information about the mechanism of injury to determine a treatment plan.[2]

Death of another occupant in the same vehicle is a valuable predictor of substantial injury from blunt trauma.[2] Therefore, any older patient involved in a motor vehicle crash where another occupant in the car has died should be transported to an appropriate trauma center. Other mechanisms that warrant consideration for transport to a trauma center after a motor vehicle crash include rollover, speed greater than 40 mph, ejection, more than 20 inches of deformity to the vehicle's body or 12 inches of intrusion into any part of the passenger compartment, and being struck by a vehicle traveling greater than 5 mph. Additionally, you should examine the interior of the vehicle for a bent steering wheel, broken (spidered) windshield, or deployed airbags—all evidence that will help anticipate the types of injuries that may have occurred as well as in making a decision as to the appropriate receiving facility for the patient (▶ **Figure 7-6**).[15]

Falls represent another blunt injury mechanism. In young patients, a fall of greater than 15 feet or 3 times the patient's height is considered to be a sufficient mechanism for referral to a trauma center. In older patients, a fall from a much lower level, including standing position, may lead to significant injuries; therefore, a thorough history and physical exam should be performed before assuming the patient has only minor injuries.

Initial Assessment

The goal of the initial assessment is to identify life-threatening conditions. The early phase of re-

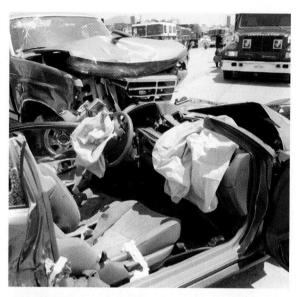

Figure 7-6 A bent steering wheel, broken windshield, or deployed airbag is evidence to help determine the types of injuries that may have occurred.

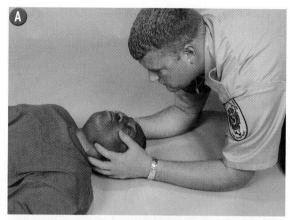

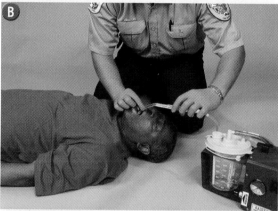

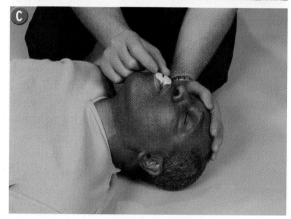

Figure 7-7 The airway should initially be addressed using simple techniques, such as (A) the modified jaw thrust, (B) suctioning, and (C) placement of an oropharyngeal or nasopharyngeal airway.

suscitation that aims to treat those life-threatening injuries occurs simultaneously with the initial assessment.[16] The initial assessment conducted for a medical patient is expanded from ABC to ABCDE, with D and E referring to disability and exposure, respectively.

Airway

Initial evaluation of the airway should be performed immediately after assessment of scene safety. A patient who is awake and able to speak clearly without significant effort is likely to have a patent airway.[17] The patient with noisy respiration or extreme difficulty speaking may have a compromised airway. For those found unconscious, the airway initially may appear secure; however, the tongue may suddenly occlude the pharynx and prevent ventilation.

Initially, address the airway using simple techniques, including the modified jaw thrust, suctioning if blood or foreign material is evident upon visual inspection, and the placement of an oropharyngeal airway in the unconscious patient, or a nasopharyngeal airway if the patient is conscious and does not display signs or symptoms of a head injury (▶ **Figure 7-7**).[17] If these techniques provide an adequate airway, continue the initial assessment to look for other life-threatening conditions.

Once other life-threatening issues have been addressed, the airway may be reassessed and more definitive treatment may be started, including intubation. If, despite the use of simple airway techniques, the airway continues to be compromised or doubtful, intubation should be performed immediately to provide a secure airway.

It is essential to keep in mind that breathing should not be evaluated or addressed until the airway has been secured or observed to be adequate.

Other factors also need to be considered when evaluating or establishing an airway. If the patient has evidence of trauma in the mouth, pharynx, or trachea, early aggressive airway management may be necessary. Additionally, soft tissue injuries to the neck can lead to swelling that potentially may obstruct the airway, and therefore early intubation may be indicated even if the airway appears adequate.

The possibility of cervical spine injury also affects airway management. When cervical spine injury is suspected, immediately immobilize the head and neck by applying a cervical collar or using manual stabilization, and ensure that stabilization is maintained. Endotracheal intubation may be performed while adequately maintaining cervical spine immobilization with the assistance of two other EMS providers.[17]

When evaluating the airway of the older patient, keep in mind that dentures and other dental accessories may be present in the patient's mouth and that they could be a source of airway obstruction. Dentures and other dental appliances that are found to be loose or poorly fitting should be removed from the mouth. This may be accomplished by opening the patient's mouth with one hand, and using the thumb and index finger of the free hand to grasp the front of the device and apply light pressure away from the patient's gums to ensure that the appliance is loose. Once the appliance is loose, it can be removed from the patient's mouth. Also, the greater likelihood of broken teeth in older patients increases the possibility of aspiration and bleeding into the airway. Because the cough reflex also may be diminished, aggressive suctioning is warranted to reduce the risk of aspiration and subsequent breathing compromise.

Patients with severe kyphosis pose a challenge for airway management. Use pads to fill any voids under the head and neck, and stabilize the spine before attempting oral intubation. Oral intubation may be extremely difficult, and nasotracheal intubation or needle cricothyrotomy may be necessary to establish an airway if it is compromised. Medical direction should be sought when airway management is necessary in patients with this condition, and transportation to the closest facility for airway stabilization may be warranted.

Breathing

After an adequate airway has been established, you must first determine whether the patient is breathing, then evaluate the quality of the breathing. Because the presence of labor-free respirations is not sufficient evidence of adequate breathing, next you should examine the neck for a midline trachea and the chest for breath sounds and excursion. Keep in mind that the goal of the assessment of breathing is to identify the presence of three life-threatening conditions: **tension pneumothorax**, puncture wounds to the chest, and flail segment.[17]

When assessing the breathing of an older patient, keep in mind that the drive to increase respiratory rate in response to injury is reduced. Therefore, patients may have a normal respiratory rate despite being hypoxic. Additionally, seemingly minor injuries to an older patient's chest, such as rib fractures, can result in substantial underlying injury to the lungs, heart, or great vessels.[18] It is very important to continue monitoring the patient's breathing using pulse-oximetry if available, inspection of the chest and neck, and frequent auscultation of lung fields.

Patients found to be severely injured or who are suspected of being seriously injured should receive high-flow oxygen; patients with only minor injuries or a low index of suspicion can receive low-flow oxygen via nasal cannula or Venturi mask. The goal for all older trauma patients is to maintain oxygen saturation greater than 95%.

If a patient reports a history of chronic obstructive pulmonary disease (COPD), it is important to monitor his or her respiratory status because these patients are occasionally driven to breathe by a low arterial partial pressure of oxygen, rather than a high carbon dioxide level. Oxygen should never be withheld from these patients if they need it. In these situations, carefully monitor the patient for signs of increased carbon dioxide retention such as lethargy, decreased respiratory drive, and changes in mental status. If these signs develop, oxygen delivery should be adjusted to maintain the respiratory drive while still attempting to maintain oxygen saturation greater than 90%. The use of a bag-valve-mask (BVM) device may be necessary for patients who have a major decrease in respiratory drive (▶ **Figure 7-8**).

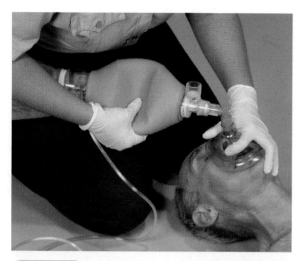

Figure 7-8 It may be necessary to use a BVM device in patients with a major decrease in respiratory drive.

Circulation

Once a patient has a secure airway and adequate breathing, you should assess the circulatory system. This is most easily accomplished by palpating the patient's pulses and noting their quality, rate, and rhythm and by obtaining a baseline blood pressure. After the blood pressure has been obtained, ask the patient about their normal blood pressure to determine if the reading is near the patient's normal level. Capillary refill time is notably unreliable in most older individuals.

You should now identify any gross bleeding and apply compression dressings or direct pressure to the site. Cardiac monitoring should also be initiated to identify life-threatening arrhythmias, and IV access should be established. If a cervical collar has not been placed on the patient by this point, one should be applied before continuing.[17] Never attempt to straighten out the patient's neck. Rather, use a cervical collar that provides the best fit for the patient's neck as is.

It is of vital importance to remember that cardiac arrest shortly following injury is most commonly the result of cardiovascular failure in the older patient. Those patients who are normally hypertensive and are found to have a blood pressure within the normal adult range should be suspected of having internal bleeding. Patients with any drop in blood pressure, even if only briefly with spontaneous return to normal, should also be suspected of having internal bleeding.

The presence of premature ventricular contractions upon the initiation of cardiac monitoring could indicate hypoxia if the patient has no past history of such and may warrant the immediate administration of high-flow oxygen or the use of airway adjuncts to achieve maximal oxygen delivery to the heart.

Disability

A rapid evaluation of the patient's neurological status is the next step. An assessment of level of consciousness may be easily accomplished by using the mnemonic **AVPU**, where **A** stands for "awake and alert," **V** for "responds to verbal stimulus," **P** for "responds to pain," and **U** for "unconscious." Do not assume that a decreased level of consciousness is the baseline mental status of an older patient. Obtain assistance with determining level of consciousness from people familiar with the patient, if available. It is often helpful to ask questions such as, "What was he like an hour ago? What was he like yesterday? Does he usually talk like this? Can he usually move his arms and legs?"

A rapid evaluation of the spine also is performed at this point by having the patient move the upper and lower extremities to assess gross motor function ▼ **Figure 7-9** . Also, comparison to previous levels of function can be helpful, particularly if the patient has a previous history of stroke.

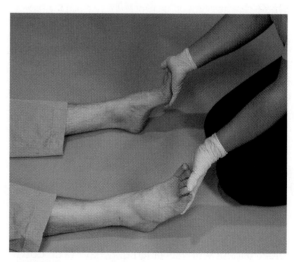

Figure 7-9 A rapid evaluation of the spine is performed by having the patient move his or her upper and lower extremities to assess gross motor function.

Exposure

Patients who are suspected of having significant injuries should be unclothed to facilitate the identification of injuries during the physical exam. Older patients are particularly predisposed to hypothermia; protective measures such as blankets and warmed IV fluids should be used to prevent this. If a patient appears to be suffering from minor injuries and only a low index of suspicion for additional injury exists, the clothing may be left intact and the physical exam may be performed by palpating through the clothing.

> ### Attitude Tip
>
> Be respectful of the older person's privacy when performing an examination.

Past Medical History

Recall from Chapter 5 that the history of the older patient is critical. Be sure to gather as much information as possible from the patient and those familiar with the patient if available.

Physical Exam

Recall that as with any trauma patient, the physical exam should be conducted in the most efficient manner possible.

Head

Palpate the head to feel for depressions and symmetry, and to determine the presence of bleeding from a laceration to the scalp. Scalp lacerations can bleed enough in older patients to cause shock. Any sites of significant bleeding should also be palpated for depressions and inspected for signs of an open head injury, such as a cerebrospinal fluid (CSF) leak or the presence of brain matter. Check the head for **Battle's sign** (bruising behind the ear) and the face for **periorbital ecchymosis** (raccoon eyes). These are later signs of head injury, and their presence may indicate a previous head injury or provide a clue as to how long an older patient who has fallen may have been down.

Inspect the ear canals for the presence of injury, blood, and CSF. Blood coming from the ear canal without the presence of an injury to the canal can

be tested for CSF by allowing it to drip onto a piece of gauze or sheet. In this quick test, a classic halo ring sign appears if CSF is present in the fluid. Once the cranium has been assessed, pupillary status should be determined. Assess pupil size, symmetry, roundness, and reactivity to light (▼ **Figure 7-10**). In older patients, the presence of cataracts and other conditions of the eye may prohibit a complete exam of the pupils or cause the patient to have a baseline pupillary asymmetry.

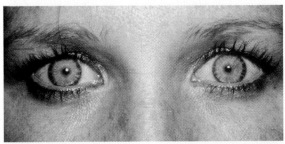
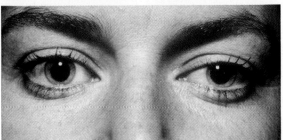
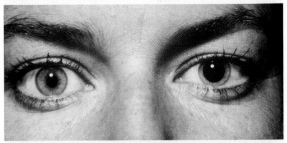
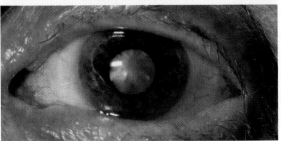

Figure 7-10 Assess the pupils for size, symmetry, roundness, and reactivity to light. The presence of cataracts could prohibit a complete examination of the pupils or cause the patient to have a baseline pupillary asymmetry. (A) Constricted pupils. (B) Dilated pupils. (C) Unequal pupils. (D) Cataracts.

As discussed in Chapter 5, the Glasgow Coma Scale (GCS) is one of the most significant determinants of the potential for a positive outcome in older patients.[19] The GCS is a method of assessing level of consciousness by scoring the patient's response to eye opening, motor response, and verbal response. Assign a score based on the GCS by asking simple questions and having the patient follow simple commands (▼ **Figure 7-11**). Any older patient with a head injury and a score of less than 15, who normally has a score of 15, should be transferred to a trauma center. Many older patients have a pre-existing decrease in cognitive function, diminished affect, and memory loss, making it difficult to determine the presence or extent of a head injury.[5] When uncertain, it is wise to triage an older trauma patient to a trauma center. Other signs and symptoms that may be present in a patient with a head injury or that indicate the possibility of such include diminished motor function on one side of the body, hypertension coupled with bradycardia and a decreased level of consciousness, a loss of consciousness for more than 5 minutes, and **retrograde amnesia** (inability to remember events leading up to injury).[2]

Face

Older patients have an increased propensity for facial and nasal fractures that may lead to bleeding into the airway. The facial region should be evaluated for bleeding, integrity of the bony structures, and other signs of injury. Inspect the mouth first for bleeding, dentures, and other objects that potentially could occlude the airway.

Continuous suctioning may be required if there is bleeding from structures within the oropharynx, to prevent aspiration and ingestion that could lead to vomiting. Examine the mandible and maxilla for crepitus and stability by palpating the area around the mouth and the patient's jaw. Any odors coming from the mouth, such as that of an alcoholic beverage or a ketone odor, should also be noted. Inspection of the oral cavity for the presence of fluids may yield useful information. Blood present in the mouth without an identifiable source of bleeding may hint at an injury to the structures of the airway or esophagus. The presence of coffee-ground vomitus may be a sign of an injury to the gastrointestinal tract.

Inspect the nose for bleeding and CSF leakage. Blood from the nose may indicate a head injury or the presence of an injury within the nasal cavity. Bleeding from the nose may not be controllable in the prehospital setting, and care should be used because the blood from the nasal cavity may be aspirated or swallowed, increasing the possibility of vomiting and airway compromise. Bleeding and a CSF leak should not be controlled, because they could lead to increased intracranial pressure. Blood or CSF leaking from the head should be either absorbed or suctioned.

Neck

Examine the neck in more detail at this point. If a collar was placed during the initial assessment, it should now be opened while another EMS provider maintains stabilization to allow for a thorough exam to be completed. Palpation of the posterior neck is done to evaluate for pain and deformity. Evaluation of the anterior aspect of the neck focuses on identifying conditions that could impact airway, breathing, and circulation. The presence of distended neck veins in an older patient may be normal if the patient has a history of heart failure or pulmonary hypertension, but could also indicate a tension pneumothorax, pericardial tamponade, or other conditions that result in impaired venous return to the heart or impaired function of the right side of the heart, such as an AMI.

GLASGOW COMA SCALE

Eye Opening	
Spontaneous	4
To Voice	3
To Pain	2
None	1

Verbal Response	
Oriented	5
Confused	4
Inappropriate Words	3
Incomprehensible Words	2
None	1

Motor Response	
Obeys Command	6
Localizes Pain	5
Withdraws (pain)	4
Flexion (pain)	3
Extension (pain)	2
None	1

Glasgow Coma Score Total	15

Figure 7-11   The Glasgow Coma Scale.

Soft-tissue injuries to the neck may develop into a life-threatening condition due to hypovolemia, airway occlusion, or the development of an air embolus. Evidence of an expanding hematoma on the anterior or lateral aspect of the neck is an airway emergency. To assist in determining the extent of injury, ask the patient if there is difficulty breathing, speaking, or swallowing.

Chest

Examine the chest wall thoroughly for crepitus, subcutaneous emphysema, and integrity of the bony structures. The chest should be exposed to allow for the most thorough examination. Secondary inspection of the chest should evaluate the chest wall for abnormal respiratory patterns, symmetry, and evidence of bruising or penetrating wounds. The presence of scars on the chest could indicate a history of heart surgery or past thoracic trauma (▼ **Figure 7-12**). The arms should be abducted as well so that the axillae may be visualized for penetrating wounds and bruising. A more thorough assessment of lung sounds should be performed to evaluate the quality of air exchange and look for evidence of a pneumo/hemothorax or other pathological conditions. Heart sounds should also be assessed for quality. Distant heart sounds, coupled with the signs and symptoms of shock, could indicate a pericardial tamponade. However, older patients with cardiac hypertrophy or COPD may have pre-existing distant heart sounds.

Blunt trauma to the chest may also cause a blunt cardiac injury. In blunt cardiac injury, the heart muscle is bruised, leading to an increased risk that the patient will develop an irregular heartbeat or reduced cardiac output. Most commonly, these patients will complain of sternal pain. The ECG will reveal sinus tachycardia and/or nonspecific changes in the ST segment.[20]

Another, often fatal, consequence of a blunt injury to the chest is a rupture of the aorta, usually caused by a deceleration injury, such as a motor vehicle crash. Older patients are at a high risk for this injury because of atherosclerosis and its effects on the elasticity of the vasculature. Complete rupture of the aorta almost always leads to rapid hemorrhage and cardiac arrest. Partial tears of the aorta often seal off temporarily, yet still lead to a 50% mortality rate in the first 24 hours following injury.[20] Patients who have an aortic injury may often have chest pain with radiation to the jaw, neck, and teeth. This pain differs from cardiac pain in that it is usually the most severe at its onset, tends to move around the patient's chest, and is often described as a "tearing," "cutting," or "ripping" pain. Patients may also complain of back pain between the shoulder blades as well as lower back discomfort. Physical findings associated with aortic rupture include differing blood pressures in the upper extremities, unequal pulses, elevated diastolic blood pressure, pulsation at the sternoclavicular joints, and hypotension.[21]

Penetrating trauma to the chest can damage many important structures (▼ **Figure 7-13**). While

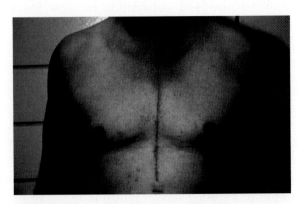

Figure 7-12   The presence of scars on the chest could indicate a history of heart surgery or past thoracic trauma.

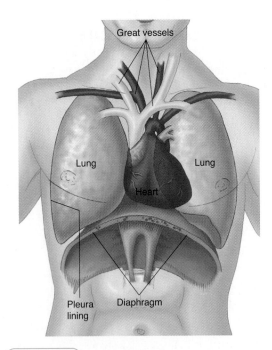

Figure 7-13   Penetrating trauma to the chest can damage many important structures.

evaluating the thorax, including the axillae and back of a patient with a penetrating wound, recall the relationships of the various organs with the anatomical features on the surface of the body. On the right, the liver may rise as high as the sixth intercostal space during exhalation, allowing it to be injured by a wound to the chest. On the left side of the chest, the lung extends several centimeters above the clavicle and could potentially be injured by a penetrating wound to the neck. Patients with a penetrating wound should be closely monitored for the development of a tension pneumothorax. At no time should a penetrating wound to the chest be probed, because it may lead to the creation of a pneumothorax.

Abdomen

The older patient's abdomen can pose substantial challenges to EMS providers because of the physical changes associated with aging. Older people tend to have an anterior abdominal wall that contains less muscle and more fat, causing it to be flaccid. As a result, stimuli from within the abdomen that normally lead to pain, spasm, and rigidity in younger patients may not produce the same findings in older patients.[22] Inspection of the abdomen may not be as useful or specific due to the looseness of the skin that allows fluid to accumulate within the abdomen without distending the anterior abdominal wall; however, it is important to inspect for ecchymosis, particularly around the umbilicus and flanks. For those patients with a flaccid abdominal wall, pressure should be applied more deeply and thoroughly about the regions of the abdomen to adequately assess for injury (▼ **Figure 7-14**).[22]

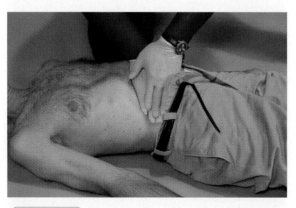

Figure 7-14   Because older patients may have a flaccid abdominal wall, pressure should be applied more deeply and thoroughly about the regions of the abdomen to adequately assess for injury.

The liver and spleen, both classified as solid organs, are the most commonly injured organs in the abdomen. The liver occupies the majority of the space in the right upper quadrant (RUQ) and in general is located under the surface of ribs six through ten. It also extends to approximately the midclavicular line of the left upper quadrant (LUQ). Unlike the liver, which occupies the anterior to posterior volume of the RUQ, the spleen is situated more posteriorly and laterally under the surface of ribs eight to ten in the LUQ. Injury to these organs commonly results from a penetrating wound to the abdomen or as the result of rib fractures that lacerate the organs. Patients with an injury to the liver or spleen may have localized or diffuse abdominal pain as well as referred pain to the shoulder. The abdomen may feel tense and distended, but recall that the older person's abdominal wall has less musculature, therefore making a negative finding less reliable. Any older trauma victim who complains of abdominal pain should be suspected of internal organ injury, even if the abdominal examination is entirely normal.

Pelvis

Determine the stability of the pelvis by applying pressure on the iliac crest directed posteriorly and superiorly. The pelvis should not be rocked because this may lead to further injury. Also palpate the symphysis pubis. Indications of an injury to the pelvis include instability with palpation, bruising in the groin and perineum, blood from the vagina or penis, rotation or shortening of the lower extremities, decreased distal pulses in the legs and feet, and neurological changes in the lower extremities.

Lower Extremities

The lower extremities may be rapidly assessed by palpating each limb from thigh to foot. This is most efficiently accomplished by placing your hands around the extremity and squeezing gently (▶ **Figure 7-15**). While moving distally, also inspect the extremity for deformities, open wounds, surgical scars, edema, and bruising. Once you have reached the feet, palpate the dorsalis pedis and posterior tibial pulses for presence and quality. In some older patients who have a history of peripheral vascular disease (PVD), assessment of the lower extremities may reveal absent or diminished pulses. A neurological exam of the lower extremities should also be performed. Assess

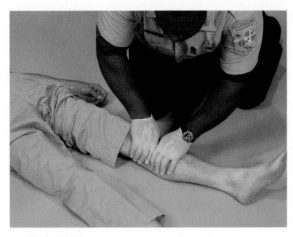

Figure 7-15 The most efficient way to assess the legs is to place your hands around the extremity and squeeze it gently.

motor function by having the patient flex and extend his or her feet against moderate resistance, and evaluate sensory function by touching the patient's feet and legs to determine if the stimuli feel normal.

Evaluation of range of motion should be performed in patients who have specific complaints in a particular limb. Evaluate range of motion by asking the patient to move the joints in question. It is important to ask patients who have a history of arthritis or previous joint replacements about their normal range of motion. Remember to avoid excessive flexion or extension of replaced joints, as this may lead to injury or damage the limb.

Communication Tip

When evaluating range of motion, it is important to ask patients who have arthritis or joint replacements about their normal range of motion.

Upper Extremities

The same technique used to assess the lower extremities is also applicable to the upper extremities. Signs and symptoms of a fractured radius include localized pain, swelling, deformity, weakness, and laceration. The patient may also have signs and symptoms of unilateral neurological or vascular

findings distal to the fracture site, including diminished pulse strength and motor and sensory function.

Back

Examination of the back may be performed prior to other activities of the physical exam to facilitate rapid spinal immobilization. Palpate the back along the midline to assess for deformity and pain. Patients who have a history of scoliosis or kyphosis may be difficult to examine. The scoliotic spine is curved in an abnormal manner to the side, and requires a thorough exam along the length of the spine throughout its course to determine the presence of pain and injury. This may require several attempts to properly identify the course of the spine and ensure the adequacy of the exam. Kyphotic patients may require additional personnel to log-roll effectively (▼ Figure 7-16). Because the patient is hunched over and cannot have his or her back straightened, providers may be needed to support the spine as well as position pillows and blankets once the patient is returned to the supine position. Patients with kyphosis should never be forced into a fully flat position, because this may lead to severe injury. Vacuum splints can be helpful in padding the patient for transport (▶ Skill Drill 7-1). Examination of the kyphotic spine may demonstrate pain and deformity that existed prior to injury and subsequently may not lead to reliable findings. While the patient is log-rolled, the back should also be inspected for

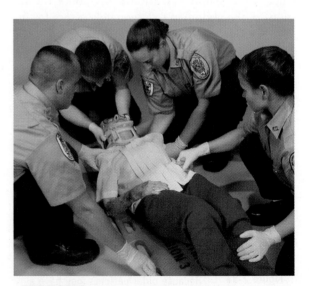

Figure 7-16 Kyphotic patients may require additional personnel to log-roll effectively.

Skill Drill 7-1 Application of a Vacuum Splint to a Wrist Fracture

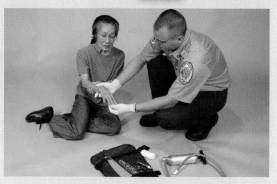

1. Assess pulse, motor, and sensory function of the extremity and cover open wounds with a dry, sterile dressing and apply direct pressure, if necessary.

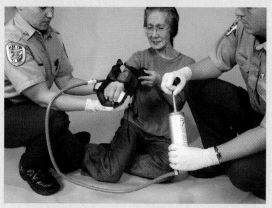

3. Apply the vacuum splint to the extremity.

   Remove the air from the splint through the suction valve with the vacuum pump until it conforms to the extremity and immobilizes the fracture.

   Reassess pulse, motor, and sensory function.

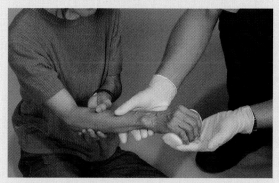

2. Move the hand into the position of function. Place a soft roller bandage in the palm.

wounds, bruising, skin integrity, and surgical scars. Posterior lung fields should also be auscultated, especially if a patient has been supine for an extended period of time.

A thorough initial assessment as well as continuous reassessment is crucial to identifying injuries that are life threatening or have the potential to become so. As the assessment progresses and new injuries and complications are identified, priorities need to be adjusted continuously to address the most important issues first. By following an orderly system of assessment and reassessment, injuries are less likely to be missed and the patient may be treated most effectively. These principles are similar to those used for the

care of younger patients, but they are even more critical in older patients because of the increased potential for rapid deterioration.

Management

The goal of prehospital management of older trauma patients is to deliver a viable patient to the most appropriate facility in the minimum amount of time. Treatment priorities should be directed at maintaining adequate ventilation and perfusion, as well as preventing further injury. Patients appearing to be stable may decompensate quickly without many warning signs due to the lack of physiological reserve. Additionally, because of the many medications and underlying diseases in older patients, complications are more likely to occur.

Principles of Care

The following principles are applicable to the treatment of all older trauma patients who have significant injuries or who have a high index of suspicion for injury based on the mechanism of injury. Significant injuries include head, spinal cord, chest, pelvis, and abdominal trauma, a single proximal long bone fracture (eg, humerus or femur), and two or more distal long bone fractures (eg, tibia or radius).

♦ Rapid initial patient assessment and physical exam with ongoing monitoring of airway, breathing, circulation, and neurological status

♦ Careful and early spinal immobilization

♦ Administration of high-flow oxygen

♦ Initiation of IV access

♦ Cardiac monitoring

♦ Prevention of hypothermia by the use of blankets and environmental controls

♦ Rapid transportation to the appropriate receiving facility

If any question exists at any time as to the best plan of management, medical direction should be obtained.

Blunt Injury

To treat older patients with blunt trauma most effectively, interventions must be performed quickly and efficiently. In cases of significant blunt injury, you should suspect spinal injury and immobilize properly. Intravenous access should be established early because of the possibility of internal bleeding, the low cardiac reserve, and the potential for development of cardiac arrhythmias (▶ **Figure 7-17**). No more than several minutes should be spent on-scene attempting to establish an IV; additional attempts, if necessary, should be made while en route to the hospital. For hypotensive patients, fluids should be given liberally providing lung sounds are clear, in an attempt to maintain a systolic pressure of 100 mm Hg. If a hypotensive patient presents with rales or

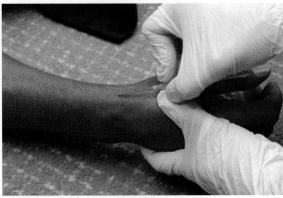

Figure 7-17   In cases of significant blunt injury, IV access should be established early because of the possibility of internal bleeding, the low cardiac reserve, and the potential for development of cardiac arrhythmias.

other evidence of CHF, prompt medical direction should be obtained to determine how aggressively fluids should be administered.

Any sites of obvious bleeding should be treated quickly with a pressure dressing. Direct pressure, even for patients who are anticoagulated, usually should be sufficient to stop the bleeding. Suspected fracture sites should be splinted while en route; do not delay transport to apply splints.

Injuries to the Spine

As with all patients, prompt spinal immobilization is an effective method of reducing further damage to the spinal cord and preserving the older patient's neurological function. The optimal method for immobilizing the spine is to secure it in the midline. Often, patients may be found in positions where the neck or body is not in the neutral position, such as the head being rotated to one side. To facilitate the application of a cervical collar, the provider should slowly return the head to the midline. At no time should these attempts continue if the patient develops changes in neurological status or complains of increasing pain. If these complaints do develop, the head should be secured in the position in which it is found by using blankets and tape to prevent further movement (▶ **Figure 7-18**).

The older patient presents several unique challenges to EMS providers when treating spinal injuries. To immobilize kyphotic patients, several

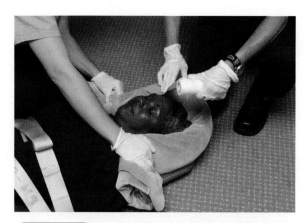

Figure 7-18 If the attempt to move a patient's head to the midline results in changes in neurological status or complaints of increasing pain, secure the head in the position in which it was found by using blankets and tape.

blankets and pillows or vacuum splints may be required to provide support to the head and upper back (▶ **Skill Drill 7-2**). The blankets and pillows or vacuum splints are placed under the cervical spine, as well as under the patient's head, to provide support, because the patient's back will not completely conform to the backboard. This technique is similar in principle to padding the void spaces under a patient's knees or lumbar spine. Once in place, secure the patient to the backboard by using straps that maintain the position of the patient as well as pillows and blankets to provide support. The head may be secured to the backboard by simply applying gauze to protect the fragile skin, and then taping over the gauze and across the cervical collar and patient's forehead.

Another situation that provides a challenge to EMS providers is the treatment of **spinal shock** in older patients. Spinal shock represents a situation in which the volume of the intravascular space dramatically increases and leads to hypotension. Patients with spinal shock should not be considered hypovolemic unless internal injuries are suspected or obvious bleeding is witnessed. Sympathetic tone typically returns within 24 hours after injury, and the intravascular space returns to normal.

The challenge for these patients is determining how aggressively IV fluids should be administered. If too much fluid is given, pulmonary edema could develop.[10] A dramatic decrease in blood pressure, however, could result in cardiac ischemia or stroke. Fluid resuscitation must be directed to prevent these systemic complications of shock. Medical consultation should be considered early in these situations.

Head Injuries

Older patients who have signs or symptoms of a significant head injury, such as a loss of consciousness, are assumed to have sustained a substantial injury even if the patient is neurologically intact at the time of exam. Additionally, patients who have sustained even minor-appearing head injuries and who are on blood thinners are suspected of having a brain injury and are treated as such. These patients may need persuading to seek medical treatment, because they may feel completely normal and may not believe medical treatment is necessary. In situations where patients refuse care yet have a high risk of brain injury, relatives or neighbors should be instructed to be aware of subtle changes in neurological status that could indicate deterioration.

Prehospital treatment of older patients with a head injury should be aimed at maintaining maximum oxygen delivery to the brain. Patients with a severe head injury may require intubation to protect the airway and provide adequate oxygen delivery. If end-tidal CO_2 monitoring is available, the level should be maintained at approximately 32 to 36 mm Hg, because recent studies indicate that hyperventilating patients to a level less than 30 may have a negative influence on the patient's outcome. In addition to airway management and oxygen supplementation, IV fluids may be required to maintain cerebral perfusion. Fluids should be given to support a systolic blood pressure of at least 100 mm Hg. Patients who have signs of head injury may also benefit from a slight

Communication Tip

In situations where patients refuse care yet have a high risk of brain injury, relatives or neighbors should be instructed to be aware of subtle changes in neurological status that could indicate deterioration.

Skill Drill 7-2 — Immobilizing a Kyphotic Patient to a Long Backboard

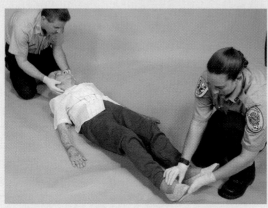

1. Apply and maintain cervical stabilization. Assess distal functions in all extremities.

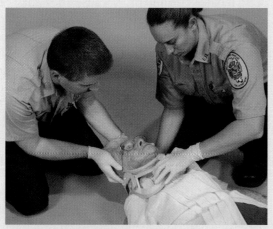

2. Apply a cervical collar. Do not attempt to straighten out the patient's neck.

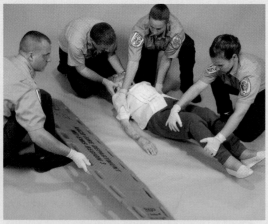

3. Rescuers kneel on one side of the patient and place hands on the far side of the patient.

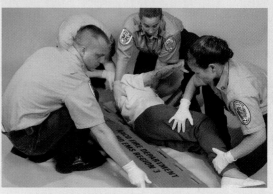

4. On command, rescuers roll the patient toward themselves,

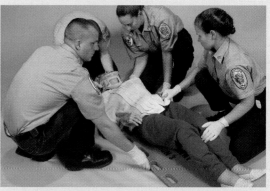

5. Quickly examine the back, slide the backboard under the patient, and roll the patient onto the board.

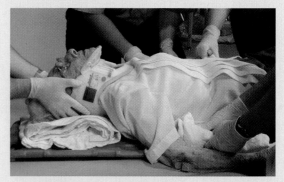

6. Pad the void space below the kyphotic region of the spine with pillows and blankets. The pillows and blankets should be as wide as the backboard to allow for effective immobilization and support.

Place rolled towels or foam padding onto the surface of the padding next to the patient's head.

(continued)

Skill Drill   7-2   Immobilizing a Kyphotic Patient to a Long Backboard (continued)

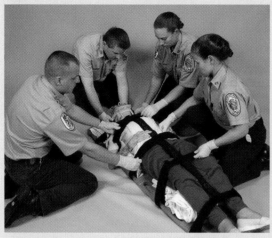

7. Secure the torso to the backboard with straps.

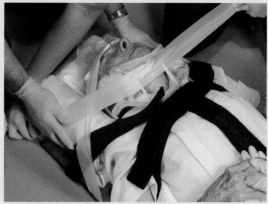

8. Secure the patient's head and padding to the backboard with 2-inch medical tape. The tape should be applied across the forehead and cervical collar and should prevent the padding from becoming dislodged.

   Immobilize the remainder of the body as normal.

elevation of the head, because this may help in reducing intracranial pressure and increasing cerebral perfusion pressure (▼ Figure 7-19).

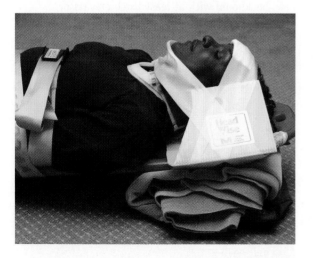

Figure 7-19   Patients who have signs of head injury may benefit from a slight elevation of the head, which may help in reducing intracranial pressure and increasing cerebral perfusion pressure.

Hip Fractures

Fractures of the hip should be treated by splinting the injured extremity with a blanket roll or long board splints. Fractures of the hip do not necessarily require the use of traction splints. The purpose of the blanket roll is to maintain the leg in a static position so that further injury does not occur, and to allow the patient's pain to be controlled (▶ Skill Drill 7-3). The blanket roll should be placed between the patient's legs and the injured extremity should be secured in the position in which it was found by using blankets and pillows. A long backboard or scoop stretcher should be used, so that the patient and the splinting material may be secured in position. These patients should have continued monitoring of the distal neurovascular status as well as for signs and symptoms of shock.

Isolated Musculoskeletal Injuries

The treatment of an isolated extremity injury without evidence or suspicion of significant systemic injury should be more deliberate. Always follow

Skill Drill 7-3 Splinting a Hip Fracture

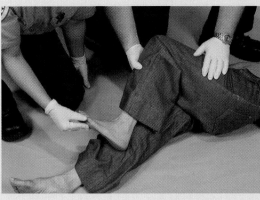

1. Assess pulse, motor, and sensory function of the extremity. Cover open wounds with a dry, sterile dressing and apply direct pressure, if necessary.

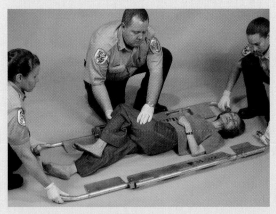

2. Place the patient onto an orthopaedic stretcher or long backboard by logrolling the patient onto the uninjured leg while having a provider support the injured extremity.

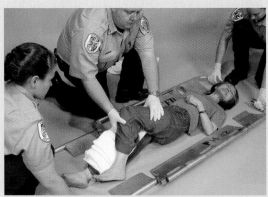

3. While continuing to support the injured extremity in its deformed position, your partner should place a blanket-roll between the patient's legs.

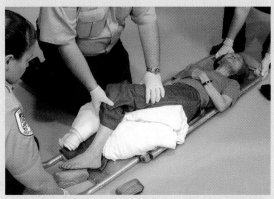

4. Place blankets and pillows under the injured extremity to provide support to fracture site in the deformed position.

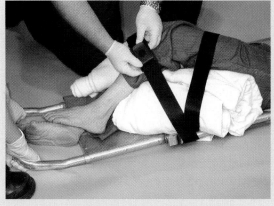

5. Secure both legs and the padding to the backboard with at least three cravats or straps.

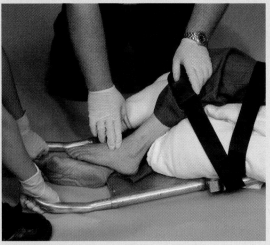

6. Reassess pulse, motor, and sensory function.

CASE STUDY 3

You are dispatched to the residence of a 76-year-old woman who was working in the yard when she tripped over a hose, causing her to fall. Her neighbor, who was bringing in her mail, witnessed the fall and reports that she did not appear to get dizzy before she fell. The patient is complaining of severe left hip pain, and a deformity with bruising is noted in the region. The patient has normal vital signs and has no evidence of neurovascular compromise distal to the injury. She advises you that she has osteoporosis, and has fallen one other time after tripping over a toy, which resulted in a broken wrist.

How should this patient's hip injury be treated?

What are the possible long-term consequences of this injury?

good splinting technique. Splinting is most optimally performed with the extremity in the neutral position. In some older patients, however, attempts to straighten the injured extremity may lead to further injury. This is particularly true in patients who have arthritis that causes a reduced range of motion in the joints of the affected limb. If, while attempting to straighten the extremity, the patient complains of increasing joint pain or you feel resistance, the injured limb should be immobilized in the position in which it is resting. At no time should an extremity be forced into any position to facilitate splinting.

Penetrating Injuries

Management of penetrating trauma to the head, body, and proximal extremities requires expedient transportation to a trauma center. The amount of time spent on-scene should be kept brief, only long enough to administer oxygen, perform an initial assessment, and search for wounds. Studies demonstrate that the survival rate of any patient with a penetrating injury corresponds with how quickly definitive care is reached.

The need for endotracheal intubation and thoracic decompression are among the acceptable reasons for delaying transport. Conversely, the placement of an IV catheter should not delay transport and is best accomplished while en route to the hospital. Spinal immobilization is neces-

sary for patients who have a penetrating wound to the neck or who demonstrate signs of a neurological injury. Spine precautions also may be warranted in patients with penetrating wounds in the chest, abdomen, and buttocks. For these patients, initiate rapid immobilization on a backboard while at the scene and perform more formal immobilization measures while en route to the hospital.

Exercise caution while administering IV fluids for the treatment of a penetrating wound. Fluid administration should be titrated to maintain a systolic blood pressure of approximately 100 mm Hg. Hypertension should not be induced by administering a large volume of IV fluid to a patient who has a normal blood pressure and who does not display signs or symptoms of shock. Excessive administration of IV fluid may lead to further blood loss and have a negative effect on the patient's outcome. Recall that the older patient cannot adapt readily to changes in blood volume; fluid overload may also lead to pulmonary edema and impaired ventilation.

Burns

Pathophysiology

Severe burn injuries lead to a multitude of complications and affect nearly every organ system in the body. Of immediate concern in the older patient is the rapid cardiovascular failure that may occur soon after injury and the onset of hypothermia. Burns lead to a loss of circulating volume, primarily in the form of blood plasma, and this loss of volume is not tolerated well by older patients. As the result of the decrease in circulating volume, vasoconstriction occurs throughout the body. Electrolytes, including potassium, are lost as the body attempts to compensate for the decrease in intravascular volume. Due to the continuous release of vasoconstricting agents, several organs, including the kidneys and liver, may fail in the older patient. If the older patient survives the acute phase, there remains an increased likelihood of death from infection. Most older patients already have a weakened and less efficient immune system, and the risk of developing an infection of the burn site and/or pneumonia is very high.

Assessment

The assessment of the burn patient follows the same approach as the assessment for all other patients. This includes an evaluation of airway, breathing, circulation, a thorough history, and a complete physical exam. An approximate body surface area (BSA) of injury should be determined by using the **Rule of Nines** as well as the degree or depth of the burn. If an agent other than heat caused the burn injury, the nature of the agent should be determined. For those patients who suffered an inhalation injury or who ingested caustic chemicals, the airway must be monitored constantly, because laryngeal edema may develop. Continuous cardiac monitoring is also indicated in the older patient, because the potential for the development of a cardiac arrhythmia exists due to the increased workload being placed on the heart.

Management

First, halt the burning process by extinguishing and removing clothing that continues to burn. In the case of a chemical burn, irrigate the sites of the chemical burn to remove any of the residual agent. Once this has been accomplished, proceed with evaluation of the patient. For patients who are found to have an inadequate airway or who are apneic, perform immediate endotracheal in-

tubation. Those who have suffered from a chemical or thermal burn to the airway may need to be transferred rapidly to the closest hospital to have the airway secured if progressive laryngeal edema is suspected. These issues are at heightened concern in the older patient because of their relatively decreased capacity, compared to younger patients, to tolerate even brief episodes of hypoxia and shock.

Intravenous access should be established rapidly because the cardiovascular system is likely to become stressed; however, as with other traumatic conditions, transport should not be delayed by more than several minutes to accomplish this. If possible, the catheter should be placed in a non-burned area proximal to any circumferential burns. A simple way to estimate how quickly fluids should be administered is to multiply the surface area burned by the patient's weight in kilograms and then divide by 8. This equation will yield the hourly rate of IV fluid infusion needed to replace the volume lost from burned tissues.[23]

A sterile, dry dressing should cover large areas of the body that have been burned **▼ Figure 7-20**). A dressing moistened with sterile water may be applied to patients who have suffered from minor burns with a total body surface involvement of less than 10%.

Treatment of patients who have been injured by lightning or sustained other electrical burns should include spinal immobilization. This is essential, particularly in the older patient, because

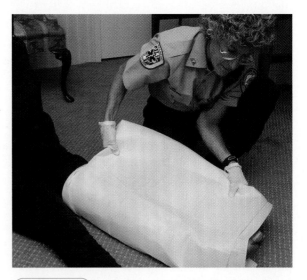

Figure 7-20   A sterile, dry dressing should cover large areas of the body that have been burned.

of the risk of associated spinal column injury.[23] The same management principles identified previously apply to high-voltage burn injuries.

The need for referral to a burn center should be based on the type and extent of burn injury. The criteria for transferring an older burn patient to a burn center include the following:

◆ Greater than 10% BSA total partial and full-thickness burns

◆ 5% BSA or greater of full-thickness burns

◆ Chemical, radiation, or electrical burns

◆ Burns to the face, airway, hands, feet, genitalia, or perineum.

Injury Prevention

Many of the injuries that older patients sustain are preventable. It is important to understand that EMS providers play a key role in preventing injury in the older population. Injury prevention may be accomplished in a variety of ways, including discussions with patients, families, and neighbors, speeches at senior centers, and by simply making recommendations to patients based on what is observed in the environment where they are encountered. The following list contains tips on how to help reduce the risk of injury for older people.

To reduce the risk of being involved in a motor vehicle incident, older people and/or their families should:

◆ Not drive if medications are being used that may impair judgment or cause drowsiness

◆ Periodically have vision and hearing checkups

◆ Monitor driving ability on a regular basis

◆ Avoid attempting to cross busy intersections and intersections that do not have crosswalks and signals

The risk of being burned may be reduced by:

◆ Checking the batteries on smoke detectors semiannually

◆ Having an escape plan

◆ Providing information to the fire department about the location of disabled family members in the house

◆ Exiting the house if there is a fire

Injuries that occur as the result of violence and elder abuse may also be preventable. Measures that can be taken by older people and/or their family members and friends to reduce the risk for these injuries include:

◆ Accompanying older people on trips outside the home, particularly at night

◆ Ensuring that doors and windows are secured

◆ Answering the door only if the person who is knocking is known by the older person

◆ Removing weapons from the home, particularly if an older person suffers from depression or mental status alterations

◆ Constantly monitoring older patients in both the in-home and long-term care facility settings for signs of neglect and abuse, such as bruises, an unkempt environment, and injuries

Specific Musculoskeletal Disorders

Osteoporosis

Clinically, **osteoporosis** is a condition that affects both men and women, and is characterized by a decrease in bone mass leading to a reduction in bone strength and a greater susceptibility to fracture. It is estimated that 15 to 20 million people in the United States over the age of 45 are afflicted with the condition, and that it leads to nearly 1.3 million fractures annually. Osteoporosis is a major public health issue and generates nearly 4 billion dollars per year in health care expenses.[24]

The body is constantly remodeling bone. Cells called **osteoclasts** absorb bone while other cells known as **osteoblasts** deposit newly formed bone in areas where it is needed. The greatest bone mass is reached at approximately age 35. After the age of 35, an imbalance develops between the activity of the two types of cells, leading to a loss of bone mass. The extent of bone loss that a person undergoes is influenced by numerous factors, including genetics, smoking, level of activity, diet, alcohol consumption, hormonal factors, and body weight. Fair-skinned, thin women have the highest risk of developing osteoporosis. The most rapid loss of bone occurs in women during the years following menopause because of decreased hormone production affecting the bones.

People with a higher body weight and who are physically active are likely to have less bone loss because there is mechanical stimulus for the body to deposit new bone. Smoking is believed to cause a reduction in bone mass because it may affect the levels of hormones responsible for maintaining bone mass. A diet poor in calcium and vitamin D, or problems of the gastrointestinal tract leading to poor nutrient absorption, are additional reasons why osteoporosis can develop. Finally, many medications can contribute to osteoporosis.

The most common fractures associated with osteoporosis are those of the spine, hip, and wrist. Fractures of the vertebral body occur more frequently in women than in men, and are typically compression (or collapse) fractures. Nearly 50% of these fractures, however, are asymptomatic; the others result in significant pain, disability, and physical deformities that affect breathing, digestion, and body image.[2,24]

Fractures of the hip affect women five times more commonly than men. Wrist fractures frequently occur as the result of attempting to brace from a fall. These fractures generally result in only short-term disability, but serve as an opportunity to identify and treat osteoporosis before more serious fractures occur.

Numerous measures may be undertaken to reduce the risk of developing osteoporosis and slow its progression. Many postmenopausal women will use hormone replacement therapy as a means to reduce the loss of bone. Calcium and vitamin D supplementation is another common treatment for the condition, because it may retard the loss of bone in both men and women. Many other medications are now available to improve bone strength in both women and men. Older people should also remain physically active by walking and performing low-impact exercises to maintain bone and muscle strength (▶ Figure 7-21).[24]

Osteoarthritis

<u>Osteoarthritis</u> is a progressive disease process of the joints resulting in the destruction of cartilage, the formation of bone spurs in joints, and joint

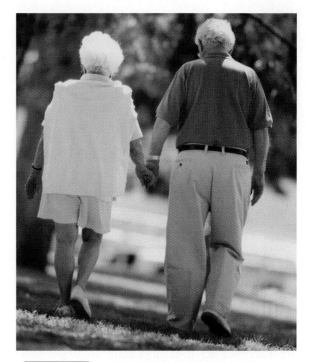

Figure 7-21 Older people should remain physically active by walking and performing low-impact exercises to maintain bone and muscle strength.

stiffness (▼ Figure 7-22).[25] This type of arthritis is thought to result from "wear and tear" and, in some instances, by repetitive trauma to the joints. The disease affects approximately 35% to 45% of the population over the age of 65, and its prevalence is equal between men and women.[25]

Typically, osteoarthritis affects several joints of the body, most commonly those in the hands,

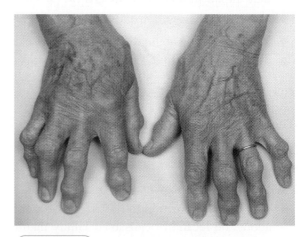

Figure 7-22 Osteoarthritis may cause substantial disfigurement.

knees, hips, and spine. Patients will complain of pain and stiffness that gets worse with exertion and tends to be worse at the end of the day. Ultimately, substantial disuse and disfigurement can occur.[25] Most commonly, patients are treated with anti-inflammatory medications and physical therapy to improve the range of motion.

Rheumatoid Arthritis

Unlike osteoarthritis, **rheumatoid arthritis** is a systemic inflammatory disease that affects the body's joints.[25] Men are 3 times less likely to be affected by the disease than women, and approximately 1% of the population is affected by this condition. To date, no specific cause has been determined for rheumatoid arthritis; however, some consider it to be an autoimmune disease.

Patients affected by rheumatoid arthritis have a variety of symptoms, most commonly inflammation in and around the joints in the hands, wrists, ankles, and feet, and less often in the knees and spine. As a result of the inflammation, joints become stiffer. In addition, the tissues supporting the inflamed joint may become unstable and result in dislocation or subluxation (sinking of the bone out of position). For this reason, one should always pay particular attention to the spine in an older trauma victim with rheumatoid arthritis.

Summary

With the population of older people increasing, the number of emergency calls for help for injured older patients can only be expected to rise. The best possible treatment plan is devised by considering the numerous changes that occur as the body ages and the patient's medical history, and integrating those factors with information gathered during evaluation of the scene and patient. It is particularly important always to remember that many injuries older patients sustain are the result of a medical condition leading to the incident. Therefore, the assessment of the older patient should always aim to identify any medical conditions that could have led to the injury as well as evaluate the specific injuries sustained.

For all older patients who have suffered a severe injury, or who have a high probability of severe injury, careful attention must be given to the cardiovascular system, because it is at an increased risk to fail. Rapid transportation as well as the use of supplemental oxygen, cardiac monitoring, and appropriate volume replacement are essentials for prehospital care of the older patient. In addition, spinal immobilization is critical for all older patients who have the potential for an injury to the spine.

Many older patients will have isolated injuries and complaints related to the musculoskeletal system. Many of these simply may be an aggravation of pre-existing conditions, such as arthritis, while others may have the potential to be severely debilitating injuries, such as hip fractures. A thorough history of the present complaint, past medical history, and physical examination will aid in determining who among these patients will need to be transported. When splinting an injured extremity in an older patient, the limb should never be forced into the "normal" position because serious injury may result.

As the role of the EMS provider expands to include not only prehospital and interhospital care, many providers will be called upon to provide education to family members about how to prevent injury. By instructing patients and family members about the various methods for reducing the risk of injury, EMS providers may play an active role not only in treating the injured older patient, but more importantly in preventing injuries from happening in the first place.

Case Study Summaries

CASE STUDY 1 SUMMARY

The most likely reason why the driver of the vehicle crashed the car is because he had a stroke while driving. This can be explained by the information gathered from bystanders pertaining to the events that occurred prior to the crash, such as failure to brake and no reason to swerve. In addition, the medical history of hypertension and the use of Coumadin place the patient at risk for a stroke, and he demonstrates typical signs of one (confusion and facial droop).

Treatment of this patient should address both the trauma and the medical condition. Therefore, the usual spinal precautions should be instituted and any obvious injuries should be treated accordingly. Just as important, however, is treating the patient for the stroke. Measures also should be established to maintain a patent airway, maximize oxygen delivery to the brain, and provide rapid transportation to an appropriate emergency department. The situation where a patient has a medical condition that leads to an injury occurs frequently, and leads to not only motor vehicle crashes, but falls and other accidents as well. It is of the utmost importance always to assess for a medical condition that has led to trauma whenever an older patient is evaluated.

CASE STUDY 2 SUMMARY

This patient is likely to have suffered from a compression fracture of her spine while she was getting up from her chair. Compression fractures are very common in older persons and often occur while doing normal activities of daily life, such as bending over to pick up something, rising from a chair, or lifting items. Often, the fractures go without notice unless significant pain is present. Most commonly, they are stable fractures that pose a low risk of permanent damage to the spinal cord. Osteoporosis is a major risk factor predisposing older persons to compression fractures.

Several risk factors are present that would indicate osteoporosis is likely. The most significant factor is a postmenopausal woman, because the greatest amount of bone density is lost shortly after menopause. Other risk factors are present as well. In a less active person, the rate of bone loss is expected to increase because the mechanical stimulus that causes bone deposition is lost. Also, a decreased appetite is likely to lead to a reduction in her calcium intake, another important factor leading to osteoporosis. Her physician's recommendation that she begin using a calcium supplement also indicates that she is likely to have osteoporosis.

CASE STUDY 3 SUMMARY

The patient's hip injury should be treated by using the blanket-roll splinting technique. This method will prevent further damage from occurring to the hip and will also improve the pain as the injury is immobilized. To best facilitate the splinting process, the patient should be rolled onto the uninjured side so that pressure is not placed onto the injured area. The majority of low-energy hip injuries do not cause significant vascular damage; therefore hypovolemia is not of great concern, but the vital signs should still be monitored carefully and the use of oxygen is warranted to provide maximal oxygen delivery to the femoral head, a region that easily becomes hypoxic after injury.

Several long-term complications are associated with hip fractures. These include death, disability, chronic infection, and the need for numerous operations. In addition to the physical consequences, numerous psychological complications often follow a hip injury. These psychological manifestations are often from the loss of independence, reduced mobility, and fear of suffering from another and possibly more devastating hip injury. As a result, the older patient with a hip injury may also present with severe emotional distress that needs to be addressed by the EMS provider. The emotionally distressed patient should be calmed and cautiously reassured by indicating that it is too early to determine that the hip is injured severely, while also not providing false hope.

Endnotes

1. National Safety Council. *Injury Facts*. Chicago: Authors; 1999: 12–13, 96, 100, 121.

2. Feliciano DV, Moore EE, Mattox KL. *Trauma*. Stamford: Appleton & Lange; 1996: 900–907.

3. Barancik, JE, et al: Motor vehicle trauma in northeastern Ohio. Incidence and outcome by age, sex, and road use category. *American Journal of Epidemiology*. 1986;13:846.

4. Schwab CW, Kauder DR. Trauma in the geriatric patient. *Archives of Surgery*. 1992;127:701–704.

5. Coodley EL, Carston D. Trauma in the geriatric patient. *Trauma*. 1985;5:7, 8, 14.

6. Tinetti ME, Speechley M, Ginter SF: Risk factors for falls among geriatric people living in the community. *New England Journal of Medicine*. 1988; 319 (26)1705.

7. Settle JAD. *Principles and Practice of Burns Management*. New York: 1996: 20, 32.

8. Lewis CB. Musculoskeletal changes with age. *Clinical Management Physical Therapy*. 1984; 4:12–15.

9. Horan MA, Little RA. *Injury in the Aging*. Cambridge: Cambridge University Press, 1998: 191–193.

10. Zuckerman JD. *Orthopaedic Injuries in the Geriatric*. Baltimore: Williams & Wilkins 1990: 213–263, 451–468.

11. Kennedy SC. Thoracolumbar fractures. *Trauma*. 1999; 6:27–37.

12. Zuckerman JD. *Orthopaedic Injuries in the Geriatric*. Baltimore: William & Wilkins; 1990:269–339.

13. Schwartz GR, et al. *Principles and Practice of Emergency Medicine*. Baltimore: William & Wilkins; 1999:378–380.

14. Hirsh HL. Pain: An overview. *Trauma*. 1988; 2:80–82.

15. Feliciano DV, Moore EE, Mattox KL. *Trauma*. Stamford: Appleton & Lange; 1996:75, 77.

16. Feliciano DV, Moore EE, Mattox KL. *Trauma*. Stamford: Appleton & Lange; 1996:126–127.

17. Schwartz GR, et al. *Principles and Practice of Emergency Medicine*. Baltimore: William & Wilkins; 1999:224–226.

18. Alexander JQ, et al. Blunt chest trauma in the geriatric patient: How cardiopulmonary disease affects outcome. *The American Surgeon*. 2000; 66:855.

19. Osler T, et al. Trauma in the geriatric. *The American Journal of Surgery*. 1988;156:539.

20. Starr DS. Emergency room treatment of blunt and penetrating chest trauma. *Trauma*. 1992; 4:5–11.

21. Tanenbaum HL. Aortic dissection. *Trauma*. 1997;2:5–11.

22. Ficarra BJ. Acute abdomen in the geriatric. 1995; 1:5–15.

23. Feliciano DV, Moore EE, Mattox KL. *Trauma*. Stamford: Appleton & Lange; 1996:938–939.

24. Bernstein MJ. Osteoporosis. *Trauma*; 5:2–5.

25. Gibofsky A, Schwartzman S. Rheumatological disorders. *Trauma*. 1991;1:19–23.

Respiratory Emergencies

1 Describe the epidemiology of pulmonary diseases in the older population, including chronic obstructive pulmonary disease (COPD), pneumonia, pulmonary embolism, acute respiratory distress, and pulmonary edema.

2 Discuss assessment of the older patient with pulmonary complaints.

3 Differentiate the lung sounds associated with various respiratory problems and conditions.

4 Identify the need for intervention and transport, and develop a treatment and management plan for the older patient with pulmonary complaints.

CHAPTER 8

James R. Webster, MD, MS

CASE STUDY 1

You are dispatched to the home of a 74-year-old man who reports being "winded and wheezy for the past two days." He is coughing, is sitting on the edge of his bed, and says he can't remember anything else, such as whether he takes medicines, what they are, or if he has had this type of problem before. His vital signs are a blood pressure of 120/80 mm Hg, a pulse of 130 beats/min, respirations of 28 breaths/min, and he has a dusky appearance. His neck veins stand out each time he exhales and his breath sounds are distant with faint, high-pitched musical sounds audible with each breath. The heart sounds are hard to hear in this man, who has a deep chest.

What should you do next?

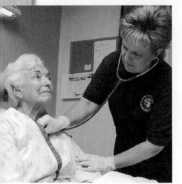

Introduction

Most older adults are generally healthy and mentally sharp. They are, however, disproportionately affected by acute illnesses due to a decrease in physiologic reserves. This is especially true with respect to heart and lung function. These patients therefore present a great opportunity to change health outcomes through early interventions. Respiratory symptoms, both acute and chronic, are very common in older adults. The findings are often nonspecific, and thus may require careful detective work, rapid problem solving, and appropriate emergency treatment to prevent a disaster. Keep in mind that age is not a big factor in outcomes for older adults. Function and disease status are. For example, older adults in the intensive care unit—even if they require mechanical ventilation—have the same outcomes in terms of morbidity and mortality as younger patients in similar clinical situations *if* both have an equal functional status.

Approach to the Older Patient with Respiratory Signs and Symptoms

There is often a history of underlying disease and predisposing factors. This information can be helpful later to the hospital staff in reaching a final diagnosis (▶ **Figure 8-1**). The onset of a respiratory problem is often acute. This offers an opportunity, with proper assessment and emergent treatment, to restore the patient to full function.

Respiratory assessment can be challenging in older patients. Atypical presentations are common in older adults, and many respiratory diseases can have overlap in their presenting symptoms. For example, pneumonia may occur in older adults without fever or cough; and pulmonary edema can be present without the need to sit up to improve breathing (**orthopnea**). Mental status changes (delirium) are often the first sign of respiratory trouble (see Chapter 10).

Frequently, decisions must be made and treatment begun without a specific diagnosis.

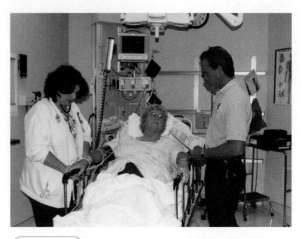

Figure 8-1 Information you discover about underlying disease and predisposing factors in the older patient with a respiratory problem will be important to hospital staff in later diagnosis and treatment.

This means that an evaluation of signs and symptoms is a crucial aspect of problem solving. Dealing with the older patient is both challenging and very rewarding.

Normal cardiorespiratory changes with age are usually benign; most significant declines in lung function result from disease or risk factors such as cigarette use or obesity (▼ **Table 8-1**). Drug side effects are often major complicating issues for older patients. For example, beta-blocker eye drops, such as timolol, can precipitate asthma, and antihistamines such as diphenhy-

TABLE 8-1 Changes in Lung Function with Aging

♦ "Normal" changes with aging are mild. These include (1) a slight reduction in lung volumes and airflow speed, (2) gradual reduction in arterial oxygen levels, (3) a decreased sensitivity to low oxygen and high carbon dioxide levels, and (4) a decreased cough response.

♦ Loss of **reserve capacity**—the body's ability to respond to increased demands under stress, such as illness or exercise—is another normal change with age and is the big problem.

♦ Cigarette use is a much more important cause of lung problems than aging.

dramine (Benadryl) can cause confusion and drying of lung secretions. (▼ Table 8-2) lists common respiratory medications.

Signs and Symptoms

Patients often present with signs and symptoms that require rapid evaluation and treatment based on your education and experience. This section covers common lung problems in older patients. Because many heart conditions can present similarly to lung conditions, these are briefly mentioned as well.

Dyspnea

It is sometimes difficult in the older patient to separate a subjective shortness of breath (dyspnea) from chest pain, and both may be present at the same time. Is it heart or lung disease? A history of past illness and current medications is often helpful in answering the question. Cough, sputum, fever, and signs of emphysema suggest lung disease. Chest tightness, sweating, or leg swelling, or a history of high blood pressure or heart disease, suggests the heart is the source of the problem.

Attitude Tip

Remember that "elderly patients over the age of 85 are more likely to present with shortness of breath than with chest pain as the initial manifestation of an acute myocardial infarction."[1]

TABLE 8-2   Common Respiratory Medications

Class of Drug	Generic Medication	Trade Name	Color of Inhaler (body/cap)*
Beta-agonist Inhalers	Albuterol	Proventil	yellow/orange
	Albuterol	Ventolin	lt. blue/dk. blue
	Metaproterenol	Alupent	grey/purple
	Pirbuterol	Maxair	blue/white
	Salmeterol	Serevent	teal/lt. teal
	Terbutaline	Brethaire	white/orange
Steroid Inhalers	Beclomethasone	Beclovent	white/brown
	Beclomethasone	Vanceril	pink/dk. pink
	Budesonide	Pulmicort	white/brown
	Flunisolide	Aerobid	grey/purple
	Fluticasone	Flovent	orange/lt. orange
	Triamcinolone	Azmacort	white/white
Other Inhalers	Cromolyn	Intal	white/blue
	Ipatropium	Atrovent	silver/green
	Nedocromil	Tilade	white/white
	Albuterol + Ipatropium	Combivent	silver/orange
Anti-inflammatory Pills	Theophylline	Theodur, Slo-bid	-
	Montelukast	Singulair	-
	Zafirlukast	Accolate	-
	Zileutin	Zyflo	-
Oral Steroids	Betamethasone	Celestone	-
	Methylprednisolone	Medrol	-
	Prednisolone	Prelone	-
	Prednisone	Deltasone	-

*Generics and other brands may differ in colors.

Hypoxia

Hypoxia (low blood oxygen, such as pulse oximeter reading less than 90%) does not usually cause dyspnea unless it is severe. Assess the patient's presentation, symptoms, and history of heart or lung disease. The most common lung problems in older adults are COPD (asthma, emphysema, and bronchitis), **acute pulmonary edema** (fluid accumulationn in the lungs), and upper airway obstruction. Other causes of low blood oxygen are pneumonia, pulmonary embolism, or heart problems. Rarely, drug overdose and brain disorders can slow breathing so much that blood oxygen is lowered.

Unless it is severe, the treatment of hypoxia is oxygen administration via nasal cannula or face mask. If possible, this should be monitored by pulse oximetry to restore the level to at least 92% to 94%. If hypoxia is severe, the patient will need to be placed on a ventilator, and prompt transport is crucial. Occasionally this may cause problems in patients with COPD by decreasing respiratory drive with a resultant increase in carbon dioxide and a decrease in consciousness.

Controversy

Administering high-flow oxygen over a long period of time can harm, or even kill, certain patients (such as those with COPD, who may lose their respiratory drive when overoxygenated). Be sure to follow your local protocol with regard to oxygen administration. If it allows a less aggressive form of oxygen administration for certain patients, be sure to consider this in the appropriate situations. All patients on high-flow oxygen should be re-evaluated; if they become drowsy or develop very slow respirations, consider decreasing the O_2 rate if your protocol allows this.

CASE STUDY 1 (continued)

This patient is in dire circumstances because of evidence of heart failure and hypoxemia, and his mental status changes suggest that he is in respiratory failure with an elevated carbon dioxide level in his blood.

The patient's wife returns from her part-time job as a school crossing guard. You ask her if he has ever been like this before, and if he is on any medicine. She says this happens every time he gets a cold that goes to his chest. She also says that he has emphysema, and that the doctor has him on a spray and some pills, which he refuses to take. Meanwhile, your partner says that the pulse oximeter shows an oxygen saturation of 89% to 90%. The spray is albuterol with the directions, "Use 2 sprays 4 times a day with spacer if breathing becomes difficult," and the pills are ampicillin 500 mg with directions, "Take one 4 times a day if you have a chest cold."

You start high-flow oxygen and use his spacer and metered dose inhaler (MDI) to administer the albuterol, while your partner starts an intravenous (IV) drip and you prepare for transport to the emergency department. In 15 minutes he appears more comfortable, his pulse is 106 beats/min, respirations are now 24 breaths/min, and his color is normal. His chest is now filled with high-pitched sounds on inspiration and expiration, and he brings up a large amount of thick greenish-gray sputum. His pulse oximeter reading is 98%. He asks for a "tonic for his nerves."

Is he better or worse?

Should you administer a sedative?

Cough

A cough may produce sputum, or may be nonproductive. A cough productive of thick sputum can be due to acute infection, such as pneumonia or bronchitis. A cough productive of thin white sputum characterizes pulmonary edema. Nonproductive coughing is most often caused by viral infections or asthma. Cough associated with eating may indicate impaired swallowing with aspiration of food or liquid, or <u>esophageal reflux</u> (regurgitation of food or acid from the stomach into the esophagus). Lying flat makes the cough from pulmonary edema or postnasal drip worse. Using these clues, the cause of the cough can often be determined by taking a careful history from the patient. Medical history sometimes reveals this sequence of events, which is especially common in older adults.

Wheezes

<u>Wheezes</u> are high-pitched musical sounds heard over the lung fields. They must be differentiated from noisier inspiratory sounds (<u>rhonchi</u>, or if severe, <u>stridor</u>) caused by secretions blocking the upper airways (▼ **Figure 8-2**). Localized squeaks over the lung fields suggest small mucus plugs or a foreign body. Although most wheezing is caused by COPD, wheezing with a nonproductive cough and <u>orthopnea</u> (difficulty breathing when lying down) is often cardiac in origin. New wheezing in a patient with known emphysema often indicates an acute infection, especially if there is an associated change in sputum, an increase in cough, or a new fever.

Hemoptysis

<u>Hemoptysis</u> most often is seen simply as streaks of blood in the sputum. It is usually not life threatening, but it is never normal. Anxiety is common in patients with even minor hemoptysis. They need to be reassured and referred expediently into the health care system for a firm diagnosis. Massive welling up of blood may be related to a ruptured blood vessel. This will require immediate and ongoing suctioning to prevent aspiration of blood and hypoxia, and may well be a life-threatening situation. Infections, foreign bodies, and cancer are the most common pulmonary causes of hemoptysis in the older age group.

Chest Pain

Chest pain, a history of heart attack (myocardial infarction), abnormal heart sounds (heart murmurs), and orthopnea may indicate heart disease. Chest pain may be continuous or may be related to breathing. The latter, called **pleuritic chest pain**, strongly suggests lung, chest wall, or other noncardiac problems, for example, a rib fracture. It may also be called pleurisy, an irritation of the membranes (pleura) that cover the lungs and internal chest wall (▼ **Figure 8-3**). Pneumonia, pulmonary

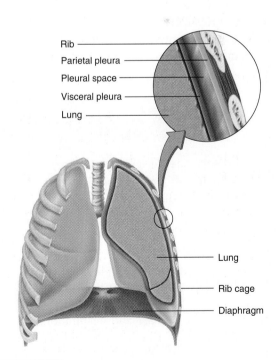

Rib
Parietal pleura
Pleural space
Visceral pleura
Lung

Lung
Rib cage
Diaphragm

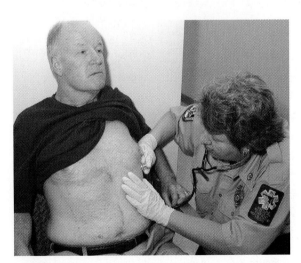

Figure 8-2 When auscultating lung sounds, it is important to differentiate wheezes from noisier inspiratory sounds (rhonchi or stridor) caused by secretions blocking the upper airways.

Figure 8-3 Pleuritic chest pain can be caused by pleurisy, irritation of the pleural membranes, or by other—usually noncardiac—lung or chest wall conditions.

embolism, and pneumothorax are all causes of pleuritic pain. The chest wall itself can be the site or cause of chest pain. For example, shingles (herpes zoster infection), which shows up as a rash with blisters in a line over nerve pathways, can give chest pain of a steady nature. Continuous, dull substernal chest pain suggests cardiac or esophageal causes.

Assessment

Respiratory assessment proceeds best with simple, traditional history and physical examination techniques. (See Chapter 5 for a more general discussion of patient assessment.)

History

The chief complaint, even if the patient is restless, agitated, or confused, will often clearly indicate the problem. For example, he or she may say, "My asthma is acting up," or, "This pain is just like my last heart attack." Asking, "Have you ever had this before?" may draw out useful information. A medication review will often help clarify the situation, and is especially important if there are any new drugs that might have caused side effects. For example, beta-blocker eye drops may trigger asthma, and sedatives can depress breathing. Questioning the family frequently turns up important data that the patient may be too agitated, confused, or anxious to provide.

> **Communication Tip**
>
> The patient's chief complaint can be very accurate in identifying the problem, even if the patient is agitated or confused.

Examination

The physical examination focuses on specifics to determine the extent of the emergency. Compare blood pressure, pulse, and respirations to the level of symptoms. Does the patient have a dusky appearance (cyanosis)? Is there evidence of upper airway obstruction? The latter is a true emergency, suggested by a history of difficulty getting air in, and exam signs such as stridor or crowing

sounds, tissue retractions between the ribs (intercostal) and above the collarbones (supraclavicular) 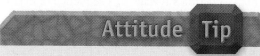 (▼ Figure 8-4), cyanosis, sweating, and—in the most severe cases—inability to speak or absence of air movement at the mouth.

Inspection of the upper airway is critical. Are there missing dentures? Is there food residue in the mouth? If there is any indication of foreign body obstruction, immediately begin steps to clear the obstruction according to current basic life support standards. Magill forceps can be used for foreign body removal.

Respiratory examination consists of four basic techniques: inspection, palpation, percussion, and auscultation (▶ Table 8-3).

> **Attitude Tip**
>
> Always let the patient and family know how much you care, not how much you know.

Inspection

Inspection of the pattern of breathing, and of the movement and symmetry of the chest wall, should be routine. Splinting is common with pleuritic pain.

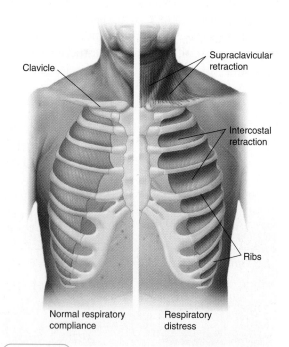

Figure 8-4   Retraction of soft tissue between the ribs (intercostal) and above the clavicles (supraclavicular) on inspiration is a sign of severe respiratory distress that may be caused by upper airway obstruction.

TABLE 8-3   Physical Findings on Chest Exam

Lung Condition	Inspection	Percussion	Auscultation
Normal	Good expansion, equal on both sides	Resonant	Soft and breezy
Pneumothorax	Decreased expansion, trachea may be deviated	Hyperresonant	Absent on affected side
Pneumonia	Decreased motion if pain is present	Dull to flat	Loud crackles, loud sounds in general
COPD (asthma, chronic bronchitis, emphysema)	Enlarged chest, restricted expansion, muscle wasting	Hyperresonant	Prolonged expiration, wheezes, decreased intensity of sounds generally
Pleural effusion (fluid around the lung)	Decreased expansion on the affected side	Dull	Decreased-to-absent sounds
Heart failure (pulmonary edema)	Unremarkable, though tachypnea and tachycardia are common	Normal to dull	Generalized fine crackles

Asymmetry of chest movements occurs with the accumulation of free fluid (**pleural effusion**) or air (pneumothorax) in the chest. Both of these decrease chest wall movement on the affected side, but the two entities can be differentiated in other ways.

Central cyanosis, seen around the mouth and on the trunk, indicates significant hypoxia that requires emergent care including oxygen administration. Peripheral cyanosis of nail beds or ear lobes may indicate circulatory problems. In the presence of **anemia** (is the patient pale?), cyanosis may not occur even if there is a low-oxygen state. Inspection of the chest involves checking for the use of accessory muscles of respiration, especially in the neck, which suggests severe respiratory distress. Retractions in the intercostal or supraclavicular areas may indicate upper airway or tracheal obstruction. Jugular venous (neck vein) distention is a sign of elevated central venous pressure (CVP) seen in heart failure.

Palpation

Palpation includes checking the trachea to see if it is displaced away from the midline and feeling the chest wall for vibrations arising in the airway when the patient breathes (caused by retained secretions). Also confirm any asymmetrical movements that were seen on inspection, and note any chest wall tenderness.

Percussion

Percussion can be used if the environment is quiet. It is performed by using the third finger of the chosen hand as a hammer to strike the third digit of the other hand, which is placed horizontally on the patient's chest wall to act as a sounding board (▼ **Figure 8-5**). Normal lungs produce a hollow, resonant sound on percussion. Dullness and flatness

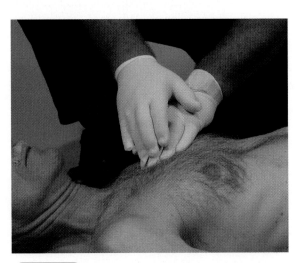

Figure 8-5   Percussion, performed by striking a finger placed on the patient's chest with a finger of the other hand, produces sounds that can indicate the condition of the lung underneath.

CASE STUDY 2

You are dispatched to the home of a 72-year-old woman. The family called 9-1-1 reporting that she had just "fainted" while attempting to have a bowel movement. She had undergone an uneventful hip replacement one week ago and had been home for less than 48 hours. You find her lying on the bathroom floor, wide awake and fully alert. Her main complaint is left-sided chest pain, which "began last night and happens every time I take a breath." She also feels short of breath. She does not remember fainting, but says that she was surprised when, just before you arrived, she spit up a small amount of bright red blood.

Is this likely a heart or lung problem?

What are your concerns?

What is your initial treatment?

are abnormal signs of fluid or congestion in the lung, or fluid in the pleural space. A hyperresonant sound like a bass drum suggests a pneumothorax.

Auscultation

Auscultation involves assessment of the breath sounds with a stethoscope. Normal sounds are "breezy," soft, and loudest during inspiration. Evaluating abnormal sounds comes with experience. <u>Crackles</u> are high-pitched popping sounds that occur during inspiration; they sound like rubbing hair near your ear. Crackles indicate fluid in the alveoli, and are heard in pneumonia and heart failure (pulmonary edema). <u>Wheezes</u> are musical, continuous sounds caused by airway obstruction. The higher the pitch, the smaller the obstructed airways. Such sounds may change after deep breathing or coughing. <u>Pleural friction rubs</u>, which usually occur in late inspiration, are loud, harsh, and short. Often associated with pleuritic pain, they result from friction between the two pleural surfaces.

Specific Lung Conditions

Chronic Obstructive Pulmonary Disease

Asthma, chronic bronchitis, and emphysema are all forms of <u>chronic obstructive pulmonary disease (COPD).</u>

Asthma

<u>Asthma</u> in older adults causes bronchospasm, edema of the lining of the air passages, and an accumulation of secretions in the airways. It is a recurrent, chronic disorder. Between attacks, the patient may feel relatively well and have near-normal pulmonary function. Attacks may be triggered by viral infections, air pollutants, esophageal reflux, cold air, allergens such as pollens, and medications. Episodes are made worse by anxiety and dehydration. The patient complains of breathlessness, most often has diffuse (scattered) wheezing and a cough, is sitting bolt upright, and is anxious. On examination, there are both inspiratory and prolonged expiratory wheezes. Distant breath sounds may indicate impending respiratory failure. Signs of life-threatening asthma also include changes in mental status, inability to speak, cyanosis, and diaphoresis.

The chest may be hyperresonant on percussion. A **pulsus paradoxicus** (a loss of more than 10 to 12 mm Hg of blood pressure during inspiration) indicates a significant asthmatic problem. To measure this, have the patient take a series of deep breaths as you deflate the blood pressure cuff between systolic and diastolic pressure, and record the variation during the two parts of the breathing cycle. A **peak flow measurement** is a simple method that patients have often been taught to check on their own status. ▶ Table 8-4 summarizes the short-term goals of asthma treatment.

TABLE 8-4   Immediate Goals of Asthma Treatment

1. Reduce the patient's anxiety by reassurance and by improving respiratory status—administer a bronchodilator and oxygen as indicated.

2. If the patient has a short-acting bronchodilator inhaler such as albuterol, assist the patient in administering it (▶ Figure 8-6). Even when not under acute stress, older patients often do not use a metered-dose inhaler (MDI) correctly, so your help will be important in effective administration. Follow these steps to assist administration:

   ♦ Ensure that the inhaler is at room temperature or warmer. Shake the inhaler vigorously several times.

   ♦ Remove oxygen mask. Hand the inhaler to the patient. Instruct the patient to exhale deeply and, before inhaling, to put his or her lips around the opening of the inhaler. Use a spacer if the patient has one.

   ♦ Have the patient depress the hand-held inhaler as he or she begins to inhale deeply.

   ♦ Instruct the patient to hold his or her breath for as long as is comfortable to help the body absorb the medication.

   ♦ Reapply oxygen. After a few breaths, have the patient repeat the dose if order/protocol allows.

3. Start oxygen by nasal cannula if hypoxia is confirmed by pulse oximetry.

4. Once the patient is stable, obtain a repeat peak flow measurement if the patient has previously been doing this.

5. During transport, provide reassurance and support, because anxiety will make a bad situation worse. Avoid sedation, which may depress respiratory drive.

Other Types of COPD

Emphysema and chronic bronchitis, the two other types of COPD, are considered together here because they are frequently present together. Both are almost always the result of prolonged

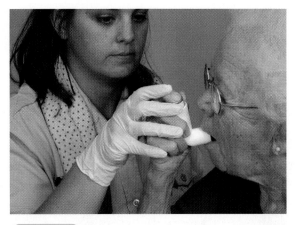

Figure 8-6   The patient having an asthma attack may have a bronchodilator medication in a metered-dose inhaler. Older patients often do not use an inhaler correctly, so your help—if your protocols allow it—will be important in effective administration.

Medication Tip

If covered in your protocols, help administer the COPD patient's inhaled bronchodilator medicine. This may improve clinical condition considerably, and you do not have to be sure what type of COPD is present to do it.

cigarette use. The bronchitic component is manifested by cough (especially in the morning) and sputum associated with inflammation of the airways. Emphysema produces lung destruction that leads to progressive dyspnea. This disorder, seen in both men and women, is the fourth leading cause of death in older patients and a common cause of disability.

Acute COPD attacks are most often due to infection. Nonadherence to COPD medications often contributes as well. Dehydration, exposure to irritating pollutants, pneumothorax, heart failure, and fever from any cause may also precipitate a decline in lung function in these patients. Medications such as sedatives, antihistamines, and beta blockers can also cause or contribute to the worsening of symptoms. Symptoms are usually gradual, even subtle: progressive breathlessness, cough with a change in sputum color, and increased volume of sputum. Use of accessory muscles of respiration in the neck is common,

0.3 mg SC (subcutaneous), or consider the administration of terbutaline 0.25 mg SC. Local protocols should be followed when considering medication administration. The patient's ECG should also be monitored.

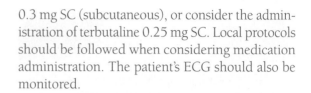

Medication Tip

Medications such as sedatives, antihistamines, and beta blockers may cause symptoms or contribute to their worsening in an attack of emphysema or chronic bronchitis.

Pneumonia and Influenza

<u>Pneumonia</u> and influenza (flu) are major killers of older adults, and greatly complicate other diseases such as COPD. The presentation may be quite different in the older adult as compared to younger patients, especially in patients who are bedridden or who live in a nursing home. For instance, fever may be absent in the older person, and cough and sputum negligible. Confusion is common. Falls, incontinence, and loss of appetite and thirst may be more prominent than cough and fever. Pneumonia may also present simply as a worsening of heart failure or COPD without apparent cause in older patients. Physical findings can include crackles, **purulent sputum** (sputum that contain pus), and loss of appetite.

Delay in hospital diagnosis and treatment are major causes of death in patients with pneumonia, so early emergency treatment and transport for definitive care are crucial. Oxygen should be given by nasal cannula or face mask. Monitor the patient for increased signs of dyspnea. Utilize pulse oximetry if available. Transport should be immediate and usually in the sitting position, which is most comfortable for the patient. Monitor the patient carefully because deterioration can be rapid and the patient may require ventilatory support. Diuretics such as furosemide (Lasix) should not be given since these patients are often already dehydrated and diuretics will only make secretions thicker and more difficult to handle, increasing the risk of kidney failure.

Aspiration pneumonia in older adults may be an acute or chronic problem. The acute episodes

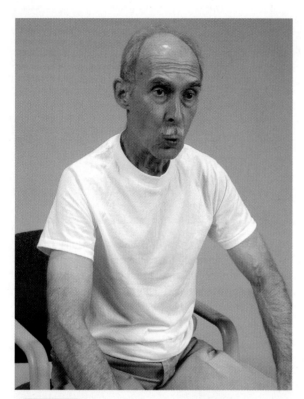

Figure 8-7   Pursed-lip breathing is a frequent sign of respiratory distress caused by a severe COPD episode.

and the patient may feel and look desperate. The expiratory phase of breathing is prolonged and breath sounds are distant. Wheezes and crackles may still be evident, even when the breath sounds are so soft that they are difficult to hear. Patients with emphysema are often breathing with their lips pursed **▲ Figure 8-7** .

Assessment should be rapid, with special attention to the time, course, and onset of the attack. It may be difficult to differentiate asthma from bronchitis or emphysema, but the management is quite similar (see Table 8-3). Administer oxygen if the patient feels short of breath or has hypoxia or tachypnea, but monitor closely for a lowered level of consciousness that can be caused by buildup of carbon dioxide precipitated by the administration of oxygen in certain patients with COPD. Once the patient is stable, with an IV in place if your level of training permits, transport to the emergency department. Consider the administration of albuterol (2.5 mg via nebulizer in 3.0 mL normal saline). With severe asthma or COPD, consider the administration of epinephrine 1:1,000

usually are related to trauma or surgery, or acute swallowing disturbances caused by drug and alcohol intoxication. These are true emergencies. Chronic aspiration is common in older adults. More than 50% of those older than 70 have abnormal swallowing and regularly aspirate food, oral secretions, or both.[2] More commonly, people who develop pneumonia and other complications from aspiration are older patients in a nursing home, often with a history of stroke, who cough when trying to eat or drink, and have periods of decreased alertness due to disease or drugs. When examined, the patient has foul breath, a poor or absent gag reflex, or scattered lung crackles. Such individuals need entry into the health care system for definitive evaluation and care. Transport status can be routine for patients with chronic aspiration unless signs of acute distress are present. Keep in mind that patients who are known to aspirate small amounts of food or fluids chronically are at very high risk for aspiration of large amounts, which is then a medical emergency.

Pulmonary Embolism

<u>Pulmonary embolism</u> is the lodging of a clot in a vessel in the lung. With or without death of lung tissue, pulmonary embolism is a life-threatening emergency that may masquerade as other diseases. Predisposing factors include recent surgery, especially an orthopaedic procedure such as a lower extremity injury or a knee or hip replacement, prior history of blood clots, obesity, and sedentary behavior, such as a recent long car trip. Medical disorders that lead to immobility, such as cancer, heart failure, or any condition associated with bed rest, can also be risk factors.

This disease causes upward of 200,000 deaths per year and is often not recognized prior to death.[3] The process begins with the development of clots in the veins of the legs or pelvis. These clots then break off and move (embolize) through the bloodstream, eventually lodging in the lungs (▶ **Figure 8-8**).

Presentation may be subtle or dramatic. Dyspnea, chest pressure or pain, cough, a brief loss of consciousness (syncope), anxiety, low-grade fever, and leg pain may all occur. Pleuritic pain may be present as a result of a lung infarct. Syncope can occur if the clots are massive and oc-

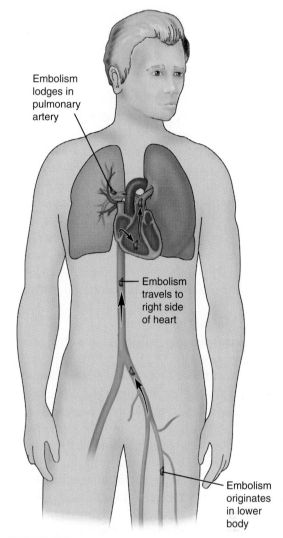

Embolism lodges in pulmonary artery

Embolism travels to right side of heart

Embolism originates in lower body

Figure 8-8 A pulmonary embolism is a clot that develops in a leg or pelvic vein, breaks loose, and travels through the venous system to lodge in the lungs.

clude a majority of the lung circulation. On examination, tachypnea, tachycardia, and lung crackles are typical, but these are nonspecific findings. Look specifically for swelling, redness, and/or tenderness of one leg that may be the source of the blood clot. However, such evidence will not be uniformly evident. If pulmonary embolism is even suspected, the patient must be transferred to a site where specific testing can be performed. Oxygen administration is appropriate since hypoxia is likely. IV access with a large-gauge needle will permit support of low blood pressure if deterioration occurs during transport.

Acute Respiratory Distress Syndrome

<u>Acute respiratory distress syndrome (ARDS)</u> is manifested by collapse, severe progressive hypoxia, and a failure to maintain adequate breathing. It often comes on after an acute insult such as an overwhelming bloodstream infection (sepsis), massive aspiration of gastric intestinal contents, extensive pneumonia involving both lungs, near drowning, or smoke inhalation. The patient appears desperately ill and is often severely dyspneic, cyanotic, and hypotensive with tachycardia and tachypnea. Diffuse crackles are audible throughout the lungs. Oxygen, IV fluids, and immediate transport to the most capable emergency department available are mandatory. Full ventilatory support is also usually required. The mortality rate for patients with this condition is high.

Chronic Respiratory Failure

<u>Chronic respiratory failure</u> is most often seen as a complication of COPD, triggered by infection, unwise use of a sedative, or some other complication. The patient has findings of COPD such as a barrel-shaped chest or clubbed fingernails, may or may not have a lowered level of consciousness, and has dyspnea, tachypnea, and tachycardia. As the situation progresses, the breathing rate may actually slow as the patient becomes too fatigued. Evaluation must include a rapid medical history to learn the cause, and pulse oximetry to determine oxygenation status (▶ **Figure 8-9**). The patient will need IV fluid administration when possible, stabilization, and transport to an emergency department for further evaluation and treatment. Such patients often require mechanical ventilation in an intensive care unit. The question of how much oxygen to administer in the field is tricky because the only thing driving the patient's breathing may be the hypoxia. If this is treated with oxygen therapy, the patient may deteriorate and require ventilatory assistance. Your system's protocols should address this situation. Be prepared to ventilate as needed.

Pulmonary Edema

The older patient in <u>**pulmonary edema**</u> may exhibit any of the following: wheezing and/or crackles, abnormal respiratory rate, rapid heart rate, stridor, grunting, cyanosis, mottled skin, altered mental status, nasal flaring, retractions,

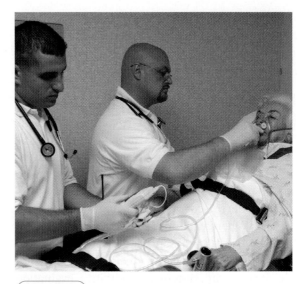

Figure 8-9   Pulse oximetry is helpful in determining a COPD patient's oxygen status. Follow local protocol regarding oxygen therapy for COPD patients.

Controversy

The question of how much oxygen to administer to a COPD patient is tricky because hypoxia may be the only thing driving the patient's breathing. Oxygen therapy could reduce that hypoxic ventilatory drive. Follow local protocols and be prepared to ventilate if needed. Never withhold oxygen from a patient in respiratory distress.

accessory muscle use, dyspnea, diminished or absent breath sounds, peripheral edema, jugular vein distention, or frothy pink sputum. Treatment by BLS providers should include positioning the patient in a high Fowler's position and administering high-flow oxygen. Transportation to the emergency department should not be delayed. Advanced airway maneuvers such as endotracheal intubation may be necessary. Intravenous access should be established. The patient's ECG should be monitored and the underlying rhythm treated accordingly. The following medications are indicated in the treatment of pulmonary edema: nitroglycerin 0.4 mg SL, Lasix 0.5 to 0.10 mg/kg, morphine sulfate 2 to 10 mg slow IV push. In those patients who are hypoten-

CASE STUDY 2 (continued)

You immediately record her blood pressure as 90/50 mm Hg, a pulse of 102 beats/min, and respirations (panting) at 32 breaths/min. The pulse oximeter reading is 88% saturation. Your further examination reveals that there is no sign of head injury, her breath sounds are normal though shallow and rapid, and her chest expands less on the left than on the right side. Her right calf is swollen, warmer, and clearly larger than her left calf. The ECG shows only sinus tachycardia.

What are the concerns that motivate your next actions?

sive, consider dopamine 2 to 20 µg/kg/min. Dosages are based on ALS guidelines, but could vary in your area. Be sure to check your local protocol regarding medication administration.

Special Techniques for Respiratory Care

Airway Control

Some airway protection can be achieved manually with standard basic life support maneuvers, and by positioning the head with a small pillow or a rolled towel behind the neck. This extends the head into the "sniffing position" so that an oral or nasal airway can be placed, and makes it easier to maintain an open airway while delivering positive pressure ventilation with a bag-valve device and mask.

Respiratory compromise and failure may raise the need for more active control of the patient's airway. Tracheal intubation is the preferred method for ALS providers trained in the procedure. Specialized multi-lumen airways such as the Pharyngeotracheal Lumen Airway (PtL) and the Esophageal Tracheal Combitube (ETC) are available to BLS personnel in some systems (▼ **Figure 8-10**). All of these devices offer effective airway control in situations of ventilatory failure due to primary lung disease, cardiac arrest, or upper airway obstruction, or in cases of bleeding or excessive secretions or gastric contents in the airway that the patient cannot handle.

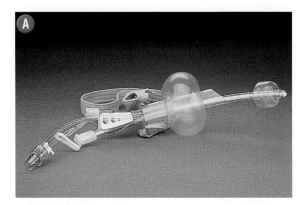
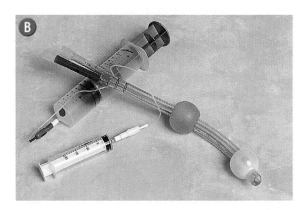

Figure 8-10   Multi-lumen airway devices such as the pharyngeotracheal lumen airway **(A)** and the esophageal tracheal combitube **(B)** are available to BLS responders in some systems to provide additional airway protection in the patient who needs airway control and ventilation.

Oxygen Therapy

Oxygen delivery for any acute illness is an important strategy to improve outcomes of older patients with breathing impairment. Indications are **hypoxia** (a pulse oximeter reading of less than 90% in most people), respiratory distress (where the respiratory rate is greater than 25), hypotension (systolic blood pressure less than 90 to 100 mm Hg), or cardiac or respiratory arrest.

There are several delivery systems suitable for field use. Nasal cannulas with the flow rate set at levels of 1 to 6 liters per minute (L/min) will give inspired oxygen levels (FIO_2) between 24% and 44%. Nonrebreathing masks cover the nose and mouth and can deliver inspired oxygen levels of up to 90% with flow rates of 10 to 15 L/min. Problems with masks include potential displacement, concealment of aspiration, and interference with talking and coughing up sputum. A bag-valve-mask device with a reservoir bag can be used manually to assist ventilation. Flooding the device with oxygen by connecting the reservoir to an oxygen tank can give an FIO_2 level of up to 100%, through a tight-fitting mask or an endotracheal tube, for such events as a cardiac arrest.

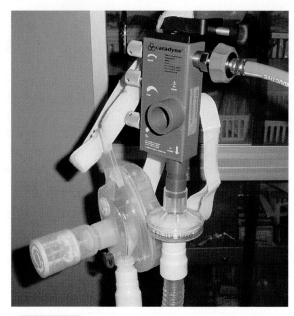

Figure 8-11   CPAP is a form of noninvasive positive pressure ventilation that can be used as a viable alternative to endotracheal intubation in the prehospital setting.

Continuous Positive Airway Pressure

Intervention for acute pulmonary edema includes oxygen, Lasix, nitroglycerin, and morphine. If these treatments fail to improve the patient's condition, continuous positive airway pressure (CPAP) can be utilized (▶ **Figure 8-11**). CPAP is a form of noninvasive positive pressure ventilation, and is proving to be a viable alternative in many patients previously requiring endotracheal intubation. Conscious intubation is a stressful event for the hypoxic patient. Noninvasive positive pressure ventilation works by raising pressure in the nose and pharynx, forcing air into the lungs during inspiration. At the end of inspiration, pressure returns to a lower level. This pressure is dependent on the end expiratory pressure setting.

CPAP transmits positive pressure into the airways of a spontaneously breathing patient throughout the respiratory cycle. It applies positive end expiratory pressure (PEEP) while the patient breathes through a system that maintains normal airway pressure fluctuations on either side of this new baseline. CPAP maintains constant positive pressure within the airways, but requires the patient to be breathing and able to protect their own airway. In pulmonary edema, CPAP improves gas exchange, reduces pulmonary shunting, improves cardiopulmonary performance, assists redistribution of extravascular lung water, increases alveolar size and recruitment, and reduces the work of breathing.

There are adverse effects associated with CPAP. These include hypotension, barotraumas, and regurgitation or aspiration owing to gastric distention. There are also a small number of patients who cannot tolerate the equipment.[4]

Inclusion criteria for CPAP in patients with pulmonary edema include: retraction/accessory muscle use, bilateral rales, a systolic blood pressure greater than 110 mm Hg, a respiratory rate greater than 25 breaths/min, a pulse oximeter reading of less than 90%. Exclusion criteria (any) are: respiratory or cardiac arrest, asthma, a systolic blood pressure of less than 90 mm Hg, unresponsiveness, the inability of the patient to maintain his or her own airway, major trauma, vomiting, facial surgery with associated swelling, sutures, or ecchymosis (bruising).

If CPAP is indicated, the patient's heart rate, respiratory rate, ECG, and pulse oximeter reading must be closely monitored and recorded every 5 minutes. If the patient's condition deteriorates during CPAP use, consider endotracheal intubation.

CPAP usage in the prehospital setting is practical with the potential for improvement in patient outcomes. A moderate amount of training is required with minimal investment in equipment. It is recommended that EMS systems wishing to utilize CPAP work closely with their medical director as well as educate the hospital emergency departments who will be receiving patients on CPAP.

Manual and Mechanical Ventilation

Breathing is controlled by a complex system of chemical receptors in the blood vessels and brain that respond to blood levels of oxygen (O_2) and carbon dioxide (CO_2), and drive the muscles of breathing. The receptors become less sensitive with increased age and in people with diseases such as COPD. There is also a wide variation in sensitivity in different individuals. In urgent respiratory failure situations, it may become necessary to take control of a patient's ventilation manually by using a bag-valve device and a mask or endotracheal tube to deliver oxygen under positive pressure (in other words, to push air into the lungs, rather than rely on the patient sucking in air).

Mechanical ventilators are machines that can work for a prolonged period to control a patient's breathing (▶ **Figure 8-12**). They can be regulated in several ways. For example, they can be preset to deliver a certain number of breaths per minute, or simply to assist and enhance spontaneous breathing. They can also be set to maintain increased pressure in the airways throughout both inspiration and expiration, to keep the alveoli (air sacs) open. Though most EMS providers will not routinely use mechanical ventilators, specialized transport services may use them, and you will likely encounter them in hospitals and nursing homes. Their use requires special training; transferring facilities must provide a trained medical escort when the patient is on a ventilator that you have not been trained to use.

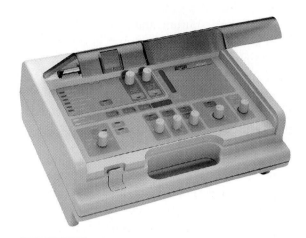

Figure 8-12   Mechanical ventilators may be used by some specialized transport services, and in hospitals and nursing homes.

Summary

We have covered the major respiratory emergencies in older patients, but in addition to providing emergency care, you can encourage prevention when interacting with older people. Prevention is the responsibility of all of us as EMS providers. We should be models for the community in all our behaviors. Older patients especially need to have their immunizations, including flu and pneumococcal vaccines, up to date. It is clear that these prevent disease, reduce hospitalizations, and save lives, and they are extremely cost effective. Their use is discouragingly low among older patients, however. The moment just following a time of emergency is a good opportunity to remind patients and families of the importance of these measures. Health care providers who have contact with the older population can also prevent flu infection in their patients by getting themselves vaccinated regularly. Some studies in nursing homes show that vaccination of the staff is even more effective in preventing flu infections in the patients than vaccination of the patients themselves. This is likely true for EMS providers as well.

Cigarette use is the major cause of lung disease (and many other causes of death) in the country today.[5] It is never too late to quit.

Patients who stop note immediate benefits: decreased cough, sputum, and dyspnea. The risk of heart attack and lung infection begins to drop almost immediately after cessation of smoking. Once the immediate stress of an acute event is resolved, take a little time to give counseling regarding prevention. A few moments dedicated to such a discussion may save a life.

Attitude Tip

Prevention is the responsibility of all health care professionals. Take a little time after an emergency to counsel patients about prevention. Though it is less dramatic than emergency care, you may save a life by doing it.

Case Study Summaries

CASE STUDY 1 SUMMARY

This patient presents with a typical exacerbation (worsening) of his COPD as a result of acute bronchitis. He was hypoxic and on the verge of respiratory failure when you arrived. The information provided by his wife was crucial. After you treated him with oxygen and the bronchodilator (albuterol), his clinical situation improved substantially. The improved airflow brought out the wheezes. Other indications of his improvement include his ability to bring up sputum to clear his airways, reduction in his pulse rate, and his blood pressure coming into a normal range. Do not give a sedative because this could slow his breathing and contribute to his confusion.

CASE STUDY 2 SUMMARY

The findings of pleuritic chest pain and hemoptysis suggest a lung problem. The shortness of breath is a nonspecific symptom that may be due to multiple causes (eg, heart, lung, anemia, anxiety may be involved). The loss of consciousness (syncope) may also be due to multiple causes.

Her recent surgery puts her at risk for infection, and for a tendency to increased blood clotting for such things as the blood clot in her leg (**deep venous thrombosis**, or DVT) that she had (the leg findings were classic) or for myocardial infarction or stroke.

The findings indicate that a blood clot (embolus) likely traveled from her leg to her left lung. She is at risk for another such event, which could result in a more severe episode of cardiovascular impairment. The increased strain on her heart results because it has to work against the obstruction in the lung due to the clot which has plugged the blood vessels in the lung. The cardiac output (volume of blood pumped per minute) is thus reduced. This chain of events is what caused her to "faint" by decreasing blood flow to the brain. She needs to be transported to the hospital because this is a potentially lethal situation.

Endnotes

1. Bosker G, Schwartz G, Jones J, Sequeira M. *Geriatric Emergency Medicine*. St. Louis: Mosby; 1990:166.

2. Terpenning MS, Taylor GW, Lopatin DE, et al. Aspiration pneumonia: Dental and oral risk factors in an older veteran population. *J Am Geriatr Soc*. 2001;49:557–563.

3. Goldharber SZ. Medical progress: Pulmonary embolism. *N Engl J Med*. 1998;339:93–104.

4. Hatlestad D. Calming the waters: Noninvasive positive pressure ventilation in prehospital care. *Emergency Medical Services*. 2002;31(5):67–71, 74.

5. Doll R, Peto R, Wheatly K, et al. Mortality in relation to smoking: 40 years' observations on male British doctors. *BMJ*. 1994;309:901–911.

Cardiovascular Emergencies

LEARNING OBJECTIVES

1 Discuss the epidemiology of cardiovascular diseases in the older population.

2 Discuss the signs and symptoms, precipitating factors, and management of cardiac events in the older patient.

3 Discuss the assessment of the older patient with complaints related to the cardiovascular system, including acute myocardial infarction, congestive heart failure, arrhythmias, hypertension, and syncope.

4 Given a list of signs and symptoms, identify the need for intervention and transport, and formulate a treatment plan for the older patient with cardiovascular complaints, including acute myocardial infarction, congestive heart failure, arrhythmias, hypertension, and syncope.

CHAPTER 9

Luis F. Amador, MD

Eric C. Nager, MD, FAAEM

Robert C. Salinas, MD, CAQ(G)

CASE STUDY 1

You are dispatched to the home of an 84-year-old man because he hasn't been feeling well for the past 24 hours. According to his wife, he had been doing well up until last night. He did not sleep well and was awake most of the night. He is now lying on the couch complaining of fatigue and shortness of breath. His wife tells you that he has a past medical history of hypertension, diabetes, arthritis, and mild memory loss. He smokes about 10 cigarettes a day and denies any alcohol use.

> **Before arriving at the scene, what are your thoughts about the patient's complaint?**
>
> **What are possible contributing factors for behavioral changes in older people?**
>
> **What medical conditions may be occurring with this patient?**

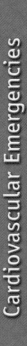

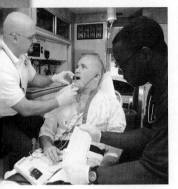

Occurrence Patterns of Heart Disease in Older Patients

Older adults represent one of the fastest growing segments of the U.S. population. It is estimated that by the year 2030, 1 in 5 persons in the United States (approximately 35 million) will be older than 65 years.[1] As the numbers continue to grow, so does the number of people living with multiple chronic diseases. Not surprisingly, cardiovascular disease leads the list of diseases that afflict older people.

Cardiovascular diseases are the most common cause of morbidity and mortality among people age 65 and older. Coronary artery disease (CAD) and congestive heart failure (CHF) are at the top of the list. Coronary artery disease accounts for approximately 70% to 80% of deaths among men and women in this age group.[2] Congestive heart failure is the most common cause of hospitalizations among older patients and the incidence continues to increase.[3, 4]

As the population increases in number and people continue to live longer, the number of new cases of heart disease is expected to increase. The normal changes in the cardiovascular system that occur with aging were reviewed in detail in Chapter 2. In this chapter, we will consider common cardiovascular disorders that occur in the older population.

Coronary Artery Disease

Coronary artery disease (CAD), the leading cause of death in older people in the United States, is responsible for more than two thirds of all cardiac deaths. About 60% of the 650,000 patients hospitalized in the United States for **acute myocardial infarction (AMI)** each year are older than 65.[5, 6] The principal feature of coronary artery disease is the buildup of fatty deposits (plaque) on arterial walls, a process called **atherosclerosis** (▶ **Figure 9-1**). Numerous risk factors make this process more likely to occur (▶ **Table 9-1**).

Hypertension, diabetes, cigarette smoking, and high cholesterol present an even greater risk

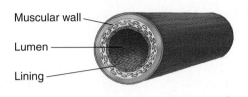

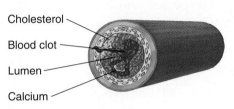

Figure 9-1   Atherosclerosis, the buildup of fatty plaque on arterial walls, may progress to the point that the plaque—or a migrating clot or a piece of plaque that broke off elsewhere—occludes the artery.

to the older patient because their effects grow worse with time. Hypertension is an important risk factor for the development of coronary artery disease in the older adult. Aggressive treatment of hypertension can reduce the morbidity and mor-

TABLE 9-1   Risk Factors for Atherosclerosis
Not Reversible
◆ Aging
◆ Male sex
◆ Genetic traits: family history of atherosclerosis before 50 years of age in a male relative or before age 60 in a female relative.*
Reversible
◆ Cigarette smoking*
◆ Hypertension*
◆ Obesity
◆ High cholesterol level*
◆ High levels of triglycerides
◆ Diabetes*
◆ Low levels of high-density lipoproteins (HDLs)
Indicates a major risk factor.

tality associated with cardiovascular disease. In patients whose blood pressure remains poorly controlled over a long period of time, the heart muscle can **hypertrophy** (called hypertensive heart disease). Hypertrophy of the heart muscle can also be a risk factor for the development of other forms of cardiac disease, such as congestive heart failure.

Smoking is a common risk factor in older people. Data from a major study found that smoking alone is associated with a 64% increase in the risk of developing cardiovascular disease.[7]

Older people with a history of diabetes may have disease involving the peripheral nervous system, the eyes, the kidneys, and the cardiovascular system. Because of involvement of the peripheral nerves in diabetes, a diabetic patient may not experience chest pain, or angina, when having an AMI. Diabetics, as well as the older population, may have a different perception of pain, and a heart attack may present with vague symptoms or may be totally symptom free.

Angina Pectoris

Clinical Presentation

When the blood circulation to the heart is compromised, some people experience chest pain as a major symptom (**angina pectoris**). It is often thought that the presentation of coronary artery disease is different in older patients, despite recent findings that angina pectoris was the presenting symptom in over 80% of older patients with a known medical history of coronary artery disease. Keep the atypical presentation of lack of chest pain in mind, however, when evaluating persons age 65 and over who have risk factors for coronary artery disease. Silent ischemia is also known to occur at a much higher rate in this population.[4]

Thus, it is important to consider symptoms other than pain that may alert you to a cardiac event. Common symptoms include dyspnea, fatigue, syncope, nausea, **anorexia** (lack of appetite), and acute confusion. **Palpitations** or sweating also may indicate a cardiac emergency. When older persons do complain of chest pain, the pain may be less localized, vague, and not the classic "crushing or squeezing." Some patients will deny experiencing pain; be sure to ask the patient about any chest discomfort, tightness, dizziness, or other symptoms.

Communication Tip

Because some older patients may not experience pain during an episode of cardiac ischemia or infarction, it is especially important to identify other signs. Ask about symptoms such as fatigue, syncope, nausea, and anorexia. In patients with a prior myocardial infarction, ask specifically whether their symptoms now are similar to those they experienced with their prior infarction.

Assessment

Angina may be difficult to distinguish from other causes of chest discomfort. Thoracic aorta dissection, pneumonia, pleurisy, gastroesophageal reflux, and pulmonary embolism all have a higher incidence of occurrence in the older population. Maintaining a high index of suspicion and carefully reviewing medications (▶ **Table 9-2**) and risk factors may help with assessment. It is especially critical to document medications the patient is taking, as failing to take the medication or taking it incorrectly may be contributing to the problem. As the older patient may be on multiple medications, bringing all of the patient's medications to the hospital is very helpful. This allows the medical staff to identify dosage, frequency, strength, and adherence to the medication and saves the EMS provider the time of having to write down drug information. Past medical history provides you with clues to the cause of the problem when the results of the physical examination are not conclusive. Some older people may find it difficult to communicate information about their past medical history. This could be the result of hearing difficulties or acute confusion. Consider asking family or neighbors who may know about the patient's medical history. Phone numbers of the patient's doctor may be on cabinets or refrigerators, along with a list of medical problems or medications.

If time permits, a 12-lead ECG should be performed on all patients with chest discomfort or suspected cardiac symptoms. Combine the ECG findings with your clinical exam to form a better picture of the disease process. As the patient's signs and symptoms may be nonspecific, an ECG may help determine if the patient is having an AMI.

TABLE 9-2 Medications Commonly Prescribed for Heart Disease

Drug Type	Examples
Angiotensin-converting enzyme (ACE) inhibitors	Captopril (Capoten); enalapril (Vasotec); lisinopril (Prinivil, Zestril); ramipril (Altace)
Angiotensin-receptor blockers (ARBs)	Irbesartan (Avapro); losartan (Cozaar); valsartan (Diovan)
Antiadrenergic agents	Clonidine (Catapres); doxazosin (Cardura); prazosin (Minipress)
Antiarrhythmics	Amiodarone (Cordarone); digoxin (Lanoxin); quinidine sulfate (Quinaglute)
Anticoagulants	Heparin; warfarin (Coumadin)
Anti-hyperlipidemic agents	Atorvastatin (Lipitor); lovastatin (Mevacor); pravastatin (Pravachol)
Antiplatelet drugs	Aspirin; clopidogrel (Plavix); dipyridamole (Persantine); ticlopidine (Ticlid)
Beta blockers	Atenolol (Tenormin); labetalol (Normodyne); metoprolol (Lopressor); propranolol (Inderal)
Calcium channel blockers	Amlodipine (Norvasc); diltiazem (Cardizem); nifedipine (Procardia); verapamil (Calan)
Diuretics	Furosemide (Lasix); hydrochlorothiazide (Hydrodiuril); spironolactone (Aldactone)
Nitrates	Sublingual, long acting, and transdermal
Potassium supplements	KCl (K-Dur, KLyte)

Management

Begin by making sure that the patient is as comfortable as possible. This may require that he or she be moved to a sitting position. Provide reassurance, because patient anxiety can increase cardiac stress, and thus exacerbate pain and heart damage. Obtain a set of vital signs to help guide therapy, and provide supplemental oxygen. In addition to the oxygen, sublingual nitroglycerin may have to be administered to help relieve chest pain (▶ **Figure 9-2**).

Start by addressing the ABCs and managing immediate life threats. Obtain a 12-lead ECG, and if there are no contraindications, begin administering nitroglycerin. Standard therapy is 0.4 mg sublingual nitroglycerin every 3 to 5 minutes as needed for chest pain. Consider aspirin 162–324 mg orally for any patient with angina. A caveat for the older population is that they tend to be on multiple medications that may interact with nitrates and aspirin. Many of the antihypertensive

Communication Tip

Patients with angina may not be able to communicate clearly about their medical history. Ask family or neighbors who may be able to give you more information.

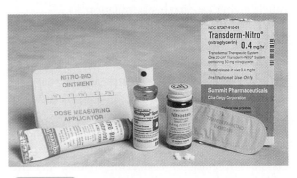

Figure 9-2 Nitroglycerin can help relieve the pain of angina attack.

agents will act in concert with nitrates and precipitously lower blood pressure. If this should occur, place the patient in Trendelenburg's position (supine with head lower than feet), administer a fluid bolus of 250 mL of a crystalloid solution intravenously if there is no chest congestion, and reassess the patient. Nitrates given sublingually may lower blood pressure for a short time. Aspirin may interact with the antiplatelet drugs or with warfarin (Coumadin), causing excessive bleeding. Consulting with medical direction regarding angina pectoris allows you to inform the ED that a critical patient is coming soon. As always, follow local protocols for medication administration.

Acute Myocardial Infarction

When an occlusion of a coronary artery occurs due to rupture and thrombosis of an atherosclerotic plaque, decreased blood flow to the heart muscle causes a decrease in oxygen perfusion to the tissue. This can produce ischemia, pain, or, if the decreased perfusion is substantial and sustained, death of the heart muscle **(myocardial infarction [MI])**. Older patients tend to be able to tolerate ischemia better than younger patients due to collateral circulation, which is the development of new blood vessels around tissue that is subjected to low flow rates of blood. The purpose of collateral circulation is to increase perfusion. The new vessels allow blood to shunt around occluded areas and supply ischemic tissue with oxygen.

Clinical Presentation

Remember that older patients can have atypical presentations in AMI (▶ **Table 9-3**). A review of the patient's past medical history, medications, and risk factors may help you focus on a cardiac problem when you suspect heart disease.

Management

As with all patients, management begins with ABCs. The patient should be placed on 100% oxygen if the airway is patent and he or she is breathing. Try to obtain a pulse oximetry reading on room air if possible.

After obtaining the blood pressure and pulse, the patient should be placed on a monitor, and intravenous access should be obtained. A focused history should be obtained from the patient, with

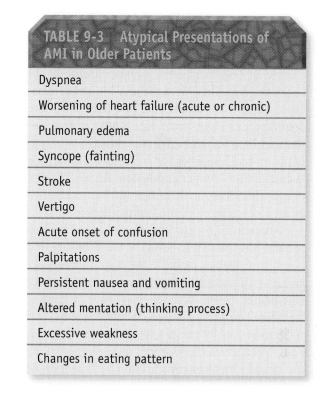

TABLE 9-3 Atypical Presentations of AMI in Older Patients
Dyspnea
Worsening of heart failure (acute or chronic)
Pulmonary edema
Syncope (fainting)
Stroke
Vertigo
Acute onset of confusion
Palpitations
Persistent nausea and vomiting
Altered mentation (thinking process)
Excessive weakness
Changes in eating pattern

special emphasis on cardiac risk factors and eligibility for thrombolytic therapy. If the patient is actively having chest pain/discomfort, nitroglycerin and aspirin should be given in accordance with local protocols. Have the patient rate the pain on a scale of zero to ten, with ten being the worst pain of his or her life and zero being none at all. This rating scale will help guide the effectiveness of your therapy, and allow you to make decisions on the next treatment to be given. A 12-lead ECG should be obtained if time, personnel, and the situation permit. Morphine should be considered in addition to care of the patient who is not responding adequately to nitroglycerin, and if morphine is dictated by local protocol.

Some locales have thrombolytic check sheets prepared so that the appropriate questions may be asked quickly, and the information assessed and relayed to the receiving ED. Important questions to ask are:

1. When did the pain begin?
2. Do you have any bleeding disorders?
3. Have you ever had brain cancer/masses or a stroke?

4. Are you on any blood thinners?

5. Have you had any recent surgery or trauma?

Clearly, an older person has a higher probability of answering "yes" to one of the above questions because these medications and problems are more common in this age group. Age is not a major contraindication for thrombolytic therapy, and patients up to 75 years of age are treated in a similar fashion to the younger population. Above 75 years of age, thrombolytic therapy is still considered to be an acceptable, safe, and useful intervention.

Attempt to contact the receiving hospital as soon as possible. This allows the ED to ensure that a bed is available, mobilize the appropriate staff, and have thrombolytic therapy ready to administer emergently. Some facilities may have a cardiac catheter team ready to open occluded vessels, and this group usually needs advance notice to mobilize. Speed is of the essence, as is suggested by the phrase "time is myocardium." Thrombolytic agents are most beneficial when given as soon after symptom onset as possible. From the time the patient enters the emergency department, most hospitals aim for administering thrombolytic agents within 30 minutes. By suspecting an AMI in the prehospital setting and relaying this information to the ED, the door to needle time can be greatly reduced, with a consequent rise in survival rates.

Congestive Heart Failure

Congestive heart failure (CHF) is a common cardiovascular condition that you will encounter in older people on a regular basis. The prevalence of this disease increases dramatically with age. CHF occurs in about 10% of people over the age of 80. It is also the most common reason for admission to an acute care hospital in people age 65 and over.[8]

Definition and Origins

Congestive heart failure is a disease process in which the heart is not able to maintain an output adequate to meet the metabolic needs of the body. Essentially, the heart muscle fails to pump sufficiently. This occurs as the aging heart and vessels undergo structural and physiological changes,

particularly stiffening of the muscle. The three leading disease processes associated with CHF in older patients are hypertension, coronary artery disease, and atrial fibrillation.

Pathophysiology

There are many ways to categorize CHF, but for prehospital purposes, the easiest is left- and right-sided heart failure. Right-sided heart failure manifests as excess fluid backing up into the body. The signs of right-sided heart failure include jugular venous distention (JVD), enlarged liver, fluid in the abdomen (**ascites**), and **peripheral edema**. The most common cause of right-sided failure is left-sided failure. Left-sided heart failure causes fluid to back up into the lungs and, eventually, to the right side of the heart. The primary sign of left-sided heart failure is **pulmonary edema**.

Assessing the Patient with CHF

History and Symptoms

Patients with congestive heart failure generally require multiple medications, so a review of medications may help you during assessment (▼ **Table 9-4**). Patients with CHF often develop problems associated with fluid overload. This could be secondary to worsening heart function from a myocardial infarction or an arrhythmia. An increase in dietary salt or failure to take medications, es

TABLE 9-4   Common Medications in Patients with CHF
Angiotensin-converting enzyme (ACE) inhibitors (Captopril and Altace)
Angiotensin-receptor blockers (ARBs) (Losartan and Hyzaar)
Digoxin (Lanoxin, Lanoxicaps)
Diuretics (Lasix, hydrochlorothiazide, spironolactone)
Nitrates (Imdur, Isordil)
Potassium supplements (K-Dur, Slow-K)

pecially <u>diuretics</u>, can also lead to worsening heart failure. The older population is at higher risk for exacerbations of CHF for multiple reasons. Memory impairment and multiple medications increase the risk of medication errors. Poor vision may also contribute to problems to taking medications properly. Drinking too much fluid or eating too much salt or processed foods (high in salt) can cause fluid overload. Fear of incontinence at public events prompts many to skip doses of their diuretics.

Medication Tip

Patients with CHF usually take multiple medications. Watch for diuretics, potassium supplements, and other medication categories listed in Table 9-4.

The most common complaint with acute or worsening CHF is shortness of breath. Patients may also experience pedal/peripheral edema, cough, or fatigue. Orthopnea (dyspnea when lying down), and dyspnea on exertion are also classic findings with CHF ▼ Figure 9-3 . Patients may report, when asked, that they have put on additional

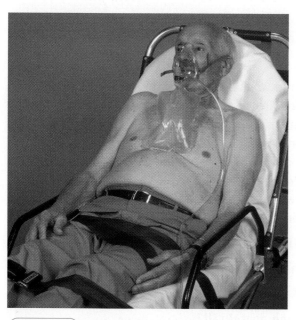

Figure 9-3 CHF patients may need to be transported in an upright position because shortness of breath and cough often worsen when they lie flat.

weight in a short period of time. Try to find out if these are new or chronic problems. Ask questions that compare this most recent episode to how the patient functioned one month ago (eg, "How far can you walk before you get out of breath? How far were you able to walk a month ago?").

Physical Exam

Patients in acute heart failure may present in acute respiratory distress. The respiratory exam is crucial in the evaluation of the CHF patient. Auscultation will reveal bilateral crackles in the patient with pulmonary edema. In isolated or severe cases, breath sounds may be diminished, or wheezes may be present (cardiac asthma). When describing lung sounds, note how high the crackles are auscultated (eg, 1/3 up, 1/2 up, etc.). Auscultation of the heart may reveal tachycardia. When checking vital signs, common abnormalities in addition to heart rate are hypertension, low pulse oximetry readings, and increased respiratory rate. A good axiom to remember is that hypertension in combination with shortness of breath is CHF until proven otherwise. When heart failure is severe, however, blood pressure will be low because the heart is not strong enough to generate a pressure. Round out your focused exam by checking for JVD, peripheral and dependent edema (the sacral area and abdominal area are common) ▶ Figure 9-4 , and enlargement of the liver.

Attitude Tip

When comparing the value and benefit of resuscitation efforts for a younger patient versus an older patient, remember that older patients *do* benefit from aggressive resuscitation efforts, from heart attack and stroke risk-reduction efforts, and from other treatment modalities, such as thrombolytics, coronary artery bypass surgery, and angioplasty.

Management

Dyspnea is usually the presenting complaint of patients with an acute exacerbation of CHF. This is due to pulmonary edema and problems with oxygenation. Vital signs should be obtained and ABCs addressed. If the situation permits, the

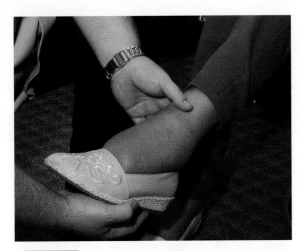

Figure 9-4 Swelling in the lower extremities, or peripheral edema, is a sign of CHF. To distinguish fluid in the lower extremities from fat, gently press a finger along the shin bone. If this leaves an indentation, it is more likely fluid in the tissues; if not, it is more likely fatty tissue.

patient should be positioned upright to allow gravity to shunt some of the fluid away from the lungs. High-flow oxygen should be started, as well as an IV line and ECG monitor.

Medical therapy should be geared at reducing preload and removing extra fluid from the body. Sublingual nitroglycerin should be considered first line therapy in treating CHF with pulmonary edema. Its main benefit is via vasodilation and preload reducing effects. Check your local protocol to determine the dosage of nitroglycerin you should administer. Furosemide (Lasix) should be given intravenously as soon as possible, usually in a 1 mg/kg dose. Again, check your local protocol. Furosemide is a mild vasodilator, so it has mild preload reducing effects, but its main action is as a diuretic. This diuretic effect may not be seen in the field; time of onset is 1 to 1½ hours. Morphine has a minor role in treatment, but it does have mild vasodilating effects. Check your local protocol regarding morphine administration. Aspirin should be considered in any CHF patient with chest pain.

Continuous positive airway pressure (CPAP) is a mechanical means of reducing preload and work of breathing in patients with pulmonary edema and may be considered. Contact medical control to inform the ED about an incoming sick patient. Consider obtaining a 12-lead ECG if the situation permits.

CASE STUDY 2

You are dispatched to the home of a 74-year-old woman whose neighbor called 9-1-1 for a woman with difficulty with breathing. You arrive at the home and find the patient sitting in a chair complaining that she cannot "catch" her breath. She also reports to you that she stopped taking her heart medications about two weeks ago. In your initial evaluation, you find an irregular heart rate of 170 beats/min, a blood pressure of 100/60 mm Hg, and a respiratory rate of 24 breaths/min. She also appears slightly cyanotic and you hear some gurgling sounds when assessing for lung sounds. Your partner finds several empty medication vials in the kitchen.

What does the initial evaluation of this patient suggest?

What types of medications do you expect to find?

What is she likely presenting with?

What could have caused her to become acutely ill?

Arrhythmias

Changes in the cardiovascular system with aging can lead to conduction system abnormalities. These conduction abnormalities result in disturbance of the heart rhythm or rate from its normal parameters. This abnormal rhythm is called an **arrhythmia** and may be asymptomatic or may present with chest pain, dyspnea, palpitations, dizziness, changes in mental status, syncope, or even sudden death. There are many types of arrhythmias, some of which are listed in (▼ **Table 9-5**). Entire textbooks have been dedicated to the recognition and management of arrhythmias, and the discussion of all of these is beyond the scope of this chapter.

Atrial fibrillation is the most common sustained arrhythmia found in the older population (▶ **Figure 9-5**). It is estimated that about 5% of people age 65 and over are afflicted with this. Because of its prevalence, and the importance of recognizing and treating atrial fibrillation with rapid ventricular response in the prehospital setting, a short discussion is worthwhile. A sum-

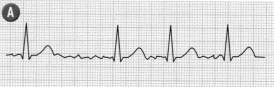
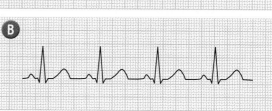

Figure 9-5   Atrial fibrillation (A) compared to normal sinus rhythm (B).

mary of possible causes can be found in (▼ **Table 9-6**).

The incidence and prevalence increase with age and so atrial fibrillation is a major contributor to stroke in the older population.[9] Atrial fibrillation is

TABLE 9-5   Common Arrhythmias
Bradyarrhythmias
◆ Sinus bradycardia
◆ Atrioventricular heart blocks (1st degree, 2nd degree, etc.)
◆ Junctional bradycardia
Tachyarrhythmias
◆ Atrial fibrillation
◆ Atrial flutter
◆ Junctional tachycardia
◆ Multifocal atrial tachycardia
◆ Supraventricular tachycardia
◆ Ventricular tachycardia
◆ Wolff-Parkinson-White

TABLE 9-6   Some Possible Causes of Atrial Fibrillation
Underlying Structural Heart Defects
◆ Conduction abnormalities
◆ Valvular heart defects
◆ Myocardial infarction (MI)
Acute Systemic Illness
◆ Pneumonia
◆ Electrolyte abnormalities
◆ Pulmonary edema (cardiogenic and noncardiogenic)
◆ Pulmonary embolism
Chronic Systemic Illness
◆ Thyroid disease
◆ Asthma
◆ Chronic obstructive pulmonary disease
◆ Chronic renal disease

usually classified as acute or chronic. At times, acute systemic illnesses such as pneumonia or electrolyte abnormalities can precipitate an episode of atrial fibrillation. Chronic, previously undiagnosed systemic problems such as thyroid disease, poorly controlled chronic obstructive pulmonary disease, or kidney failure can also contribute to atrial fibrillation.

Prehospital treatment focuses on recognition of atrial fibrillation and control of a rapid ventricular response. Cardioverting the patient back into a sinus rhythm may be required. Remember that although a rhythm strip is helpful, a 12-lead ECG is also helpful in determining the cause of the arrhythmia.

 Medications for rate control of atrial fibrillation may include beta blockers, calcium channel blockers, and digoxin. Those patients who are considered to be at minimal risk for medication interaction, adherence issues, or falls may also require treatment with an anticoagulant such as warfarin (Coumadin). Aspirin is a good alternative to warfarin to prevent stroke.

Hypertensive Emergencies

Hypertensive emergencies are generally regarded as elevated blood pressure occurring with evidence of organ damage. Common organs affected are the heart, eyes, brain, and kidneys. Damage would manifest as chest pain, visual changes, mental status changes, or urinary abnormalities, respectively. Blood pressure cutoffs vary from textbook to textbook, and as such there are no set-in-stone criteria for the level of blood pressure needed to create a hypertensive emergency. Previous teachings stressed that blood pressure needed to be lowered as rapidly as possible, to low or "normal" levels to protect the patient. Subsequent studies have shown this to be potentially harmful to the patient. Rapid lowering of the blood pressure can result in stroke, MI, or death. Newer thinking dictates lowering blood pressure about 30% from the initial mean arterial pressure.

 The agents of choice for this are labetalol (Normodyne), sodium nitroprusside (Nipride), or intravenous nitroglycerin. With relatively short transport times, it is important to realize that rushing to lower a patient's blood pressure with an inferior drug may be harmful to the patient. Using one of the aforementioned drugs in the prehospital setting, or contacting the hospital early to have the appropriate medications available upon arrival, will be more likely to benefit the patient.

Syncope

Syncope becomes increasingly common with aging and the older patient with syncope is much more likely to be injured than a younger patient with syncope. Syncope in older people can be attributed to many causes, but those of most concern involve neurologic and cardiac causes. While vasovagal syncope may be the most common culprit in the younger population, the older population tends to have a wider variety of causes. Keep in mind that older patients may be much more sensitive to dehydration and antihypertensive medications than their younger counterparts. The most important cardiac problems to investigate are myocardial infarction, arrhythmias, and valvular disease. A history of cardiac disease is a very important clue to a cardiac cause, and the absence of a history of heart disease makes this cause extremely unlikely. A myocardial infarction may cause enough damage to pump action to decrease blood flow to the brain and precipitate syncope. An MI may also precipitate an arrhythmia which produces syncope. Heart rates going too slow or too fast may decrease blood flow to the brain to the point when it becomes inadequate to sustain consciousness. Aortic stenosis (stiffening of the aortic valve, thereby impairing the left ventricle's ability to pump blood) is a common serious cause of cardiac syncope in the older patient.

Summary

Cardiac emergencies tend to happen with greater frequency in the older population than in any other age group. The signs and symptoms do not always conform to the classic presentation we read about in textbooks. Remember to take a detailed medical history, try to bring all medications with you to the hospital, and pay close attention to what the patient tells you. Strongly consider the use of a 12-lead ECG in all cardiac emergencies.

The patient may have very vague complaints that do not necessarily point to a cardiac cause. By keeping an open mind and looking a little deeper, you may be surprised to find a cardiac problem where you did not initially suspect it.

Chapter Resources

Case Study Summaries

CASE STUDY 1 SUMMARY

The husband is experiencing a change in behavior that could indicate acute confusion or delirium. Possible contributing factors include his age, living alone with his wife, his multiple medical problems, possibility of multiple medications, multiple risk factors for vascular disease, and lack of sleep. The husband could be experiencing acute confusion secondary to not sleeping, problems with hyperglycemia or hypoglycemia, problems associated with his vascular system such as stroke or heart ischemia, overmedication, undermedication, or a combination of problems, given his multiple risk factors.

CASE STUDY 2 SUMMARY

The initial evaluation suggests cardiopulmonary distress. The exam is consistent with congestive heart failure, but with the unusual presentation of hypotension. Her irregular rhythm and rapid rate suggest atrial fibrillation with rapid ventricular response. She is clearly unstable, and this is most likely secondary to her heart rate.

After applying high-flow oxygen and establishing an IV, cardioversion should be attempted to resolve the patient's compromised hemodynamic state. Her situation may have been caused by nonadherence to her medications. Medications you might expect to find would be digoxin, diuretics, and perhaps a calcium channel blocker. Without these medications, the patient's heart rate would climb, her heart would not beat as strongly, and extra fluid would accumulate. You might also expect potassium supplements and nitrates.

Treatment in the field would be dictated by the response to cardioversion. Her congestive heart failure and atrial fibrillation could have also been caused by an AMI. A 12-lead ECG and early medical direction to alert the emergency department of this critical patient are essential.

Endnotes

1. Wei JY, Gersh BJ. Heart disease in the elderly. *Curr Probl Cardiol.* 1987;12:1–65.

2. Cannon LA, Marshall JM. Cardiac disease in the elderly population. *Clin Geriatr Med.* 1993;9: 499–525.

3. Ghali JK, Cooper R, Ford E. Trends in hospitalization rates for heart failure in the United States, 1973–1986: Evidence for increasing population prevalence. *Arch Intern Med.* 1990;150: 767–773.

4. O'Connell JB, Bristow MR. Economic impact of heart failure in the United States: Time for a different approach. *J Heart Lung Transplant.* 1993; 13:S107–S112.

5. National Center for Health Statistics. Advance report of final mortality statistics, 1988. In: *Monthly Vital Statistics Report.* 39(7). Hyattsville, MD: Public Health Service; 1990:1–48.

6. Graves EJ. Summary, 1989 National Hospital Discharge Survey: Advance Data from Vital Statistics, No 199. Hyattsville, MD: National Center for Health Statistics; 1991:1–12.

7. Umachandran V, Ranjadayalan K, Ambepityia G, et al. Aging, autonomic function, and the precipitation of angina. *Br Heart.* 1991;66:15–18.

8. Wolf PA, Abbott RD, Kannel WB. Atrial fibrillation: A major contributor to stroke in the elderly. *Arch Intern Med.* 1987;147:1561–1564.

9. Follman DF. Aortic regurgitation: Identifying and treating acute and chronic disease. *Postgrad Med.* 1993;93:83–90.

Neurological Emergencies

LEARNING OBJECTIVES

1 Discuss abnormal changes with age of the nervous system.

2 Discuss the epidemiology of nervous system diseases in the older population, including stroke, dementia, delirium, Alzheimer's disease, Parkinson's disease, seizures, and aggressive or assaultive behavior.

3 Discuss assessment of the older patient with complaints related to the nervous system.

4 Identify the need for intervention and transport, and develop a treatment and management plan for the older patient with complaints related to the nervous system.

Matthew J. Belan

Marian P. LaMonte, MD, MSN

CASE STUDY 1

You are dispatched to the home of a 73-year-old woman by her son. The son, who was on location upon your arrival, stated that he does not live with his mother but received a telephone call from her about an hour ago. When the son answered the phone, he stated that there was no one talking. The caller ID identified the caller as his mother, but he did not hear his mother's voice.

When he arrived, he discovered that his mother was unable to speak and seemed to have trouble moving her right arm. Your assessment reveals a patient who is conscious, appearing alert, but unable to verbalize. You note some weakness in the patient's right arm. There is no significant history associated with this patient.

What is your impression?

What are your treatment priorities?

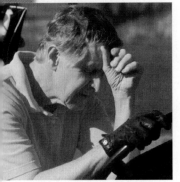

Introduction

Aging produces changes in the nervous system that are reflected in the neurological examination. Changes in thinking (cognitive) speed, memory, and postural stability are the most common normal findings in an older person. Often, these changes are not evident to the patient or family members, and they cannot recall a precise date or time when these changes began. In contrast, diseases of the neurological system tend to produce acute changes in neurological function and frequently have a sudden onset with a more rapid and noticeable decrease in neurological function. Additionally, certain disease states that are common in the older population increase the chance for secondary problems that can further damage the nervous system. (For example, a patient with Parkinson's disease may fall and sustain an injury.)

The nervous system is a complex organ system with central (brain and spinal cord) and peripheral (outside the brain and spinal cord) components (▶ **Figure 10-1**). Disease-related changes in one component alone can produce an emergency state. The neurological examination measures the function of these two component parts. A brief examination that highlights each part of the nervous system can localize the major site of dysfunction, which narrows the list of potential causes. This enables the examiner to focus on the urgent possibilities when making decisions about immediate treatment.

Normal Age-related Changes in the Nervous System

Normal age-related changes are defined as progressive and irreversible changes in the findings on neurological examination that develop with advancing age in most individuals without obvious disease.[1] The following sections discuss these changes in regard to various functions and body systems.

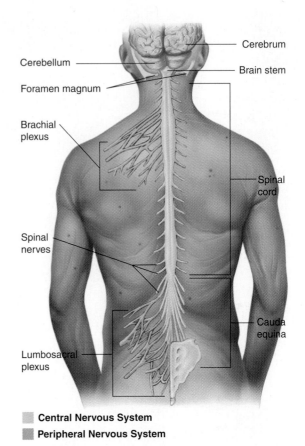

Central Nervous System
Peripheral Nervous System

(**Figure 10-1**)   The nervous system is a complex organ system with central and peripheral components.

Mental Function and Status

Studies have documented age-associated decline in mental function, especially slower central processing of sensory stimuli and language, and longer retrieval times for short- and long-term memory. Together, these typically affect performance on the mental status portion of the neurological examination. Common findings may include slow responses to questioning, or requests to repeat a question. Note that these normal changes can be confused with the symptoms associated with diseases such as Alzheimer's disease or other forms of dementia, depression, **encephalopathy** (any acute disease of the brain), or Parkinson's disease and related disorders.

The main features of normal age-related cognitive disorders are that they are relatively isolated (not associated with multiple abnormal neurological findings that suggest specific disease states) and that the onset and any progression of these findings are "in time" with the individual's aging process; that is, the findings are not sudden or extreme, and do not extend to other abnormalities.

Cranial Nerve Function

The cranial nerves provide both motor and sensory function to various parts of the head and neck including the ears, eyes, tongue, face, and muscles used for facial expression and movement of the head. The most common changes associated with deteriorating cranial nerve function include decline in vision, hearing, range of eye movements (especially vertical movements), and diminished range of both facial expression and cervical motion. Pupil size and response to light decrease progressively with age (▼ **Figure 10-2**). Age-related changes are mild, slow in onset, and progress gradually as the patient ages. It is important to distinguish these from more exaggerated changes associated with dis-

ease states. Three features in particular—diminished eye movements, facial expression, and cervical movement (along with other neurological exam changes such as tremor and limb rigidity)—might suggest Parkinson's disease or another parkinsonian-like disorder.

Motor Function

Changes in motor function take place in both the central and peripheral nervous systems. As these changes occur, the individual cannot initiate movement as quickly or sustain it as well, so coordination of movement declines. Mild coordination problems also result from reduced nervous system functions such as vision and balance. Nervous system deterioration that causes a decrease in muscle bulk, and possibly strength, can also affect motor function.

Another common finding is benign "senile" tremor, which may be **idiopathic** (of unknown cause) or inherited. This tremor is symmetrical and mainly affects the upper limbs, hands, head, and voice. Age-associated changes of motor function are generally symmetrical, mild, and—as in other systems—gradual in their development. One-sided, severe, or sudden symptoms more likely indicate a specific disease state such as stroke, Parkinson states, or acute inner ear disorders.

Sensation and Reflexes

Changes in sensation and reflexes involve decreased sensitivity to vibration and reduction or loss of ankle jerk reflex. Along with declining vision, these make the older patient susceptible to falls from misplacement of the feet, because vibration and position sense are main contributors to balance. In addition, visual acuity declines, and changes in the inner ear cause hearing loss.

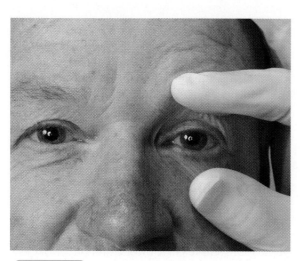

Figure 10-2   Pupil size and response to light decrease progressively with age.

Communication Tip

Difficulty in communicating with older patients is often a result of normal effects of the aging process on sensory functions. Remember that there is little the patient can do about this.

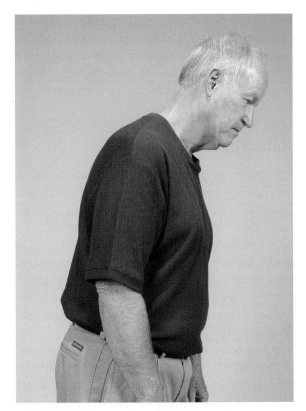

Figure 10-3   Age-related spinal changes typically result in a slightly stooped stance.

TABLE 10-1   Origins or Mechanisms of Nervous System Pathophysiology
Mnemonic: **VITAMINS C & D**
Note: some categories overlap.
V   *Vascular:* stroke, brain embolism
I   *Inflammation:* inflammation of the blood vessels in the brain (<u>vasculitis</u>)
T   *Toxins:* carbon monoxide poisoning *Trauma:* concussion, intracerebral hemorrhage *Tumors:* primary brain tumor, or <u>metastasis</u> (developed elsewhere and spread to the brain)
A   *Autoimmune:* production of immune system components against a normal structure in the central nervous system
M   *Metabolic:* liver or renal failure, hypoglycemia, hyperglycemia, hypothyroidism, <u>nonketotic diabetic acidosis</u>
I   *Infection:* meningitis, encephalitis
N   *Narcotics and other drugs:* many possibilities, with a higher chance of mental status changes if there is pre-existing brain disease
S   *Systemic:* sepsis, hypoxia
C   *Congenital:* seizures
D   *Degenerative:* Alzheimer's disease and other dementias, Parkinson's disease

Posture and Gait

With aging, changes to the spinal canal typically produce forward thrusting of the head and a flexion of the thorax that result in a slightly stooped stance (▲ **Figure 10-3**). Changing features of the **gait** (a person's manner of walking) are shortened step, wider base, and decreased arm swing, and in general, walking is slower and looks "stiff." The decreased vibration and position sense in the lower legs (mentioned above) causes older people to take smaller, more cautious steps, and produces more postural sway.

Pathophysiology and Occurrence Patterns of Nervous System Diseases

Though the underlying disease processes involved in neurological conditions can seem complex, there are ways to simplify the hunt for a cause. (▲ **Table 10-1**) presents a mnemonic that is a helpful reminder of the possible origins and mechanisms. It begins with the type of signs present, and lists what might be causing them. This approach is particularly useful when the patient has neurological symptoms that might have multiple causes.

Primary Neurological Disorders

Stroke and Cerebrovascular Disease

Of the primary neurological problems in the older population, stroke is the most common. Stroke is a leading cause of death. Stroke occurs approximately one third as often as myocardial infarction and other severe manifestations of cardiac disease in both men and women. The risk of stroke doubles with every decade over the age of 55. The main risk factors for stroke are both preventable and treatable. Hypertension, cardiac disease (especially atrial fibrillation), smoking, diabetes, and high levels of fats in the blood, including cholesterol, are the most common and significant contributors to risk for stroke. Other important risk factors are also controllable, such as obesity and sedentary (inactive) lifestyle.

There are two main types of stroke: ischemic and hemorrhagic. About 70% to 80% of all strokes are ischemic, and the other 20% to 30% are hemorrhagic. Hemorrhages occur when a blood vessel within the brain tears and produces bleeding in or around the brain. Although hemorrhagic stroke is less common than ischemia, it is more often lethal. Ischemic stroke typically occurs when a clot obstructs blood flow in an artery that supplies a portion of the brain (▼ **Figure 10-4**). The clot may have formed within the artery at a specific site, or developed elsewhere—in the heart, for instance—and broken off, traveled, and finally lodged in an artery serving part of the brain. Brain tissue supplied by this artery is thus deprived of oxygen and glucose, resulting in immediate brain tissue death.

A vitally important concept in the pathophysiology of ischemic stroke is that of the **penumbra**, the tissue surrounding the central area of stroke. Because this tissue is still viable if treated within a few minutes to hours, it is critical to quickly transport all patients with suspected stroke to the closest center that specializes in the care of stroke patients. The main thrust of ischemic stroke research is devoted to salvaging the penumbral tissue and thus minimizing the damage done by the stroke.

The symptoms of ischemic stroke include:

♦ Weakness (hemiparesis) or paralysis (hemiplegia) on one side of the body
♦ Numbness on one side of the body
♦ Dysarthria (slurred speech)
♦ Aphasia
♦ Confusion
♦ Convulsions
♦ Visual disturbances
♦ Incontinence
♦ Numbness of the face
♦ Headache
♦ Dizziness

The symptoms of hemorrhagic stroke include:

♦ Headache (often described as the worst headache of the patient's life)
♦ Nausea and vomiting
♦ Change in mental status; patient may become restless, agitated, or confused. Mental status changes may progress from alert to lethargic.

Ischemic stroke may develop slowly, whereas hemorrhagic stroke may develop abruptly. Both forms of stroke can be life threatening. However, ischemic stroke rarely leads to death within the first hour, whereas hemorrhagic stroke can be rapidly fatal. It is vital that the EMS provider attempt to determine from the patient (if possible) or from the family or caregiver the exact time of onset of symptoms. Often, the patient will awake in the morning presenting with signs of ischemic stroke. Determine when the patient was last known to be normal (the patient's baseline mental status) to establish the time of onset.

A **transient ischemic attack (TIA)**, often referred to as a "mini-stroke," is an episode of cerebral dysfunction that lasts from minutes to hours. The patient recovers from these symptoms within 24 hours with no permanent neurological damage. A TIA is an important indication of an impending stroke. The signs and symptoms of a TIA are the same as those of a stroke—weakness, paralysis, speech disturbances, and numbness to the face.

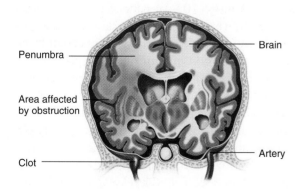

Penumbra
Brain
Area affected by obstruction
Clot
Artery

Figure 10-4   A clot that blocks an artery serving part of the brain causes immediate brain tissue death. Saving tissue in the penumbra is the goal of immediate stroke care.

EMS providers play a pivotal role in the outcome of stroke patients. The American Stroke Association has developed a Stroke Chain of Survival consisting of four components:

1. *Rapid recognition and reaction to stroke warning signs:* This component emphasizes the recognition of the warning signs of a stroke by the general public and its rapid entry into the EMS system by calling 9-1-1.

2. *Rapid start of prehospital care:* This component emphasizes early assessment and prehospital care by EMS providers.

3. *Rapid EMS system transport and hospital notification:* This component emphasizes rapid transport and notification to an appropriate emergency department.

4. *Rapid diagnosis and treatment at the hospital:* This component emphasizes prompt evaluation and treatment at the hospital.

On looking at the components of the Stroke Chain of Survival, it is clear that EMS providers can significantly impact stroke survival through public education, early recognition, and rapid transport to the appropriate facility.

Dementia and Its Consequences

Dementia is a general term to describe a brain disorder that produces memory impairment as well as significant loss of mental abilities without an alteration in level of consciousness. The most common primary type of dementia is Alzheimer's disease. Secondary causes include the effects of multiple strokes that have damaged neurons within the brain, certain nutritional deficiencies (eg, vitamin B_{12}), chronic alcoholism, and brain tumor or other specific brain disease. Loss of memory, loss of abstract thinking, and loss of judgment eventually lead to dependence on others to carry out activities of daily living (ADLs), though this decline occurs over many years. Thus, many patients with early stages of dementia may not appear impaired for quite some time. Psychiatric symptoms become evident as these losses progress and the individual has an impaired ability to understand the surrounding world. Anxiety, depression, delusions, and hallucinations may lead to aggressive behavior. The total dependence of the severe dementia patient and

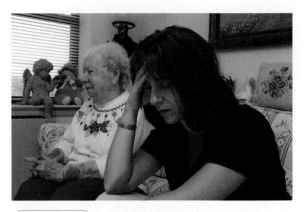

Figure 10-5 The stress of long-term care for an older person with dementia can exhaust the caregiver. This situation can end in abuse.

the stress of providing long-term care for someone so dependent may emotionally exhaust the patient's caregiver; these patients can be the victims of abuse (▲ **Figure 10-5**). See Chapter 14 for more information about elder abuse.

Parkinsonism

Parkinsonism is a general term for brain dysfunction that causes loss of flexibility and fluidity of posture and movement, and development of a tremor in the hands. Patients with signs of Parkinsonism, regardless of the cause, typically have a decreased level of function of the neurons that produce the neurotransmitter dopamine in the brain. The most common primary source of this dysfunction is Parkinson's disease, a condition caused by the loss of dopamine-producing nerve cells in the brain. The four cardinal signs of Parkinson's disease are resting tremors (the most common, affecting almost 70% of patients), rigidity, slowness of movement (bradykinesia), and postural instability.[2] Possible secondary causes include exposure to carbon monoxide, multiple strokes, brain injury such as that which occurs with boxing, and the use of antipsychotic medications to treat schizophrenia (haloperidol and other dopamine antagonists). The difference between Parkinsonism and Parkinson's disease is that Parkinsonism is a group of signs and symptoms associated with a decreased level of dopamine in the brain, while Parkinson's disease is a primary cause for the decreased levels of dopamine in the brain. The occurrence rate of Parkinsonism increases dramatically in patients older than 55.

Seizure Disorders

Seizures are defined as an intermittent derangement of the central nervous system due to a sudden, excessive, disorderly discharge of cerebral neurons. The discharge results in an almost instantaneous disturbance of sensation, convulsive movements, altered or impaired cognition, or a combination. Although seizures originating in patients aged 65 and older were once considered rare, they are remarkably frequent. With the exception of neonates, the highest incidence of new-onset seizures occurs in the population aged 65 and older.

Clinically, seizures in older people are not different from those in children, adolescents, and younger adults, except for petit mal seizures, which almost never occur in older persons. The onset of seizures after age 65 years is more often symptomatic and associated with injury. The incidence of late-onset seizure progressively increases with each decade beyond age 60. The cause of this occurrence depends to a large extent on age and cognitive integrity. Patients with advanced Alzheimer's disease are at six times the risk of experiencing an unprovoked seizure.

The most common causes of seizures in older people include cerebrovascular disease, brain cancer, head trauma, Alzheimer's disease, metabolic disorders, central nervous system infection, or multiple causes. Also, seizures are the third most common cause of neurological disorder in older people, with cerebrovascular accidents being the most common precipitant of the seizure.[3]

Secondary Neurological Disorders

Secondary neurological disorders are disorders of the central nervous system (CNS) that are caused by the influence of factors originating from outside the CNS. These disorders may be caused by toxins, hypoxia, diseases such as cancer that have spread to the CNS, and trauma to the brain.

Metabolic Encephalopathies from Systemic Illness

Nervous system response to bodywide (systemic) disorders is by far the most common secondary cause of neurological problems in older persons. Disorders in other organs of the body can produce secondary effects on any part of the nervous system. For example, patients with liver or kidney failure may accumulate toxins in the blood, leading to profound effects on the brain, such as confusion and stupor. Cardiovascular disorders may also present with nervous system dysfunction as the principal symptom. Patients with hypertension may complain of headache, dizziness, or confusion, and those who have cardiac disease may present with syncope. Patients with diabetes may have signs and symptoms of central and/or peripheral nervous system dysfunction. Blood glucose levels outside the normal range may cause a change in the patient's behavior or level of consciousness.

Drug Interactions and Toxins

Drug interactions and toxin exposure are significant problems for the older population. As multiple medical problems develop, treatment often involves medications that are metabolized in the liver. Prior liver disease, or liver damage from chronic use of alcohol, can thus lead to elevated blood levels of these medications and a higher risk of adverse reactions and dangerous interactions (▼ **Figure 10-6**). In addition, because of normal declines in liver and kidney function with aging, doses of medications that are safe in younger adults can build up to toxic levels in older adults.

Medication Tip

Liver disease or damage puts patients at higher risk of a variety of problems with medications metabolized in the liver.

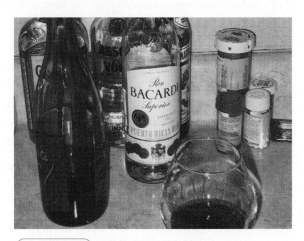

Figure 10-6 Chronic alcohol use is one cause of liver damage that can lead to elevated blood levels of liver-metabolized medications.

Chronic alcohol use or abuse results in many possible secondary neurological disorders. Both acute intoxication and delirium tremens can be deadly because of their effects on the nervous system itself, or because they lead to trauma. Alcohol withdrawal, for instance, can produce life-threatening seizures. Chronic alcohol use contributes to a higher risk of stroke and leads to dementia, acute encephalopathy, memory loss, balance disorder due to specific effects on the cerebellum, and neuropathy and myopathy (damage to cardiac and skeletal muscle) that result in pain and weakness.

Many cancer therapies (chemotherapies) are toxic to the various components of the nervous system (▶ Figure 10-7). Some of the toxic effects are not reversible.

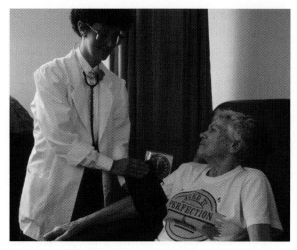

Figure 10-7 Many cancer therapies (chemotherapies) are toxic to the various components of the nervous system.

CASE STUDY 2

You are dispatched to the scene of an 80-year-old man who has fallen down a flight of stairs. When you arrive, his caregiver tells you the man has Alzheimer's disease, requires 24-hour supervision, and gets confused. You find him at the bottom of the steps, face up, and conscious but confused as to what happened and what the date is. He knows the place is "home." His sentences are simple and repetitive, but clear. His vital signs are a blood pressure of 110/58 mm Hg, a heart rate of 78 beats/min, and respirations of 20 breaths/min. He does not have facial weakness, and although he seems warm to the touch and a bit stiff, he can symmetrically squeeze with both hands and vigorously wiggle his feet on command. He has multiple bruises, and you notice that he has been incontinent of urine.

The caregiver tells you that he tripped going down the stairs. She says that it is common for him to repeat sentences, and "mess himself," and that she has not been out of his sight for months. As you logroll him onto the backboard and place a cervical collar, you ask about his medicine. She gives you bottles of Prozac, Aricept, haloperidol, lisinopril, and HCTZ. You head to the nearest trauma center, thinking of the many possible problems because—with older patients—there are frequently multiple factors involved.

What portions of the nervous system are most vulnerable in falls?

Is his mental status reassuring?

What is the significance of the incontinence of urine?

What are the other common neurological causes of falls in the older population?

Disorders Related to Trauma

Trauma to the head and spine results in needless disability and consumes a large portion of medical costs in the older population. Like stroke and dementia, brain and spinal cord injury often result in the need for long-term care due to the loss of ability to perform ADLs. Many factors contribute to injury in the older population, including diminished sensations, mental response, and physical agility. Medical disorders, depression, and drug side effects add to the older person's risk of trauma.

Infections

Systemic disorders that occur frequently in the older population and affect nervous system function include pneumonia, urinary tract infection, cellulitis, sepsis, **meningitis**, and **encephalitis**. Each can result in a change in mental status, presenting with signs ranging from confusion to coma. Patients who have a localized infection in the brain, such as an abscess, may present with general or focal neurological dysfunction.

Cancer in the Nervous System

Most malignant tumors within the brain of adults and older patients result from metastases from other parts of the body to the brain. Tumors of the brain, whether malignant or benign, may result in general or focal neurological dysfunction due to the effect that the mass has on the surrounding structures. Brain cancer might first manifest as headache or symptoms suggestive of stroke.

Assessing Complaints Related to the Nervous System

The following section is organized to highlight aspects of general patient care procedures, and assessment of mental status and airway, breathing, and circulation (ABCs) for specific categories of neurological impairment. Categories are arranged from a symptom point of view, similar to the way a patient with neurological impairment might present to EMS. Once the chief problem is recognized, key history questions and key exam features, including those directed at identifying the mechanism of neurological injury, are presented.

Attitude Tip

Don't just project a caring, interested, supportive and compassionate attitude to your older patients—embrace it and live by it! Remember that seniors do not like to be patronized or treated like children. Treat them like responsible adults, with dignity.

General Guidelines for Performing a Neurological Examination

The neurological examination begins as soon as contact is made with the patient by determining the patient's level of consciousness using the AVPU (ie, alert, verbal or painful stimuli, unresponsive) scale (▼ **Table 10-2**). Once airway, breathing, and circulation have been assessed and deemed adequate, a more focused neurological examination may begin. While assessing the patient, it is also essential to obtain as much information as possible about the history of the incident, as well as the patient's medical history, medications, and allergies. The focused neurological examination begins by evaluating the patient's mental status in more detail. This includes asking the patient simple questions, such as the date or location, and determining if the patient's comments are logical and appropriate. During this time, a general impression of the patient's behaviors and actions should also be formed.

The neurological examination continues by examining the structures of the face for symmetry, including the eyelids, mouth, and pupils. The pupils should be evaluated with a penlight to

TABLE 10-2   Assessing Level of Consciousness: AVPU
Alert
Responds to **V**erbal stimuli
Responds to **P**ainful stimuli
Unresponsive

determine if there is an equal and symmetrical reaction to light in both pupils. Next, the function of the nerves and muscles that control eye movements should be assessed by having the patient follow a penlight in both horizontal and vertical directions. Sensation of the face may be quickly examined by touching both sides of the face above the eyes, below the eyes, and along the mandible, and asking the patient if the sensation is equal and normal on both sides. The nerves that control motor function for the face may be assessed by having the patient close his or her eyes, smile, and protrude the tongue. All of these actions should produce symmetrical movements, and the tongue should not deviate to either side. Additional techniques for evaluating cranial nerve and motor function of the face are included in the sections below.

Once the face has been examined, an examination of neurological function of the extremities may be conducted. Begin by inspecting the extremities for muscle bulk, tremors, and abnormal movements such as rapid, uncontrolled movement of an arm. Then, the upper extremities should be examined by having the patient flex and extend at the elbow against a provider's hand supplying light resistance. Next, grip strength should be evaluated bilaterally and simultaneously so that differences in strength may be detected. Sensation may then be evaluated by touching the patient's arms at various points to determine if the stimulus is felt and if it feels normal. The lower extremity examination is similar to that of the upper extremities. The patient should flex and extend the knee and **dorsiflex** (toes toward the head) and **plantar flex** (stepping on the gas) the feet against mild resistance provided by a provider's hands. Sensation may then be examined in a manner similar to that of the upper extremities.

Stroke

Assessment of the older patient with suspected stroke is the same as for all other patients experiencing an acute emergency—adequate maintenance of ABCs. With severe symptoms of hemorrhagic stroke, patency of the airway and adequate circulation are vital. Be prepared to provide ventilatory support. Time of symptom onset is crucial; this will be especially important when considering interventions. In addition to abnormal findings during the neurological examination, another tool to aid the EMS provider in assessing a possible stroke patient is the use of a stroke scale. The simplest and easiest to use is the Cincinnati Prehospital Stroke Scale (▼ **Table 10-3**). This scale tests speech, facial droop, and arm drift. To test speech, ask the patient to repeat a simple phrase such as "The sky is blue in Cincinnati." If the patient is able to do this correctly, the patient can understand and repeat speech. To test facial movement, ask the patient to show his or her teeth or to smile. Observe whether both sides of the face around the mouth move equally. If only one side is moving well, there may be weakness to the muscles that control the other side. To test arm movement, ask the patient to hold both arms in front of his or her body, with palms facing up, eyes closed, and without moving. Over the next

TABLE 10-3 Cincinnati Stroke Scale		
Test	**Normal**	**Abnormal**
Facial Droop (Ask patient to show teeth or smile.)	Both sides of face move equally well.	One side of face does not move as well as the other.
Arm Drift (Ask patient to close eyes and hold both arms out with palms up.)	Both arms move the same, or both arms do not move.	One arm does not move, or one arm drifts down compared with the other side.
Speech (Ask patient to say, "The sky is blue in Cincinnati.")	Patient uses correct words with no slurring.	Patient slurs words, uses inappropriate words, or is unable to speak.

ten seconds, watch the patient's hands. If one side drifts toward the ground, there is weakness on one side of the body. If both arms drift toward the ground, the patient may be experiencing a problem other than stroke.

Controversy

At present, not enough data exists to gauge the effectiveness of stroke scales in the field. Stroke screening tools for EMS providers should be as simple as possible and provide a descriptive output, not a numerical assessment. The scale should establish a baseline and then permit evaluation of symptom improvement or worsening.

The importance of obtaining a history of the stroke patient cannot be overemphasized. Inquire of the patient (if possible), family, or caregiver about any history of cardiovascular disease, hypertension, diabetes, previous stroke, sickle cell disease, and cigarette smoking.

Loss of Consciousness

History

History is especially important in older patients who have lost consciousness (▼ **Figure 10-8**). In particular, conditions for which the individual is being treated and prescribed drugs can give significant clues to the cause. Be sure to ask about those conditions listed below, and bring all medication bottles with the patient. (▶ **Table 10-4**) lists key questions to ask.

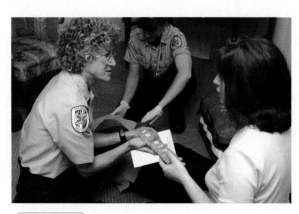

Figure 10-8   History is especially important in older patients who have lost consciousness.

TABLE 10-4   Loss of Consciousness: Key Questions

- ◆ Is there any possibility of trauma?

- ◆ Has there been or is there an infection?

- ◆ Does the patient have risk factors for cerebrovascular disease (hypertension, atrial fibrillation, diabetes, smoking, heart disease, high cholesterol)?

- ◆ Did the patient complain of a sudden, severe headache?

- ◆ Is there a known immunocompromised state, such as HIV, cancer, organ transplant, or other serious chronic disease?

- ◆ Does the patient have a seizure disorder?

- ◆ Could the individual have had a drug overdose or toxin exposure, or have a problem with alcohol abuse?

- ◆ Is there a history of an unstable medical condition, such as:
  - ◆ Myocardial infarction or insufficiency?
  - ◆ Diabetes?
  - ◆ Liver or renal failure?
  - ◆ Chronic obstructive pulmonary disease (COPD) with increased carbon dioxide levels?
  - ◆ Electrolyte and acid-base disorders?

Physical Examination

Assess Airway, Breathing, and Circulation
Look for airway patency, chest wall motion and adequacy of breathing, and pulse. If any of these are insufficient, follow standard BLS and ALS procedures.

Assess Level of Consciousness
Assess mental status using the AVPU scale.

Assess for Trauma
Inspect the head and neck for evidence of trauma such as lacerations, **Battle's sign** (bruising behind an ear) or other hematomas, and contusions, and palpate the skull for fracture (▶ **Figure 10-9**). Also check the nose and ears for leaking cerebrospinal fluid or blood. Check for fever or rash

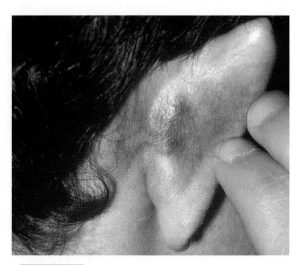

Figure 10-9   Inspect the head and neck for evidence of trauma such as lacerations, Battle's sign (shown here), or other hematomas or contusions.

suggestive of meningitis or encephalitis, and if no trauma can be assured, check for a stiff neck by having the patient touch the chin to the chest.

Assess Further for the Origin of Unresponsiveness

Examine the pupils for size and reactivity. Small, reactive pupils and respiratory depression suggest narcotic overdose. If a narcotic overdose is suspected, administer naloxone (Narcan) according to local protocol. Unequal pupils may indicate **brain herniation** (protrusion of the brain through the opening at the base of the skull) from a space-occupying lesion, such as an intracerebral hemorrhage, in which swelling causes a rapid rise in intracranial pressure (▼ **Figure 10-10**). This

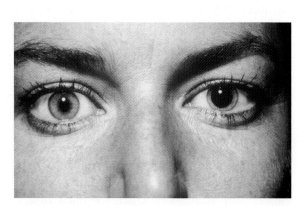

Figure 10-10   Unequal pupils may indicate rising intracranial pressure caused by brain herniation.

may also appear as two fixed (unreactive) and dilated pupils if intracranial pressure is increasing on both sides. All brain herniation syndromes ultimately result in depressed or absent respirations and fluctuations in blood pressure and heart rate. (An increase in systolic pressure, widened pulse pressure, decrease in pulse, and irregular respiratory pattern is known as Cushing's triad.) Never underestimate a patient with lowered level of consciousness, as the changes can occur rapidly. With proper management, however, they may be reversible. Conditions that can produce brain herniation are intracerebral hemorrhage, trauma, and brain tumor or abscess.

Altered Mental Status

Altered mental status describes a patient who shows abnormal mental signs such as confusion, forgetfulness, agitation, or excessive sleepiness. Altered mental status can be caused by virtually any medical illness or trauma, particularly drugs, low oxygen, abnormal electrolytes, and infections.

Delirium vs. Dementia

Distinguishing delirium from dementia in the prehospital setting may be difficult. The key difference is that delirium presents with a new onset and dementia is progressive. Delirium is an abrupt disorientation to time and place, usually with illusions. The mind wanders, speech may be incoherent, and the patient is in a state of mental confusion. Dementia is a slow, progressive loss of awareness of time and place, usually with the inability to learn new things or remember recent events. Remote memories may be intact. Total loss of function and a regression to an infantile state may result. Delirium is an acute, reversible, potentially life-threatening problem that requires extreme emergency care. Dementia, on the other hand, is very slowly progressive and requires support.

How do you differentiate between delirium and dementia? Ask a family member or caregiver, "How was the patient yesterday? One hour ago?" An acute, rapid deterioration signals delirium. A slow progression signals dementia. (▶ **Table 10-5**) lists the differences of delirium versus dementia.

If you suspect that a patient is experiencing delirium, the DELIRIUMS mnemonic in (▶ **Table 10-6**) will help in determining the cause.

CASE STUDY 3

You are dispatched to the residence of an 84-year-old woman by her family. The patient's daughter states that she took her mother to the pharmacy earlier in the day to renew her prescriptions. The daughter further states that her mother was fine all day but suddenly became confused and began speaking inappropriately. When you inquire as to the patient's normal mental status, level of functioning, and past medical history, you are told by the patient's daughter that her mother has "borderline diabetes," previous MI, and mild dementia. The daughter adds that her mother's activities have slowed down over the past several months, but that her mother still goes out shopping once or twice a week.

Your assessment reveals a conscious patient who appears alert. There are no signs of trauma. When questioned or asked to repeat a phrase, the patient responds with inappropriate words or doesn't seem to pay attention to your questions. There is no sign of facial droop or arm drift. The patient is slightly warm to touch. Vital signs are a blood pressure of 168/100 mm Hg, a pulse of 92 beats/min, respirations of 18 breaths/min, a blood glucose level of 104, and oxygen saturation on room air of 96%.

What is your impression?

What actions should you take?

---

the patient's head, and may lead to respiratory insufficiency or aspiration of stomach contents from the loss of the ability to cough. Myasthenia gravis is a condition where patients complain of rapid muscle fatigue and loss of strength following the use of a muscle or group of muscles. It occurs because of the formation of immune system antibodies to the patient's own neurotransmitter (acetylcholine) receptors that allow muscles to receive the signal to contract.

Even without initial signs of respiratory trouble, patients with a new complaint of weakness may deteriorate quickly. Be ready to provide oxygen and ventilatory support as needed. If ventilatory status is inadequate and worsening, patients in this category may benefit from intubation to protect the airway by preventing aspiration and to provide ventilatory support for patients who may no longer be capable of breathing without assistance.

Paraplegia and Quadriplegia

Paraplegia and **quadriplegia** are major, severe neurological deficits that require immediate and full attention. Paraplegia is paralysis of the lower half of the body, while quadriplegia is paralysis of all four limbs. Though most often injury related, an acute onset of paraplegia or quadriplegia may occasionally appear in the absence of trauma when an infection or other disease process affects the spinal cord.

History

If the patient is alert, ask if there is pain in a specific area of the spine. If the onset of the neurological deficit is not related to trauma, other causes should be explored, such as an infection along the spinal column, cancer, or a progressive disease process such as Guillain-Barré syndrome. A history of fever, weight loss, pain along the spinal column, or decreasing strength over the past several days may suggest a medical cause for the patient's neurological deficit. Regardless of the suspected cause of the deficit, all patients who present with paraplegia or quadriplegia should be moved using the logroll technique.

Physical Examination

ABCs may show signs of either respiratory compromise (high spinal cord injury) or neurogenic shock (mid- to low cord injury). Carefully look for protru-

---

TABLE 10-5 Delirium vs. Dementia	
Delirium	**Dementia**
Abrupt onset	Gradual onset
Reduced attention	Impaired recent memory
Disorganized thinking	Regression
At least two of the following:	
Reduced level of consciousness	Disjointed thinking
Perceptual disturbances (hallucinations, illusions)	Poor judgment
Increased or decreased psychomotor activity	Loss of mental function

History

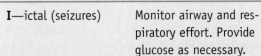 ▼ Table 10-7 lists important questions to ask about altered mental status.

Physical Examination

Assess Airway, Breathing, and Circulation
Many patients with drug intoxication, overdose, or mental status changes related to drug combinations and side effects will also have compromise of vital

TABLE 10-7 Altered Mental Status: Key Questions
♦ Was there exposure to alcohol, drugs, or toxins?
♦ What is this person normally like? When was he or she last seen normal?
♦ Did the patient complain of headache, or does the patient have a headache now?
♦ Was there a preceding infection?
♦ Was there or has there been a fever?
♦ Have there been any falls?
♦ Is the person feeling ill in any way?
♦ Is the patient adequately nourished?

TABLE 10-6 DELIRIUMS Mnemonic	
Potential Cause	**Management**
D—drugs and toxins	Manage symptoms depending upon the specific drug and naloxone (Narcan) for respiratory depression.
E—emotional (psychiatric)	Provide emotional support.
L—low PO_2 (carbon dioxide poisoning, COPD, CHF, AMI, pneumonia, pulmonary edema)	Provide oxygen and bronchodilators (albuterol) as necessary and according to local protocol.
I—infection (pneumonia, UTI, sepsis)	Provide IV fluids as necessary for hypotension.
R—retention of stool or urine	Provide supportive care.
I—ictal (seizures)	Monitor airway and respiratory effort. Provide glucose as necessary.
U—under nutrition/ dehydration	Provide IV fluids and glucose as necessary.
M—metabolism (thyroid/endocrine, electrolytes, kidneys)	This cause will often be unknown in the prehospital setting, as lab values are needed to determine this as the cause. If the cause of delirium cannot be determined, vital signs should be supported, glucose monitored (if possible), dextrose administered, ECG monitored, and an IV established.
S—subdural hematoma (An estimated 50% of people with dementia do not remember falling.)	Treat all injuries and immobilize the patient. Consider referral to a trauma center, depending on other presenting symptoms.

functions and vital signs. For example, an overdose of some types of seizure medications will produce a decreased level of consciousness as well as changes in heart rate, ECG, blood pressure, and respiratory rate. Therefore, vital signs should be monitored closely in any patient who has overdosed on a medication to identify potentially fatal changes in blood pressure, heart rate, and respiratory status.

Assess Mental Status

As with loss of consciousness, examination of the patient with altered mental status centers on the AVPU scale.

Assess Possible Causes

Give special consideration to the patient with an abnormal level of consciousness and any one of the signs and symptoms listed below.

♦ Fever
♦ Headache
♦ Neck stiffness
♦ Body rash

These patients most likely have a **subarachnoid hemorrhage** (bleeding between the arachnoid and the pia mater in the brain), meningitis, encephalitis, or other infections of the CNS that may be transmitted to EMS providers or future patients via respiratory droplets or contact with contaminated equipment.

If a patient is suspected of having an infection of the CNS, appropriate protective equipment, such as masks, should be used and the ambulance should be thoroughly cleaned after the patient is transferred to the hospital staff. It may also be prudent to leave a contact number with the hospital staff, in case the patient is diagnosed with an infectious disease that could potentially infect EMS providers, so that measures may be taken to reduce the likelihood of developing the disease.

Sudden Loss of Focal Neurological Function

Examples of loss of focal neurological function include loss of vision, language expression, or comprehension; dysarthria (slurred speech); facial or unilateral weakness (▶ **Figure 10-11**); or loss of balance in conjunction with one of these. Any patient with an abrupt, one-sided loss of a

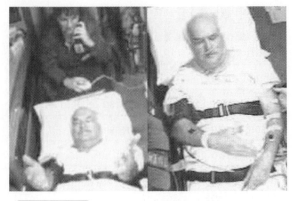

Figure 10-11   Over an 8-minute period, this patient's left arm dropped, indicating weakness from an evolving stroke. The patient survived thanks to rapid recognition and transport by EMS providers, and appropriate treatment at the hospital.

neurological function should be considered a potential stroke patient. All such patients must be transported with priority to the nearest medical center specializing in stroke care.

History

(▼ **Table 10-8**) lists questions specific to focal neurological loss.

TABLE 10-8   Loss of Focal Neurological Function: Key Questions
♦ When was the patient last known to be normal? (Not the time the patient was *discovered* to be abnormal.)
♦ Are risk factors for stroke present, such as hypertension, coronary artery disease, high cholesterol, diabetes, smoking, prior stroke or **transient ischemic attack (TIA)**? Did the patient have a previous "mini-stroke" or have previous brief loss of vision suggestive of a TIA? (Think stroke as cause of deficit.)
♦ Is there a history of preceding trauma? (Think brain contusion or intracerebral hemorrhage.)
♦ Is there a known or previously treated cancer, or an immunocompromised state caused by cancer or chemotherapeutic drugs or HIV disease? (Think brain metastasis, primary tumor, or abscess.)
♦ Is there a preceding or current infection? (Think meningitis or encephalitis.)

Physical Examination

Assess Airway, Breathing, and Circulation
Most patients with one-sided neurological deficits will be able to manage ABCs, but they may not be able to protect their airways from secretions.

Assess Mental Status
If the patient is alert, can the patient speak and understand commands? The patient who is alert but not responsive may have a language deficit known as **aphasia,** which can be caused by stroke. See Chapter 3 for information on communicating with patients with aphasia.

Assess Possible Causes
The following tests help to get a better idea of what may be causing the patient's problem.

♦ *Speech and language:* Have the patient repeat "take me out to the ballgame," and check for slurred speech. This test evaluates the patient's ability to understand commands and formulate speech.

♦ *Facial strength:* Have the patient smile widely, or "show me all of your teeth." If the patient's face appears asymmetrical while performing this task, it suggests a stroke on the opposite side of the brain.

♦ *Body strength:* Have the patient squeeze both hands, and raise both arms and legs, equally. This evaluates the ability of the patient to perform and coordinate gross motor functions.

Communication Tip

An older person's communication can convey signs about various social, environmental, and medical issues, even when you are not evaluating the patient's speech for specific neurological deficits.

Acute General Weakness

History

(▶ **Table 10-9**) provides questions to ask the patient who has a new complaint of general motor weakness.

Physical Examination

After ABCs, assess further for respiratory weakness, because this is the area of motor compromise that can most quickly create an emergency.

TABLE 10-9   Acute General Weakness: Key Questions
♦ Was there exposure to alcohol, drugs, or toxins?
♦ Was there preceding trauma? (Think spinal cord damage.)

Check for evidence of severe respiratory compromise, such as paradoxical breathing where the patient's chest moves out while the abdomen moves in during inhalation (▼ **Figure 10-12**). Some acute toxin exposures, and unusual diseases such as **Guillain-Barré syndrome** and **myasthenia gravis**, are common causes of respiratory muscle weakness. Guillain-Barré syndrome typically occurs after a patient has had a viral respiratory illness. It begins with weakness in the lower extremities that progresses toward

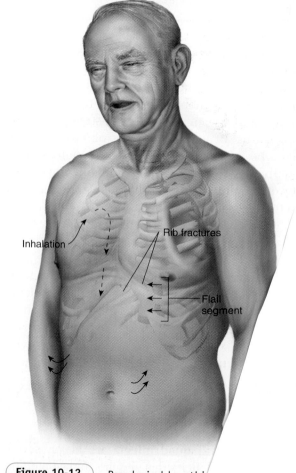

Inhalation

Rib fractures

Flail segment

Figure 10-12   Paradoxical breathi severe respiratory compromise.

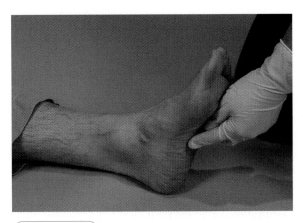

Figure 10-13   Test sensation in all four limbs with your fingertips.

sions or areas of trauma in or around the spine. Ask if the patient has sensation in the arms and legs, and test with your fingertips (▲ **Figure 10-13**). Check also if the patient can wiggle toes and fingers. When spinal cord injury is suspected, begin full-spine immobilization as soon as it is practical, using a cervical collar and backboard or other full-spine device. *Because curvature of the spine is common in the older patient, forcing the patient to lie flat may lead to further injury.* Instead, immobilize with pillows, rolled blankets, and tape.

Seizures

History

(▼ **Table 10-10**) lists important questions to ask about a patient who has had a seizure.

TABLE 10-10   Seizures: Key Questions
◆ Was there preceding trauma?
◆ Has the patient had a prior stroke?
◆ Does the patient have a known immunocompromised state (cancer, chemotherapy, organ transplant, HIV)?
◆ Is the patient diabetic? (Think hypoglycemia.)
◆ Does the patient have other organ failure such as renal or liver failure, or myocardial infarction? (Think hypoxia or electrolyte abnormality.)
◆ Does the patient use alcohol? If so, when was the last drink? (Think withdrawal.)

Physical Examination

Assess the level of alertness. A period of confusion for minutes to hours after a seizure (the postictal period) accompanies all generalized seizures, but may not be present for partial seizures. Examine the patient for head and body trauma. Assess for fever and skin rash, because these may be clues to meningitis. Assess the pupils; they may be of varying size and reactivity, but should be equal both in size and reactivity. Unequal pupils may be a sign of a serious underlying brain condition. When the patient is alert, examine for any speech, language, and motor deficit as you would for a possible stroke patient. A focal deficit is a sign of a serious underlying brain disorder; however, patients who have had a partial seizure may show a deficit in the part of the body supplied by the area of the brain where the seizure occurred, such as the eyes or an extremity. Immobilize the neck and spine if head or neck trauma may have occurred during a fall produced by the seizure.

Head and Spine Trauma

History

Determine the nature and mechanism of the injury. For instance, if this was a motor vehicle crash, was the patient the driver or a passenger, in the front or back seat, belted or unbelted, and did the airbag deploy? Did the patient fall? Was the fall caused by altered mental status, a seizure, or poor vision or balance (▶ **Figure 10-14**)? Was the individual behaving normally before the trauma? If not, what were the preceding events and behavior? If the patient is conscious, ask if there is a specific area of pain.

Physical Examination

Assess ABCs and mental status (AVPU). Check for **raccoon eyes** (bruising around the eyes), Battle's sign, blood draining from the ears, or clear spinal fluid leaking from the nose, any of which may indicate a basilar skull fracture. Check for size and symmetry of pupils and reaction to light. Ask the patient to repeat a sentence to assess language and speech, then to smile or show all of the teeth to evaluate facial movement. Assess sensation by testing the hands and legs with light touch. Ask about specific areas of numbness. Check whether the patient can wiggle the toes and fingers. While examining, maintain spinal alignment by using

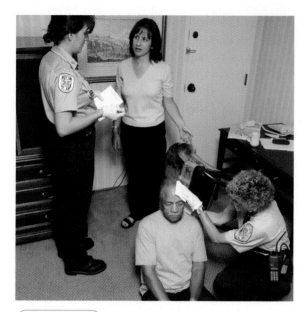

Figure 10-14   Determine the mechanism of injury. Was the fall caused by altered mental status, a seizure, or poor vision or balance?

the logroll technique to move the patient, and apply a cervical collar and full spinal immobilization according to standard protocol. Transport to the nearest neurosurgical trauma center, if one is available.

Intervention, Management, and Transport: Nervous System Complaints

General Principles

All patients who are suspected of having a neurological disorder should be transported to the closest appropriate hospital in a manner that is appropriate for the severity of the condition. Oxygen should be administered to all patients with a suspected neurological disorder to maximize oxygen delivery to the tissues of the CNS, and measures should be taken to reduce the risk of further injuries or complications while transporting the patient to the hospital. As with all patients, ABCs and vital signs should be continuously monitored in case the patient's status declines rapidly. If available, monitor the patient's ECG and establish IV access. If a question or concern ever develops regarding patient care, communications should be established between the

hospital and the EMS provider so that it may be resolved and the best possible care may be provided to the patient. It may also be of value to notify the receiving hospital of all high-priority patients so that the appropriate staff may be standing by for the patient's arrival.

Stroke

One of the most important management considerations for the stroke patient is rapid recognition of symptoms, early hospital notification, and rapid transport to an appropriate facility. The patient's ABCs must be managed. Paralysis of the muscles of the throat, tongue, and mouth can lead to airway obstruction. Be prepared to suction the patient's airway. Provide supplemental oxygen and ventilatory support. Establish IV access and monitor the patient's ECG. If available, obtain a glucose level reading. The patient's vital signs should be monitored frequently and recorded. A repeat neurological examination should be conducted in order to gauge the progression of symptoms.

Controversy

Management of hypertension in the prehospital setting is not recommended for stroke patients.

Attitude Tip

A stroke is a traumatic and emotional event for the patient. A sensitive and compassionate approach is essential. Even though these patients may not be able to communicate with you, they may be able to understand. Communicate with them as you would any other patient—in a calm and reassuring manner.

Lowered Level of Consciousness

The major concerns for patients with a lowered level of consciousness are airway protection and support of ventilation when needed. Lowered level of consciousness may result from several causes, including trauma to the head, hypoglycemia, drug overdose, or expanding lesions within the cranium

TABLE 10-5 Delirium vs. Dementia	
Delirium	**Dementia**
Abrupt onset	Gradual onset
Reduced attention	Impaired recent memory
Disorganized thinking	Regression
At least two of the following:	
Reduced level of consciousness	Disjointed thinking
Perceptual disturbances (hallucinations, illusions)	Poor judgment
Increased or decreased psychomotor activity	Loss of mental function

History

(▼ Table 10-7) lists important questions to ask about altered mental status.

Physical Examination

Assess Airway, Breathing, and Circulation
Many patients with drug intoxication, overdose, or mental status changes related to drug combinations and side effects will also have compromise of vital

TABLE 10-7 Altered Mental Status: Key Questions
◆ Was there exposure to alcohol, drugs, or toxins?
◆ What is this person normally like? When was he or she last seen normal?
◆ Did the patient complain of headache, or does the patient have a headache now?
◆ Was there a preceding infection?
◆ Was there or has there been a fever?
◆ Have there been any falls?
◆ Is the person feeling ill in any way?
◆ Is the patient adequately nourished?

TABLE 10-6 DELIRIUMS Mnemonic	
Potential Cause	**Management**
D—drugs and toxins	Manage symptoms depending upon the specific drug and naloxone (Narcan) for respiratory depression.
E—emotional (psychiatric)	Provide emotional support.
L—low PO$_2$ (carbon dioxide poisoning, COPD, CHF, AMI, pneumonia, pulmonary edema)	Provide oxygen and bronchodilators (albuterol) as necessary and according to local protocol.
I—infection (pneumonia, UTI, sepsis)	Provide IV fluids as necessary for hypotension.
R—retention of stool or urine	Provide supportive care.
I—ictal (seizures)	Monitor airway and respiratory effort. Provide glucose as necessary.
U—under nutrition/ dehydration	Provide IV fluids and glucose as necessary.
M—metabolism (thyroid/endocrine, electrolytes, kidneys)	This cause will often be unknown in the prehospital setting, as lab values are needed to determine this as the cause. If the cause of delirium cannot be determined, vital signs should be supported, glucose monitored (if possible), dextrose administered, ECG monitored, and an IV established.
S—subdural hematoma (An estimated 50% of people with dementia do not remember falling.)	Treat all injuries and immobilize the patient. Consider referral to a trauma center, depending on other presenting symptoms.

functions and vital signs. For example, an overdose of some types of seizure medications will produce a decreased level of consciousness as well as changes in heart rate, ECG, blood pressure, and respiratory rate. Therefore, vital signs should be monitored closely in any patient who has overdosed on a medication to identify potentially fatal changes in blood pressure, heart rate, and respiratory status.

Assess Mental Status

As with loss of consciousness, examination of the patient with altered mental status centers on the AVPU scale.

Assess Possible Causes

Give special consideration to the patient with an abnormal level of consciousness and any one of the signs and symptoms listed below.

◆ Fever

◆ Headache

◆ Neck stiffness

◆ Body rash

These patients most likely have a **subarachnoid hemorrhage** (bleeding between the arachnoid and the pia mater in the brain), meningitis, encephalitis, or other infections of the CNS that may be transmitted to EMS providers or future patients via respiratory droplets or contact with contaminated equipment.

If a patient is suspected of having an infection of the CNS, appropriate protective equipment, such as masks, should be used and the ambulance should be thoroughly cleaned after the patient is transferred to the hospital staff. It may also be prudent to leave a contact number with the hospital staff, in case the patient is diagnosed with an infectious disease that could potentially infect EMS providers, so that measures may be taken to reduce the likelihood of developing the disease.

Sudden Loss of Focal Neurological Function

Examples of loss of focal neurological function include loss of vision, language expression, or comprehension; dysarthria (slurred speech); facial or unilateral weakness (▶ **Figure 10-11**); or loss of balance in conjunction with one of these. Any patient with an abrupt, one-sided loss of a

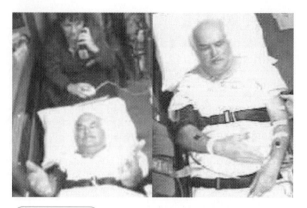

Figure 10-11   Over an 8-minute period, this patient's left arm dropped, indicating weakness from an evolving stroke. The patient survived thanks to rapid recognition and transport by EMS providers, and appropriate treatment at the hospital.

neurological function should be considered a potential stroke patient. All such patients must be transported with priority to the nearest medical center specializing in stroke care.

History

(▼ **Table 10-8**) lists questions specific to focal neurological loss.

TABLE 10-8   Loss of Focal Neurological Function: Key Questions
◆ When was the patient last known to be normal? (Not the time the patient was *discovered* to be abnormal.)
◆ Are risk factors for stroke present, such as hypertension, coronary artery disease, high cholesterol, diabetes, smoking, prior stroke or **transient ischemic attack (TIA)**? Did the patient have a previous "mini-stroke" or have previous brief loss of vision suggestive of a TIA? (Think stroke as cause of deficit.)
◆ Is there a history of preceding trauma? (Think brain contusion or intracerebral hemorrhage.)
◆ Is there a known or previously treated cancer, or an immunocompromised state caused by cancer or chemotherapeutic drugs or HIV disease? (Think brain metastasis, primary tumor, or abscess.)
◆ Is there a preceding or current infection? (Think meningitis or encephalitis.)

Physical Examination

Assess Airway, Breathing, and Circulation

Most patients with one-sided neurological deficits will be able to manage ABCs, but they may not be able to protect their airways from secretions.

Assess Mental Status

If the patient is alert, can the patient speak and understand commands? The patient who is alert but not responsive may have a language deficit known as **aphasia,** which can be caused by stroke. See Chapter 3 for information on communicating with patients with aphasia.

Assess Possible Causes

The following tests help to get a better idea of what may be causing the patient's problem.

- *Speech and language:* Have the patient repeat "take me out to the ballgame," and check for slurred speech. This test evaluates the patient's ability to understand commands and formulate speech.

- *Facial strength:* Have the patient smile widely, or "show me all of your teeth." If the patient's face appears asymmetrical while performing this task, it suggests a stroke on the opposite side of the brain.

- *Body strength:* Have the patient squeeze both hands, and raise both arms and legs, equally. This evaluates the ability of the patient to perform and coordinate gross motor functions.

Communication Tip

An older person's communication can convey signs about various social, environmental, and medical issues, even when you are not evaluating the patient's speech for specific neurological deficits.

Acute General Weakness

History

▶ Table 10-9 provides questions to ask the patient who has a new complaint of general motor weakness.

Physical Examination

After ABCs, assess further for respiratory weakness, because this is the area of motor compromise that can most quickly create an emergency.

TABLE 10-9   Acute General Weakness: Key Questions

- ◆ Was there exposure to alcohol, drugs, or toxins?

- ◆ Was there preceding trauma? (Think spinal cord damage.)

Check for evidence of severe respiratory compromise, such as paradoxical breathing where the patient's chest moves out while the abdomen moves in during inhalation ▼ Figure 10-12. Some acute toxin exposures, and unusual diseases such as **Guillain-Barré syndrome** and **myasthenia gravis**, are common causes of respiratory muscle weakness. Guillain-Barré syndrome typically occurs after a patient has had a viral respiratory illness. It begins with weakness in the lower extremities that progresses toward

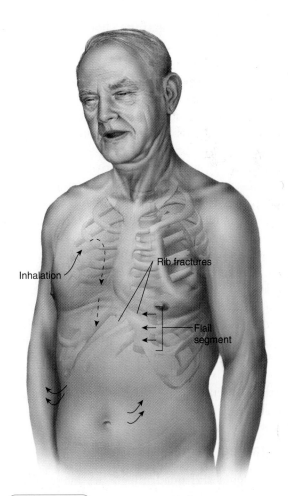

Inhalation

Rib fractures

Flail segment

Figure 10-12   Paradoxical breathing is a sign of severe respiratory compromise.

CASE STUDY 3

You are dispatched to the residence of an 84-year-old woman by her family. The patient's daughter states that she took her mother to the pharmacy earlier in the day to renew her prescriptions. The daughter further states that her mother was fine all day but suddenly became confused and began speaking inappropriately. When you inquire as to the patient's normal mental status, level of functioning, and past medical history, you are told by the patient's daughter that her mother has "borderline diabetes," previous MI, and mild dementia. The daughter adds that her mother's activities have slowed down over the past several months, but that her mother still goes out shopping once or twice a week.

Your assessment reveals a conscious patient who appears alert. There are no signs of trauma. When questioned or asked to repeat a phrase, the patient responds with inappropriate words or doesn't seem to pay attention to your questions. There is no sign of facial droop or arm drift. The patient is slightly warm to touch. Vital signs are a blood pressure of 168/100 mm Hg, a pulse of 92 beats/min, respirations of 18 breaths/min, a blood glucose level of 104, and oxygen saturation on room air of 96%.

What is your impression?

What actions should you take?

the patient's head, and may lead to respiratory insufficiency or aspiration of stomach contents from the loss of the ability to cough. Myasthenia gravis is a condition where patients complain of rapid muscle fatigue and loss of strength following the use of a muscle or group of muscles. It occurs because of the formation of immune system antibodies to the patient's own neurotransmitter (acetylcholine) receptors that allow muscles to receive the signal to contract.

Even without initial signs of respiratory trouble, patients with a new complaint of weakness may deteriorate quickly. Be ready to provide oxygen and ventilatory support as needed. If ventilatory status is inadequate and worsening, patients in this category may benefit from intubation to protect the airway by preventing aspiration and to provide ventilatory support for patients who may no longer be capable of breathing without assistance.

Paraplegia and Quadriplegia

<u>Paraplegia</u> and <u>quadriplegia</u> are major, severe neurological deficits that require immediate and full attention. Paraplegia is paralysis of the lower half of the body, while quadriplegia is paralysis of all four limbs. Though most often injury related, an acute onset of paraplegia or quadriplegia may occasionally appear in the absence of trauma when an infection or other disease process affects the spinal cord.

History

If the patient is alert, ask if there is pain in a specific area of the spine. If the onset of the neurological deficit is not related to trauma, other causes should be explored, such as an infection along the spinal column, cancer, or a progressive disease process such as Guillain-Barré syndrome. A history of fever, weight loss, pain along the spinal column, or decreasing strength over the past several days may suggest a medical cause for the patient's neurological deficit. Regardless of the suspected cause of the deficit, all patients who present with paraplegia or quadriplegia should be moved using the logroll technique.

Physical Examination

ABCs may show signs of either respiratory compromise (high spinal cord injury) or neurogenic shock (mid- to low cord injury). Carefully look for protru-

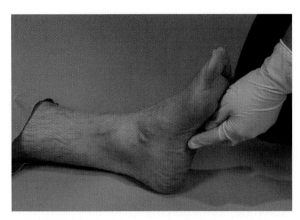

Figure 10-13   Test sensation in all four limbs with your fingertips.

sions or areas of trauma in or around the spine. Ask if the patient has sensation in the arms and legs, and test with your fingertips (▲ **Figure 10-13**). Check also if the patient can wiggle toes and fingers. When spinal cord injury is suspected, begin full-spine immobilization as soon as it is practical, using a cervical collar and backboard or other full-spine device. *Because curvature of the spine is common in the older patient, forcing the patient to lie flat may lead to further injury.* Instead, immobilize with pillows, rolled blankets, and tape.

Seizures

History

(▼ **Table 10-10**) lists important questions to ask about a patient who has had a seizure.

TABLE 10-10   Seizures: Key Questions
◆ Was there preceding trauma?
◆ Has the patient had a prior stroke?
◆ Does the patient have a known immunocompromised state (cancer, chemotherapy, organ transplant, HIV)?
◆ Is the patient diabetic? (Think hypoglycemia.)
◆ Does the patient have other organ failure such as renal or liver failure, or myocardial infarction? (Think hypoxia or electrolyte abnormality.)
◆ Does the patient use alcohol? If so, when was the last drink? (Think withdrawal.)

Physical Examination

Assess the level of alertness. A period of confusion for minutes to hours after a seizure (the postictal period) accompanies all generalized seizures, but may not be present for partial seizures. Examine the patient for head and body trauma. Assess for fever and skin rash, because these may be clues to meningitis. Assess the pupils; they may be of varying size and reactivity, but should be equal both in size and reactivity. Unequal pupils may be a sign of a serious underlying brain condition. When the patient is alert, examine for any speech, language, and motor deficit as you would for a possible stroke patient. A focal deficit is a sign of a serious underlying brain disorder; however, patients who have had a partial seizure may show a deficit in the part of the body supplied by the area of the brain where the seizure occurred, such as the eyes or an extremity. Immobilize the neck and spine if head or neck trauma may have occurred during a fall produced by the seizure.

Head and Spine Trauma

History

Determine the nature and mechanism of the injury. For instance, if this was a motor vehicle crash, was the patient the driver or a passenger, in the front or back seat, belted or unbelted, and did the airbag deploy? Did the patient fall? Was the fall caused by altered mental status, a seizure, or poor vision or balance (▶ **Figure 10-14**)? Was the individual behaving normally before the trauma? If not, what were the preceding events and behavior? If the patient is conscious, ask if there is a specific area of pain.

Physical Examination

Assess ABCs and mental status (AVPU). Check for **raccoon eyes** (bruising around the eyes), Battle's sign, blood draining from the ears, or clear spinal fluid leaking from the nose, any of which may indicate a basilar skull fracture. Check for size and symmetry of pupils and reaction to light. Ask the patient to repeat a sentence to assess language and speech, then to smile or show all of the teeth to evaluate facial movement. Assess sensation by testing the hands and legs with light touch. Ask about specific areas of numbness. Check whether the patient can wiggle the toes and fingers. While examining, maintain spinal alignment by using

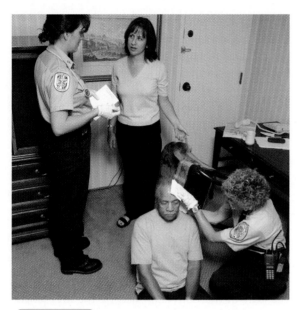

Determine the mechanism of injury. Was the fall caused by altered mental status, a seizure, or poor vision or balance?

the logroll technique to move the patient, and apply a cervical collar and full spinal immobilization according to standard protocol. Transport to the nearest neurosurgical trauma center, if one is available.

Intervention, Management, and Transport: Nervous System Complaints

General Principles

All patients who are suspected of having a neurological disorder should be transported to the closest appropriate hospital in a manner that is appropriate for the severity of the condition. Oxygen should be administered to all patients with a suspected neurological disorder to maximize oxygen delivery to the tissues of the CNS, and measures should be taken to reduce the risk of further injuries or complications while transporting the patient to the hospital. As with all patients, ABCs and vital signs should be continuously monitored in case the patient's status declines rapidly. If available, monitor the patient's ECG and establish IV access. If a question or concern ever develops regarding patient care, communications should be established between the

hospital and the EMS provider so that it may be resolved and the best possible care may be provided to the patient. It may also be of value to notify the receiving hospital of all high-priority patients so that the appropriate staff may be standing by for the patient's arrival.

Stroke

One of the most important management considerations for the stroke patient is rapid recognition of symptoms, early hospital notification, and rapid transport to an appropriate facility. The patient's ABCs must be managed. Paralysis of the muscles of the throat, tongue, and mouth can lead to airway obstruction. Be prepared to suction the patient's airway. Provide supplemental oxygen and ventilatory support. Establish IV access and monitor the patient's ECG. If available, obtain a glucose level reading. The patient's vital signs should be monitored frequently and recorded. A repeat neurological examination should be conducted in order to gauge the progression of symptoms.

Controversy

Management of hypertension in the prehospital setting is not recommended for stroke patients.

Attitude Tip

A stroke is a traumatic and emotional event for the patient. A sensitive and compassionate approach is essential. Even though these patients may not be able to communicate with you, they may be able to understand. Communicate with them as you would any other patient—in a calm and reassuring manner.

Lowered Level of Consciousness

The major concerns for patients with a lowered level of consciousness are airway protection and support of ventilation when needed. Lowered level of consciousness may result from several causes, including trauma to the head, hypoglycemia, drug overdose, or expanding lesions within the cranium such as an epidural hematoma. Brain herniation is a particularly dire condition that may progress from mild lethargy to coma and respiratory insufficiency in minutes. For patients who are suspected of having brain herniation, it is essential to protect the patient's airway, and provide aggressive ventilation with supplemental oxygen by nonrebreathing mask or bag-valve-mask device, as well as to provide IV fluids to maintain a systolic blood pressure of 100 mm Hg. Hyperventilating the patient can help reverse—or at least slow—the increase in intracranial pressure.

Many conditions that lead to a lowered level of consciousness are amenable to successful treatment if recognized early. Conditions that may be rapidly reversible if recognized and treated early are meningitis, encephalitis, subarachnoid hemorrhage, drug overdose, hypoxia, carbon monoxide poisoning, hypoglycemia, hypothermia, and alcoholic encephalopathy. For successful treatment, EMS providers must recognize the need to provide immediate treatment in the prehospital setting and/or the need for rapid transport to the hospital.

After attending to ABCs and providing supplemental oxygen, consider determining the patient's blood glucose if a glucometer is available. If the blood glucose is low, glucose or dextrose should be administered to the patient. When a glucometer is not available and the cause of the lowered level of consciousness is unknown, consider administering glucose or dextrose and naloxone (Narcan) to the patient. After appropriate therapy has been provided in the prehospital setting, patients with a continued lowered level of consciousness should be transported emergently to the closest appropriate medical facility.

Motor Weakness

Unilateral Weakness
Sudden loss of vision, language expression or understanding, dysarthria (slurred speech), facial or unilateral arm or leg weakness, and sudden loss of balance are signs of acute stroke that may need treatment with the same type of thrombolytic (clot-dissolving) medicine often used for myocardial infarction. Just as with heart attack, the patient whom you believe to be having a stroke, or "brain attack," must have symptoms called in and must be transported to the nearest emergency department equipped to evaluate and treat the patient with this medication. In some locations, a

checklist for thrombolytic therapy may be carried on the ambulance to allow for more rapid administration of thrombolytic medication once the patient has arrived at the hospital. This checklist identifies conditions that may not allow the patient to receive this type of medication because of the risk for serious complications. As much of this information should be completed as possible before arriving at the hospital, provided that it does not delay transportation.

General prehospital care includes oxygen, gentle handling, and reassurance **▼ Figure 10-15** . Patients should be transported emergently to the hospital in a comfortable sitting position if conscious and alert. For patients who have a decreased level of consciousness or who cannot maintain the sitting position, transportation should be accomplished by placing the patient onto the side of the body with the deficit and providing slight elevation for the head. This lateral position allows the airway to be monitored and more easily maintained in the event that the patient vomits and also protects the patient's body from injury.

Generalized Weakness
Patients may have generalized weakness either because of a primary neurological disease or a general medical illness. In many cases, the weakness will be progressive and lead to a decreased ability to breathe and possible exhaustion from expending so much energy to do so. These patients are extraordinarily sensitive to any medication that interferes with the metabolism or function of nervous system tissue. Do not give respiratory depressants

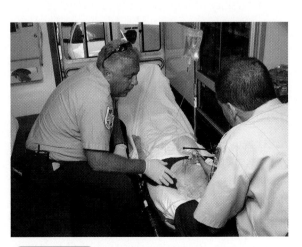

Figure 10-15   Care for patients with one-sided weakness, a possible stroke sign, includes oxygen, gentle handling, and reassurance.

(sedatives, narcotic pain relievers) to any patient with motor weakness unless you are prepared to intubate and provide ventilatory assistance.

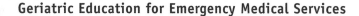

Medication Tip

Remember that generalized weakness can be caused or worsened by certain medications.

Altered Mental Status

Always assume that an older individual who is behaving erratically, unreasonably, irrationally, or aggressively is suffering from an organic (physical) disorder until proven otherwise. It is uncommon for mental disorders of strictly psychiatric origins to begin in late life. Most commonly, even in older individuals with a known or long-standing psychiatric disorder, a change in the usual pattern of behavior or thinking that brings the patient to the attention of EMS is a "red flag" for a medical problem. In addition, recall that when headache, fever, or stiff neck accompanies confusion or a change in behavior, the most likely cause is meningitis, encephalitis, or subarachnoid hemorrhage. In the older patient with an altered mental status, prehospital treatment should include ensuring the adequacy of the ABCs. Provide supplemental oxygen. Assess for the presence of a stroke or recent trauma as a possible cause for the altered mental status. Hypotension should be managed with IV fluids. Be alert for signs of fluid overload. Lung sounds should be monitored prior to fluid therapy and frequently thereafter. Consider the possibility of hypoglycemia or a narcotic overdose. Monitor the patient's blood glucose level and provide dextrose as necessary. If a narcotic overdose is suspected, administer naloxone (Narcan) per local protocol.

Seizures

Patients who have an abnormal neurological examination after a seizure should be transported with urgency, especially those with fever, stiff neck, unequal pupil size, or focal motor weakness, because this may indicate the presence of an underlying medical condition that is causing the seizure, such as meningitis. Remember that there will be a postictal period following the seizure when the patient becomes gradually more alert and oriented, but continues to be confused and acts in an awkward manner. All patients who are actively seizing should be protected from further injury by removing objects from around the patient and by preventing the patient from falling. Patients who are seizing should never be forcefully restrained as this may lead to injury. Once the seizure has stopped, oxygen should be given to the patient. If the patient is uncooperative, which is likely because of postictal confusion, the oxygen should be delivered by having a provider hold a nonrebreathing mask near the patient's face. Hypoglycemia may also cause seizures, and blood sugar should be determined if a glucometer is available. If blood glucose levels are found to be low, dextrose or glucose should be administered in accordance with local protocols. An IV should also be established on seizure patients, in case the patient develops multiple seizures without a return to full level of consciousness between each seizure, a potentially fatal condition known as **status epilepticus**. For patients who are determined to be in status epilepticus, the administration of diazepam (Valium) should be considered based upon local protocols, and these patients should be emergently transported to the closest appropriate hospital with pillows and blankets padding all hard objects near the patient.

Controversy

The use of restraints is not recommended in older patients. Restraints can injure an older person's fragile skin, and can threaten their sense of control and independence, which is often already a major concern. However, if you are alone with a violent patient who is a threat to himself or herself, or you, on a long transport, and you have tried to calm the patient without success, restraints may be considered as a last resort. This is only an option if you have exhausted all other avenues and you or the patient will be harmed as a result of not using restraints. When using restraints, place them on the patient with extreme gentleness and care. Continue to try to calm the patient by looking the patient in the eye and addressing him or her in a low-pitched, soothing voice. In general, the use of restraints is not condoned and is a last-resort measure.

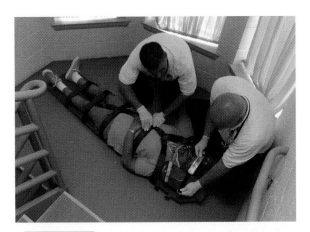

Figure 10-16   Always assume that both the brain and spinal cord have been injured when an older individual falls or is "found down."

Head and Spine Trauma

Emergency care of head and spine trauma is covered in Chapter 7. Remember to always assume that both the brain and the spinal cord have been injured when an older person falls or is found on the ground ▲ **Figure 10-16**.

Intervention, Management, and Transport: Behavioral Emergencies

Behavior That Is Potentially Threatening to the Patient

The first step in intervention and management of self-directed aggressive behavior is recognition. Be vigilant for signs of depression, such as depressed mood and somber affect. All patients suspected of depression should be assessed for suicidal thoughts. Ask in a tactful but direct manner whether they have thoughts of doing self-harm, if they have a plan to enact such thoughts, and if so, whether they have a means by which to enact the plan. (For example, "Do you think you might harm yourself?" "Have you thought about how you might harm yourself?" "Do you have a type of weapon?") Provide reassurance to the patient and stay within arm's length of a patient who has suicidal thinking, or closer if the patient is actively attempting self-harm. Chapter 11 addresses depression and suicide in more depth.

Behavior That Is Potentially Threatening to the Caregiver

Older individuals with severe depression or dementia may react with aggressive behavior toward caregivers. Patients with advanced brain disease may become aggressive or severely agitated because they do not perceive the world normally. Aggressive behavior is often the result of internal fears that are outwardly directed. Assess the situation and the patient's response to a calm, nonthreatening manner and verbal reassurance. If the patient does not respond to these primary strategies, consider giving medication prior to transport. If the situation is potentially explosive, call for police assistance. A "show of force" by a backup team provides realistic and visual assurance to the patient that aggression will be controlled, and may be all that is needed to encourage the patient to abandon the aggressive attitude.

Controversy

Sedating violent patients ("chemical restraint") is a procedure to use carefully in a limited number of circumstances—particularly in older patients who may be at higher risk than most of adverse reactions to the sedative. Some EMS systems do not allow it at all. If yours does, follow local protocol and monitor the patient closely.

Uncooperative Patients and Refusal of Transport

When faced with an obviously ill patient who is uncooperative with the history and examination, the EMS provider will need to assess the environment and question those near the patient for information. Important information can be ascertained from environmental clues and witnesses. Be sure to examine the area for any medications. If head or spinal trauma is suspected in the uncooperative patient, use a cervical collar and backboard.

A typical example is the intoxicated patient who has fallen. When a patient appears ill and refuses transport, make a quick assessment of the patient's ability to make appropriate judgments ▶ **Figure 10-17**. For instance, a patient with dementia may not be able to make good judgments

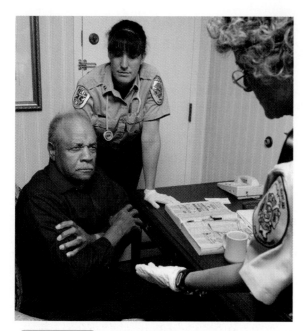

Figure 10-17 When a patient appears ill and refuses transport, make a quick assessment of the patient's ability to make appropriate judgments.

about his or her safety. Relay this information to the appropriate supervisor or individual responsible for assisting with these decisions. In extreme cases, assistance from police officers may be appropriate.

Prevention

Trauma

Many falls result from disorders of gait, balance, or vision. Point out obstructions and hazards in the environment to patients with unsteady gait or problems with balance and vision, and recommend or help with obvious solutions. Reinforce the use of assistive walking devices and proper footwear and eyewear.

Motor Vehicle Crashes

Reinforce to older individuals the practice of periodic driver safety training and hearing and vision testing. Encourage older patients to use seat belts at all times. Also encourage patients, particularly those with vision problems or dementia, to ask their doctor if it is still safe for them to drive, or if they need to modify their driving.

Physical Abuse

Provide a nonconfrontational, nonjudgmental message that physical abuse is not acceptable and should not be tolerated or condoned. Provide information on local shelters or safe houses for abused persons. All victims of abuse should be treated with dignity and sensitivity and transported to the nearest medical center with special expertise in this physical and psychosocial disorder. Elder abuse is covered in detail in Chapter 14.

Stroke

Remind patients that regular medical examinations result in the detection of risk factors for stroke, and that the risk factors are treatable. Encourage the use of all medications as prescribed by the physician, healthy dietary choices, and an active lifestyle including routine exercise.

Toxicities

Metabolic and Systemic
Encourage daily maintenance of the routine medical plan prescribed by a physician for chronic metabolic and systemic illnesses such as diabetes and renal disease.

Attitude Tip

Your role in caring for older patients can be an even more valuable one if you look for opportunities to counsel them about prevention.

Drug Interactions
Encourage older individuals to ask questions of their physician and pharmacist about their medications. Strongly recommend that the patient maintain one pharmacist who will be aware of all medication changes and who can provide information about drug interactions. Educate patients that they should never take more medication than prescribed by their doctor, and should never take someone else's prescription medications. Patients on multiple medications or on blood thinners should check with their health care provider before starting any new medicines, including cold remedies and vitamins. If available, medical

history cards should be offered to older patients who are being treated for numerous medical conditions, to allow rapid access to the patient's list of medications and medical conditions (see Appendix B for an example). This may also prevent an interaction from occurring if medications need to be administered in the prehospital setting.

Poisonings and Medication Misuse

Denial of illness and loss of vision, reading skills, memory, and income all contribute to medication misuse and accidental poisoning. Suggest organizational strategies such as noting when medications are taken on a calendar, and using inexpensive weekly pillboxes (▶ **Figure 10-18**). If necessary, suggest that another individual check in with the patient to ensure medications are taken properly.

Addiction

Provide a nonconfrontational, nonjudgmental message that illicit drug use is not acceptable and should not be tolerated or condoned. Provide information on local treatment centers for addicted persons and also assure the patient that there is no need to be embarrassed about seeking help with a drug or alcohol problem.

Depression and Suicide

Depression is treatable, yet the nature of this disorder tends to prevent those who have it from seeking treatment. If you suspect depression or

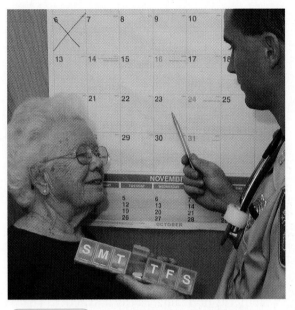

Figure 10-18 To help prevent medication misuse, suggest organizational strategies such as noting when medications are taken on a calendar, and using inexpensive weekly pillboxes.

suicide potential (see Chapter 11), refer the patient to a health care provider who can give support by helping the patient recognize the disorder and accept treatment. Encourage routine follow up as advised by the physician or mental health worker, and adherence to daily medications as prescribed.

Case Study Summaries

Your assessment reveals a 73-year-old woman who appears alert, but unable to speak, and who has weakness in the right arm. She has no significant history and takes no medications, but is allergic to penicillin. You learn from the son that he received the telephone call from his mother within the hour. He states that his mother is normally healthy and active. The patient's vital signs are a blood pressure of 160/100 mm Hg, a pulse of 92 beats/min, and a respiratory rate of 12 breaths/min.

Treatment for this patient should include high-flow oxygen (90%–100%), IV access, and ECG monitoring. Consultation should be made with the closest appropriate emergency department as soon as possible—ideally with a facility that specializes in stroke treatment or offers thrombolytic therapy. From the presentation and history, this patient is likely experiencing evolving stroke manifesting with, among other things, aphasia. This is evidenced by the patient's inability to verbalize. You have learned from the son that the patient was healthy and active until an hour ago. This patient is likely to benefit from aggressive and rapid treatment, which must begin in the prehospital setting.

The brain and the spinal cord are the portions of the nervous system that are most vulnerable in falls, but individual nerves that are proximally located to bone fractures are also vulnerable.

The patient's mental status is reassuring in that he is awake and seems to have an examination similar to his baseline. However, it is not reassuring because an epidural hematoma may result from the fall, giving rise to a normal or baseline mental status examination at outset, but followed by rapid deterioration to lethargy and coma.

It is possible that there is no significance to the incontinence of urine; Alzheimer's patients are frequently incontinent. It could also be a clue to a seizure due to meningitis, encephalitis, subarachnoid hemorrhage, serotonin syndrome, or to a focal brain lesion such as tumor, or the result of a urinary tract infection leading to sepsis. Do not forget that the patient's diagnosis of dementia requiring 24-hour supervision is handled with variable degrees of patience and frustration by caregivers, and incontinence may have led to abusive caregiver behavior inciting the fall. Check for varying stages of healing of the body bruises, which can give you a clue about prior abuse.

Common neurological causes of falls in the older population include disorders of posture and gait such as parkinsonism, prior stroke with residual disability, new onset stroke, neurogenic syncope, Guillain-Barré syndrome; chronic and acute effects of alcohol, medications, or toxins on the nervous system; and the effects of acute systemic medical illness on the nervous system such as sepsis, myocardial infarction, heart failure, and metabolic derangements such as hypoglycemia, and nonketotic hyperosmolar hyperglycemia.

Your assessment reveals a patient who is conscious and alert, but speaks inappropriately when questioned or asked to repeat a phrase. You were told that this episode had a sudden onset. The initial presentation of this patient could lead you to think of several possibilities, such as hypoglycemia, acute stroke onset, delirium, or a progression of the patient's dementia. Knowing the patient to be "borderline diabetic," you obtained a glucose reading of 104. You noted that the patient had no facial droop or arm drift. This should lead you to think that the patient's emergency is due to either delirium or the progression of dementia.

From this chapter, you know that dementia progresses gradually. This patient had a sudden onset of symptoms, evidenced by the daughter's description that the patient was fine all day but suddenly became confused and began speaking inappropriately. She also has difficulty sustaining attention to your questions. The sudden onset and the difficulty with attention are hallmarks of delirium. People who have dementia can have some fluctuation in their thinking,

however, so it is imperative to confirm with the caregiver that this is different from her usual behavior. People with dementia can very easily become delirious, so history of pain from someone who knows the patient well is very useful in diagnosing delirium in a patient with dementia.

Using the DELIRIUMS mnemonic, you can attempt to determine a probable cause (though recognition of delirium is the most important step—definitive diagnosis can be made later at the emergency department). Treatment should include oxygen, establishment of an IV, ECG monitoring if available, and transportation to the emergency department with notification to the receiving physician. Often, delirious patients are very frightened and may quickly become agitated; be certain to approach them slowly, make eye contact, and explain everything that is happening in a clear, nonthreatening voice. Sometimes family members can be invaluable in keeping the patient calm.

This patient was diagnosed with a urinary tract infection and admitted for treatment.

Endnotes

1. Olney RK. The Neurology of aging. In: Aminoff MJ, ed: *Neurology and General Medicine*. 3rd ed. Philadelphia, PA: Churchill Livingstone; 2001.

2. Hauser R, Zesiewicz, T. *Parkinson's Disease: Questions and Answers*. 3rd ed. Merit Publishing International; 2000.

3. Smith M, Burns D, Robinson D. Geriatric seizures, letter to the editor. *J Am Geriatr Soc*. 2002;50(5): 974–975.

Psychiatric Emergencies

1 Describe the epidemiology of depression, suicide, and substance abuse in older people, including incidence, morbidity/mortality, risk factors, and prevention strategies.

2 Identify the need for intervention and transport and develop a treatment and management plan for the older patient experiencing a psychological emergency.

3 Discuss assessment findings and management considerations for older patients who have abused drugs or alcohol.

CHAPTER

James R. Pierce, LCDR, NC, USN

Christopher Schmidt, LCDR, NC, USN

You are dispatched to the home of a 78-year-old man complaining of weakness and difficulty breathing. Upon receiving the address, you recognize it as the same apartment you have responded to three times in the past week; twice the patient elected not to be transported after a normal physical assessment. This retired Army officer's history of lung cancer, hypertension, and coronary artery disease is well known to you and your partner. You arrive and find the patient sitting in a chair and in no apparent distress. Vital signs are normal. Physical exam is unremarkable except for the odor of alcohol on the patient's breath. Scene assessment reveals an apartment in complete disarray, with dirty laundry, dishes, and trash scattered about. The patient is disheveled in appearance, wearing dirty clothes, and in need of a bath. In your interview, you learn that the patient's wife of 50 years recently died. Children are grown and live out of state. He tells you he doesn't mean to be a burden and you "probably shouldn't bother" taking care of him.

Should you transport this patient to the emergency department even though his physical exam is normal?

Is there anything in your initial assessment that causes you concern regarding the risk of suicide?

Psychiatric Emergencies

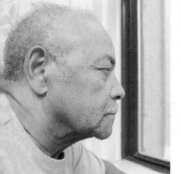

Introduction

For the majority of older people, the later years are ones of fulfillment and satisfaction with a lifetime of accomplishments. Children are grown up, grandchildren are a blessing, and one's life work is mostly completed. For some older adults, however, later life is characterized by physical pain, psychological distress, doubts about significance of life's accomplishments, financial concerns, loss of loved ones, dissatisfaction with living conditions, and seemingly unbearable disability. When these factors lead to hopelessness about the possibility for positive change in their lives, depression, substance abuse, and unfortunately even suicide are possible outcomes. Substance abuse, particularly alcohol and drug abuse and misuse, often is underestimated, underdiagnosed, and undertreated among older adults. The EMS provider is often the first health care professional to have contact with an older adult suffering these afflictions. This chapter discusses epidemiology, causes, recognition, and clinical management of depression, suicide, and alcohol or substance abuse to assist the EMS provider in recognizing the significance of identifying and caring for these specific psychiatric emergencies in the older adult.

Depression

<u>Depression</u> is a common, often debilitating, psychiatric disorder experienced by approximately 2 million older American adults. Older adults residing in skilled nursing facilities are even more likely to be depressed, with as many as 30% suffering from some degree of clinical depression.[1] Depression is diagnosed three times more commonly in women than in men. In contrast to the normal emotional experiences of sadness, grief, loss, or temporary "bad moods," depression is extreme and persistent and can interfere significantly with an older adult's ability to function. It is impossible to predict which older adults will develop depression, but studies indicate that substance abuse, isolation, prescription medication use, and chronic medical conditions all contribute to the onset of significant depression

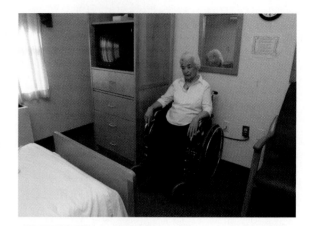

Figure 11-1   Isolation and chronic medical problems are among the factors that contribute to depression in older adults.

▲ **Figure 11-1** . The American Psychological Association lists these nine symptoms of major depression[2]:

1. Depressed mood most of the day, nearly every day, as indicated by either patient saying so (patient reports feeling sad, empty, "blue") or observation made by others.

2. Markedly diminished interest or pleasure in all, or almost all, activities.

3. Significant unintended weight loss or gain (more than 5% change in body weight over 1 month).

4. Insomnia or hypersomnia nearly every day.

5. Either physical agitation such as pacing, shaking, or rocking, or physical immobility nearly every day (observable by others, not merely subjective report of restlessness or lethargy).

6. Fatigue or lack of energy nearly every day.

7. Feelings of worthlessness or excessive or inappropriate guilt nearly every day.

8. Diminished ability to think or concentrate, or indecisiveness nearly every day.

9. Recurrent thoughts of death (not just fear of dying).

These can also be remembered by the mnemonic OPQRST:

♦ Orientation—Is the patient oriented to time, person, place, and event?

♦ **P**rovokes/palliates—What does the patient enjoy? Why were you called?

♦ **Q**uality of life—Does the patient have a recent or pending loss?

♦ **R**elationships/reassurance—Does the patient have family, friends, or support groups?

♦ **S**uicidal ideation/past attempts—Does the patient make references to suicide? Does the patient have plans and the means to commit suicide?

♦ **T**ime/treatment history—When did the symptoms begin, and how long have they lasted? Has the patient been treated?

Suspect depression when the patient has problems with four or more of these symptoms.

Most of these symptoms require a great deal of time, a quiet environment, and a well-established relationship to assess adequately. Other health care providers are rarely afforded the luxury of time or control over the older patient's environment, so it is vital that EMS providers are vigilant in making observations and aware of certain "red flags" indicating depression.

Red Flags: Possible Depression

♦ *Frequent non-urgent EMS calls.* All EMS systems have clients who appear to overuse the system. These "frequent fliers" are a source of great frustration for many EMS providers, and more importantly, divert valuable resources away from more urgent patient needs. These habitual users also represent one of the most dangerous traps for EMS providers. A sense of complacency when caring for the same non-urgent patient multiple times is natural ("Oh, it's just Mr. Jones again; he's never really sick,"), but very risky for EMS providers. For the older adult, frequent contact with caring, competent professionals may be an important part of the social support network. If an older adult begins to call frequently for EMS response, especially for non-urgent complaints, the health care team must assess for the presence of significant depression. Non-urgent complaints may be this person's desperate call for help, even if he or she is unaware of it.

♦ *Frequent visits to emergency department or physician's office.* Many older adults are able to

gain access to health care on their own. Any older adult who seeks contact with the health care system frequently, but has no chronic or complicated medical problem, must be considered for the possibility of depression.

♦ *Severity of complaint does not match physical findings.* Patient complaints of pain or discomfort that seems disproportionate to the amount of abnormality on physical examination can be troubling to the EMS provider. In the older adult, complaints of pain that seem more severe than the injury or condition should produce may be a sign of depression (▼ **Figure 11-2**). The EMS provider must guard against discounting the patient's complaints of pain and remain cognizant of the personal, subjective aspects of pain perception.

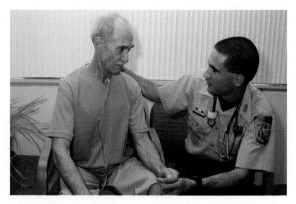

Figure 11-2 Do not automatically discount pain complaints that are out of proportion to physical exam findings. This may be a sign of depression.

♦ *Poor personal hygiene or neglect of home cleanliness and order.* Older adults suffering from depression often lose interest in keeping their environment clean and orderly. Personal hygiene is frequently neglected due to a lack of energy or a sense that "it doesn't matter."

♦ *Lack of social support network.* It is important for EMS providers to assess an older adult's support network. A patient who reports no contact with family, friends, or social or religious organizations is at a significantly higher risk of clinical depression than one who does have such contacts.

♦ *Anhedonia.* **Anhedonia**, or the sense that nothing is enjoyable anymore, is an important sign of significant depression that EMS providers can easily ask about. A simple question like, "What do you do for fun?" will often elicit an answer that alerts the provider to serious depression.

Impact

Major depression, a significant predictor of suicide in older adults, is a widely underrecognized and undertreated medical illness. In fact, several studies have found that many older adults who commit suicide have visited a primary care physician very close to the time of the suicide: 20% on the same day, 40% within one week, and 70% within one month.[3] These findings illustrate the importance of identifying older adults suffering from depression and initiating some meaningful intervention. Emergency personnel who are astute and aware of the symptoms listed earlier can be instrumental in this identification, and can help prevent deterioration to suicidal intent. Suicide in the older population is discussed in more depth later in this chapter.

Suicide can be the ultimate, tragic outcome of untreated clinical depression, but the depressed older adult suffers from other problems as well. Several studies have found that a depressed older adult has a significantly higher mortality from *all* causes. Some of this increase in mortality may be due to the tendency of depressed older adults to be less adherent to health practices such as diet and medication regimens, but good evidence exists that physiologic changes associated with severe depression degrade both the immune and cardiovascular systems. Studies of trauma victims also suggest that depressed older adults have a higher incidence of all forms of trauma, especially falls (▼ Figure 11-3). Major depression will almost always lead to cognitive impairment, most markedly memory loss. Dementia, Alzheimer's disease, and "senility" have often been diagnosed in older adults when the real origin of their memory loss and inability to function independently was clinical depression.

Screening for Depression

The Geriatric Depression Scale (▶ Table 11-1) can be used to assess an older adult's level of depression. A score of 5 or above in the older patient may indicate depression. Though use of the full scale may not be practical in the prehospital environment, the concepts can still be valuable in spotting signs of depression during patient assessment.

Treatment

Treatment of severe depression in the older adult usually consists of psychological counseling, medication, or a combination of both. For many older adults, simply reestablishing relationships with the community or with family is enough to lessen the severity of the illness. Senior citizen centers, community meeting places, social clubs, and other community outreach programs offer older adults a chance to build social networks that are extremely helpful in combating depression. Many older adults find participation in an organized

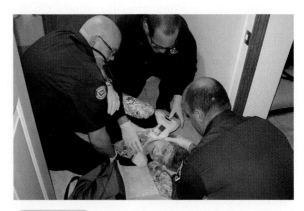

Figure 11-3　Depressed older adults have a higher incidence of trauma, especially falls.

TABLE 11-1 Geriatric Depression Scale Short Form

1. Are you basically satisfied with your life?	(no)
2. Have you dropped many of your activities and interests?	(yes)
3. Do you feel that your life is empty?	(yes)
4. Do you often get bored?	(yes)
5. Are you in good spirits most of the time?	(no)
6. Are you afraid that something bad is going to happen to you?	(yes)
7. Do you feel happy most of the time?	(no)
8. Do you often feel helpless?	(yes)
9. Do you prefer to stay home most of the time rather than go out and do new things?	(yes)
10. Do you feel that you have more problems with memory than most?	(yes)
11. Do you think it is wonderful to be alive now?	(no)
12. Do you feel pretty worthless the way you are now?	(yes)
13. Do you feel full of energy?	(no)
14. Do you feel your situation is hopeless?	(yes)
15. Do you think that most persons are better off than you?	(yes)

Scoring:
Score one point for each response that matches the yes or no answer after the question. Scores of 5 or greater indicate probable depression. These patients should be referred for more extensive evaluation and treatment.

Adapted from the University of Rochester from Yesavage. Use of Self-Rating Depression Scales in the Elderly. In: LW Poon, ed. *Handbook for Clinical Memory Assessment of Older Adults*. Washington, DC: American Psychological Association; 1986.

religion to be especially helpful. One large study showed that pet ownership significantly reduced the incidence of depression in older adults. It seems that any activity that increases social support and relieves isolation is helpful in fighting depression. In addition, physical exercise may also combat depression, and in one study was as effective as antidepressant medication.

Communication Tip

Any activity that increases social support and relieves isolation is helpful in fighting depression.

Antidepressant medications are widely used and effective treatments for depression. Antide-

pressant drugs influence the functioning of certain chemicals (neurotransmitters) in the brain. Tricyclic antidepressants and monoamine oxidase inhibitors are very effective drugs, but can have serious side effects. The newer antidepressants—selective serotonin reuptake inhibitors (SSRIs)—are very effective in treating depression and are associated with much lower levels of side effects. The key to any drug therapy for depression is to encourage adherence, especially at the onset of therapy when effects are less noticeable. Table 11-2 lists medications used to treat depression in older people.

EMS providers should become aware of the senior services available in their area of coverage. Most communities have outreach programs in place to keep older adults in contact with social

TABLE 11-2	Medications Used to Treat Depression in Older People
Medication Type	**Generic Name (Brand Name)**
Tricyclic antidepressants	Amitriptyline (Elavil, Endep); Desipramine (Norparmin); Nortriptyline (Aventyl, Pamelor); Protriptyline (Vivactil)
Monoamine oxidase (MAO) inhibitors	Phenelzine (Nardil); Tranylcypromine (Parnate)
Selective serotonin reuptake inhibitors (SSRIs)	Citalopram (Celexa) Fluoxetine (Prozac) Fluvoxamine (Luvox) Paroxetine (Paxil) Sertraline (Zoloft)
Other	Bupropion (Wellbutrin) Nefazodone (Serzone) Mirtazapine (Remeron) Trazadone (Desyrel) Venlafaxine (Effexor)

systems (eg, Meals On Wheels), contact that has been shown to be vital in both the treatment and prevention of clinical depression (▼ Figure 11-4), and many resources are available for psychiatric counseling and treatment.

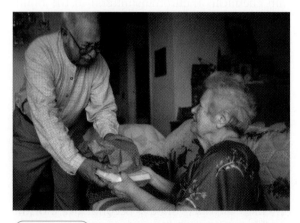

Figure 11-4 Social services with outreach programs provide contact that is valuable in preventing and treating depression.

Suicide

Older adult males have the highest suicide rate of any age group in the United States. In 1999, older adults made up 12.7% of the population, but committed 18.8% of the suicides.[4] In that same year, one older person committed suicide every hour and 35 minutes in America. That equals 5,489 deaths of older Americans that may have been avoided if those at risk had been identified and intervention initiated, though it is believed that some depression may be resistant to treatment. It is also estimated that as many as half of all suicides committed by older people go unreported, mistakenly classified as accidents, death by natural causes, or some other form of trauma.[4]

Equally concerning is the fact that older persons who attempt suicide choose much more lethal means than younger victims and generally have diminished recuperative capacity to survive an attempt. For the young, it is estimated that there are 100 to 200 attempts for every completed suicide; in the older population, that figure drops to only four attempts to one completion.[4] Over 71% of completed suicides in older persons involve firearms, as compared to just over 55% in the general population (▼ Table 11-3).[4]

Males of all age groups are more than four times as likely to complete suicide than females, yet females attempt suicide three times as often. This discrepancy in the attempts-to-completions ratios arises because males tend to use firearms over 60% of the time, whereas females use other, less lethal means in most of their attempts. Wid-

TABLE 11-3	Methods of Completed Suicides in Older Persons
Firearms	71%
Poisoning/overdose	19%
Motor vehicle crashes	3%
Jumps/falls	2%
Other (eg, hanging, carbon monoxide inhalation)	5%

Source: National Institutes of Health, 1999.

owed white males are at particularly high risk, with suicide rates almost double the average for all groups.

Etiology of Suicide

Suicide can happen in any family, regardless of socioeconomic class, culture, race, or religious affiliation. Research suggests that some circumstances increase the risk of suicide in the older adult.

Death of a Loved One

As adults reach later years of life, loss of significant people in their lives, including family, friends, and spouses, becomes inevitable. Often the surviving person is left with feelings of abandonment, guilt, fear, and loneliness. Loss of a spouse or significant other, often one who has shared the person's life for decades, can be especially devastating (▼ **Figure 11-5**).

Physical Illness

Physical illnesses common in older adults can affect mood, self-esteem, independence, and sense of well-being. Along with the psychological pressures associated with physical illness often come economic insecurity and reliance on some form of public assistance (eg, Medicare, Medicaid), which may deepen the feelings of diminished self-worth and dependency.

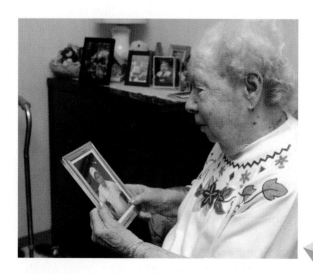

Figure 11-5   Death of a spouse or significant other can increase the risk of suicide.

Depression and Hopelessness

As discussed earlier in this chapter, depression is a very common, serious problem for many older adults. Research suggests that lifetime risk of suicide in the general population is about 1%, compared to 15% in persons suffering from depression.[4]

Although usually difficult to assess and even more difficult to quantify, hopelessness seems to be the biggest risk factor for suicide in all age groups. No matter how bad a current situation appears, if one can see the "light at the end of the tunnel" and has a reasonable expectation that life will improve, suicide becomes less of an option. Multiple studies of suicide-attempt survivors have revealed almost universal feelings of hopelessness prior to the attempt. The older adult who truly feels that his or her life circumstances are hopeless is at an extremely high risk of imminent suicide.

Attitude Tip

The older adult who feels that his or her life circumstances are hopeless is at extremely high risk of suicide. Keep this in mind during your assessment.

Isolation

Many older adults have difficulty with mobility due to physical illness. This can lead to social isolation and feelings of diminished self-worth. Death of friends and relatives may further isolate older people. Loneliness resulting from social isolation has also been shown to contribute to suicidal thoughts.

Alcohol Abuse and Dependence

A direct relationship exists between alcoholism and suicide. Studies indicate that risk of suicide in alcoholics is 50% to 70% greater than in the general population. Between 40% and 60% of the alcoholics suffer from depression as well as alcoholism; the combination of these risk factors is especially concerning.

Loss of Meaningful Life Roles

Significant changes in life's roles often result in feelings of hopelessness and low self-esteem associated with suicide. Retirement, moving out of long-time family homes, and inability to continue in community projects and work often contribute to a sense of isolation experienced by many older adults.

Screening for Suicide Potential

Frequently, the EMS provider is the first-line, and for some older patients, the only health care contact. Keep in mind that only a small percentage pursue medical treatment for psychological issues. Not only do many fail to seek care, but they frequently deny the problem when questioned. These conditions cross the entire socioeconomic spectrum. Afflicted older adults may be found in nursing homes, their own homes or apartments, prisons, homeless shelters, and on the street ▼ **Figure 11-6** .

Sections earlier in this chapter provide screening tools to help detect depression in older persons, and later sections describe tools to detect harmful drinking. It is equally important to screen for suicide. The following text discusses important warning signs every EMS provider should be aware of when interacting with the older patient.

Talking About or Seeming Preoccupied with Death

It is common for older adults to contemplate the end of life and try to "get their affairs in order." When an older adult begins to talk excessively about death, especially at the expense of other

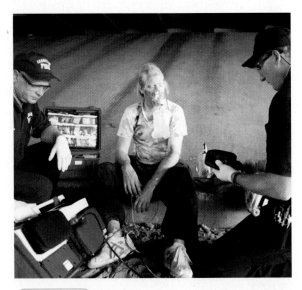

Figure 11-6 Substance abuse and depression cross the entire socioeconomic spectrum, affecting the older population in their own homes, in institutions, and among the homeless.

topics that used to interest them, their risk of suicide must be assessed.

Giving Away Prized Possessions

The older adult contemplating suicide will often give family heirlooms, photographs, and other keepsakes away. EMS providers are seen as caring, concerned professionals who are always there to help, and therefore may also receive gifts. Gifts that are expensive or represent some significant personal event in the patient's life are the provider's clues to <u>suicidal ideation</u> (thoughts or plans). Distributing prized possessions to family members can also be a last attempt at maintaining some control over life circumstances and avoiding "causing trouble" with their suicide.

Taking Unnecessary Risks

Suicide carries a certain stigma among many people. In fact, many religions teach that anyone who takes his or her own life has committed the ultimate "sin." One way to avoid an active role in one's own death is to put yourself at unnecessary risk through behavior. Walking alone in unsafe neighborhoods, driving with excessive speed without wearing a seat belt, and seeking confrontation with police or other imposing figures are all examples of behavior that may be an attempt to end life in a more "acceptable" way than suicide.

Increased Use of Alcohol or Other Drugs

In an attempt to lessen the feelings of hopelessness and depression associated with suicidal ideation, many older adults will turn to alcohol or other drugs as a means of escape. If EMS providers witness evidence of excessive alcohol or drug use at the scene of a response for an older adult, the patient must be assessed for suicide risk.

Nonadherence to Medical Regimens

Failure to take prescribed medications, follow special diets, or perform other basic health care needs may result in frequent EMS calls and generally poorer health. This is often also a sign that an older adult has "given up" and may be contemplating suicide ▶ **Figure 11-7** .

Acquiring a Weapon

Most suicides committed by older adults involve firearms. The older adult who suddenly purchases a firearm but had no prior interest in guns should alert caregivers to the potential for self-harm.

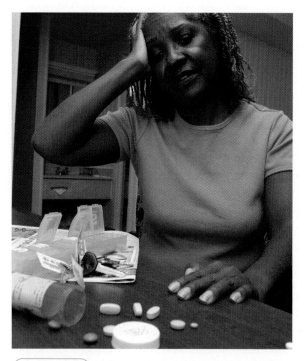

Figure 11-7 Failure to take medications or attend to other health needs can be a sign that an older adult has given up and may be contemplating suicide.

Many who are not contemplating suicide acquire a weapon to protect their family and home, but any older adult who purchases a firearm should be questioned in regard to motivation.

DOs and DON'Ts for Patients at Risk of Suicide

1. DO transport any older adult about whom you have concerns regarding suicide, regardless of your physical assessment findings.

2. DO voice your concerns to the emergency department staff, both verbally and in your run documentation.

3. DO take any verbal statements by the patient seriously. Seemingly meaningless comments about suicide may be the only warning sign before a serious attempt.

4. DO protect the patient from any further attempts. Secure potentially dangerous items in the home, the ambulance, and the emergency department.

5. DO ask directly if he or she is thinking about suicide. Bringing up the topic of suicide will not "plant the seed" and cause a nonsuicidal person to consider it. On the contrary, a direct question and a professional response to any answer conveys trust and a genuine concern for the patient's welfare.

6. DO be nonjudgmental. Never debate whether suicide is right or wrong, or feelings are good or bad. Lectures on the value of life to a suicidal patient are not helpful.

7. DO offer hope that alternatives are available.

8. DON'T let the mechanism of injury (suicide attempt) cloud your clinical judgment. Trust your training in the initial assessment and physical exam. Physical injury takes precedence over psychological intervention.

9. DON'T leave the actively suicidal patient unattended, even for a brief period.

10. DON'T be sworn to secrecy. Seek support from colleagues, emergency department staff, and outside agencies if needed.

Take Care of Yourself

Responding to a completed suicide is one of the most difficult tasks faced by an EMS provider. It is vital that some form of incident or stress debriefing be made available to allow the provider to deal with the normal feelings of frustration, anger, helplessness, and possibly guilt associated with these cases. The professional stoicism often displayed by EMS providers serves them well while at the scene, dealing with loved ones or calming an upset patient, but the emotional stress resulting from responding to a suicide must be acknowledged and coped with. Staff in most hospitals that treat critically ill and injured patients have a mechanism in place to care for one another after stressful incidents. EMS providers at times need to avail themselves of these resources and constructively deal with the feelings normally generated by responding to disturbing calls.

Chemical Dependency and Substance Abuse

Chemical dependency and **substance abuse** are problems among the older population. It is forecast that, as the number of people over age 65 in our country increases, this dilemma too will grow. Chemical dependency can include addiction to both alcohol and drugs. It may also involve abuse of prescription or over-the-counter (OTC) medications or unlawful street drugs. An **addiction** occurs when an older adult has an overwhelming desire or need to continue using a substance at whatever cost, with a tendency to increase the amount or dose.[5]

Epidemiology

Research estimates that approximately 10% of the older population, or up to 3 million people over the age of 60, suffer from chemical dependency—alcohol-related problems in particular—at a cost to hospitals of $60 billion annually.[6] One study noted the rate of alcohol-related admissions for older adults to be comparable with that of cardiac events (heart attack).[7] Unfortunately, alcohol and drug abuse in the older patient are often not identified, and thus not reported. Several factors contribute to this phenomenon. Symptoms of alcoholism or medication misuse or abuse may be mistaken by the EMS provider, physician, or family member as signs of dementia or depression. Surprisingly, some family members believe their older relative's drinking is the only "cure-all" to combat loneliness or depression. Family members may also be ashamed or embarrassed about their older relative's addiction, and as a result, fail to help the patient seek medical care (▼ **Figure 11-8**).

Compared to younger adults, older alcoholics are less likely to have criminal background records or difficulties with the police. They are seldom menacing or disorderly. They have lower rates of divorce, financial problems or bankruptcy, violence, and involvement in motor vehicle collisions while driving under the influence of alcohol. Many live alone, are isolated, and lack the assistance of a support system. As a result, the older person is less likely to be identified and referred for treatment.

Substance abuse has the potential of affecting the older person's ability to care for chronic medical conditions. The afflicted older patient may have difficulty keeping routine doctor appointments, complying with medication directions, or seeking medical help when it is needed.

Men are five times more likely than women to drink, become heavy drinkers, and become alcoholics.[8] Additionally, men are more apt to become heavy drinkers early in life (▼ **Table 11-4**). Women who drink are more likely to start later in life. Most disturbing is the fact that alcohol and depression correlate closely with suicide in the older adult.

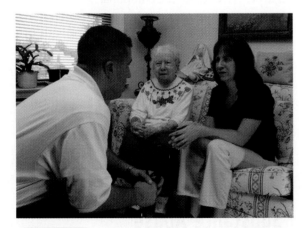

Figure 11-8 Family members of an older adult with a substance abuse problem may be ashamed to help the patient seek care.

TABLE 11-4   Early-onset Versus Late-onset Drinking

Early Onset	Late Onset
Drinking prior to age 60	Drinking mostly after age 60
Numerous medical conditions	Precipitated by a stressful event (death, loss of job, retirement)
Majority are socially isolated	More likely to have psychosocial support of family, friends
High rate of nonadherence to treatment	More responsive to rehab, therapy
More men than women	More women than men
Higher mortality rate	

Medication Misuse and Abuse

Medication or substance misuse and abuse may be considered by some to be interchangeable terms; however, they have very different meanings. **Medication misuse** is an unintentional or willful use of a medication in a way that differs from its prescribed dose or intent. Examples include the following:

◆ Taking several old or unused antibiotic pills for a sore throat from last year's prescription for strep pharyngitis, with the thought that this sore throat is also strep pharyngitis.

◆ An individual ingesting double or triple the dose of over-the-counter Tylenol for a headache, thinking a higher dose of the medication will improve symptoms more quickly.

◆ Failing to take the entire course of antibiotics.

On the other hand, **medication or substance abuse** is a deliberate use of a drug for nonmedicinal reasons. Most often, it occurs because the individual is trying to produce some desired effect. This is common with use of alcohol and illicit drugs.

Prescription and over-the-counter (OTC) medication misuse is the most common form of substance abuse by the older adult. Older adults constitute 13% of the U.S. population but use 25% to 30% of all prescription medications and 40% of OTC medications (▼ Figure 11-9).[9]

To understand the potential for medication problems, consider the variety of medications prescribed to treat chronic medical problems in older adults. Cardiovascular medications, tranquilizers, diuretics, sedatives, antidepressants, and anti-inflammatories are all frequently prescribed to manage conditions including hypertension, depression, elevated cholesterol levels, heart disease, arthritis, and diabetes. Surprisingly, 30% of patients older than 65 take eight or more prescription medications on a daily basis.[10] These numbers make it easy to see the potential for abuse and misuse.

Medication Tip

Thirty percent of patients older than 65 take eight or more prescription medications daily, a reminder of the potential for misuse and abuse.

Medication Tip

Cardiovascular medications, tranquilizers, diuretics, sedatives, antidepressants, and anti-inflammatories are frequently prescribed to treat chronic medical problems in older adults.

Older women are less likely to abuse alcohol, but more apt to abuse or misuse prescription or OTC medications. Fortunately, the use of illegal or street drugs is minimal in this population.

Risk Factors for Substance Abuse

Alcohol

The EMS provider must be familiar with several factors making the older person vulnerable to alcohol and medication misuse or abuse. Physical ailments, limited financial resources, loss of a job, or loneliness causing depression can place the older adult at risk. Shifting from a busy, productive career to a time of unwanted or unplanned retirement can produce boredom and unnecessary stress. Alcohol and medications may be used to suppress this anxiety. Older women alcoholics often had alcoholic spouses or suffered the loss of a spouse, triggering problem drinking.

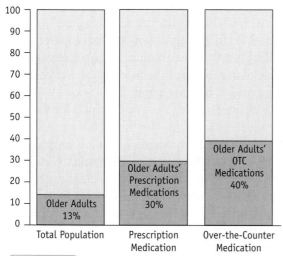

Figure 11-9   Older adults make up about one eighth of the population but use nearly one third of all prescription medications.

Medications

Many variables place the older patient at significant risk for medication misuse or abuse. A significant number of older persons take medications on a continual basis for conditions such as sleeping problems, chronic pain, and mood disorders, including depression or anxiety. This chronic use opens the door for drug tolerance and potential abuse. Many older adults require two or more medications that strengthen or counteract one another. Often, these adults "doctor shop," acquiring the same medication from different physicians who may not know the medicine has already been prescribed to the patient. Some patients are unaware of the hazards of mixing alcohol with mood-altering, pain-relieving, or muscle-relaxing medications. This is especially dangerous and potentially fatal in those who mix alcohol with the sedative-hypnotic drugs, including benzodiazepines and barbiturates. Others suffer short-term memory loss, and just cannot recall if and when they took their last dose.

Patients with visual impairment may not be able to read prescription directions properly. Some older adults, who fear loss of independence or are simply embarrassed, are reluctant to ask family, friends, and their medical provider for help in clarifying medication directions, thus further increasing risk of abuse or misuse. Given that most medications are prescribed to older adults, it is not startling that more than 50% of the medication overdoses or adverse reactions requiring hospitalization occur in older persons **▶ Figure 11-10** .[10]

Alarmingly, one must consider that some older adults know exactly what they are doing when abusing their medications. Medication abuse with true intention to do self-harm may be a cry for help—an actual suicide attempt. A list of medications and their potential side effects (signs and symptoms) secondary to overdose appears in **▶ Table 11-5** .

Pathophysiology of Substance Abuse in Older Adults

As the body ages, several physiological changes occur throughout various organ systems. These changes make the older adult much more vulnerable to potential harmful effects of drugs and alcohol. It is important to remember

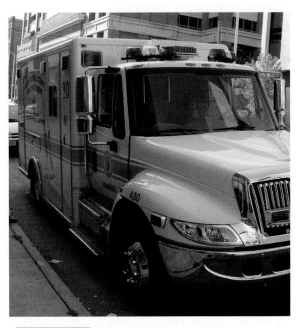

Figure 11-10   More than half of medication overdoses and adverse reactions that require hospitalization occur in older patients.

that alcohol is a powerful CNS depressant. It is both a **sedative**, a substance that decreases activity and excitement, and a **hypnotic**, meaning that it induces sleep. Alcohol and several prescription medications dull the sense of awareness, slow reflexes, and reduce reaction time.[11] Abuse of alcohol and other substances can have effects on most of the major organ systems **▶ Figure 11-11** .

Cardiovascular System

Alcohol depresses not only an older person's reactions, but also cardiac muscle, resulting in a decreased cardiac output (amount of blood pumped out of heart in one minute). Alcohol elevates the level of fatty acids in the bloodstream. High blood pressure, or **hypertension**, is worsened by excessive alcohol intake. Most importantly for the EMS provider, alcohol has the potential to mask more serious medical problems including **angina pectoris** (chest pain caused by **ischemia**). Older persons unable to interpret this warning sign that heart muscle needs additional oxygen are at greater risk for **myocardial infarction** (heart attack).

Respiratory System

The natural drive to breathe is slowed by alcohol. Inadequate oxygenation of the brain may result in marked mental confusion, especially in patients

TABLE 11-5   Toxidromes: Typical Signs and Symptoms of Specific Drug Overdose

Drug Class	Examples of Drug	Signs and Symptoms
Opioid	Butorphanol (Stadol) Codeine Fentanyl derivatives ("China White") Heroin Hydrocodone (Hycodan) Hydromorphone (Dilaudid) Meperidine (Demerol) Methadone (Dolophine) Morphine Oxycodone (Percodan) Pentazocine (Talwin) Prophoxyphene (Darvon)	Hypoventilation/respiratory arrest Pinpoint pupils (miosis) Sedation/coma Hypotension
Sympathomimetics	Amphetamines Benzedrine Cocaine Crack cocaine Ecstasy Methamphetamine ("ice") Phentermine (Adipex-P, Fastin, Ionamin)	Hypertension Tachycardia Dilated pupils (mydriasis) Agitation/seizures Hyperthermia
Anticholinergics	Atropine Diphenhydramine (Benadryl) Jimsonweed Some tricyclic antidepressants (amitriptyline [Elavil], imipramine [Tofranil])	Tachycardia Hyperthermia Hypertension Dilated pupils (mydriasis) Dry skin and mucous membranes Sedation/agitation/seizures/coma/delirium Decreased bowel sounds
Cholinergics	Organophosphate insecticides Certain wild mushrooms	Excess defecation/urination Muscle fasciculations Pinpoint pupils (miosis) Excess lacrimation/salivation Airway compromise Nausea/vomiting

Adapted from American Academy of Orthopaedic Surgeons. *Emergency Care and Transportation of the Sick and Injured.* 8th ed. Sudbury, MA: Jones and Bartlett; 2002:435–445.

already afflicted with respiratory disorders such as chronic obstructive pulmonary disease (COPD).

Hepatic System

The function of the liver is greatly decreased by chronic alcohol use. The effects of alcohol and drugs may then be prolonged because they are not metabolized by the damaged liver, and circu- late throughout the body for an extended time. Also, the liver controls essential blood clotting factors that are altered by heavy drinking, which increases the risk of bruising and significant bleeding. <u>Cirrhosis</u>, a chronic disease of the liver resulting in degenerative changes and death of functioning liver cells, causes an increased resist- ance to the flow of blood through the organ,

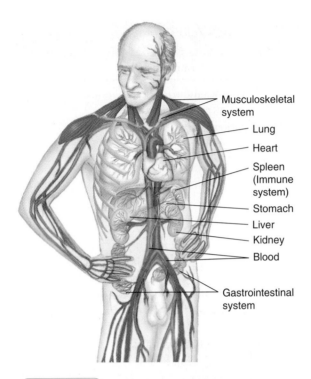

Musculoskeletal system
Lung
Heart
Spleen (Immune system)
Stomach
Liver
Kidney
Blood
Gastrointestinal system

Figure 11-11 Abuse of alcohol and other substances can have effects on most of the major organ systems.

resulting in a dangerous condition known as **portal hypertension**. As the blood continues to back up in the portal venous system, fluid is displaced in the abdomen, the liver enlarges, and esophageal varices (discussed below) may develop.

Gastrointestinal System

Long-term alcohol use results in inflammation or erosion of cells lining the esophagus or stomach. Abdominal pain and diarrhea from gastritis, **peptic ulcer disease**, or **pancreatitis** may be common complaints verbalized by the older patient. Bright red blood in feces, or dark tarry stools known as **melena**, indicates bleeding somewhere in the gastrointestinal tract. Continued alcohol abuse may result in cancers of the upper digestive tract. Persistent portal hypertension (discussed above) creates enlarged venous channels in the esophagus, known as **esophageal varices**. These have the potential to rupture, causing uncontrolled, life-threatening bleeding and possibly compromising the airway.

Musculoskeletal System

Bone density decreases with age. Muscle tissue, which is composed mostly of water, wastes away over time. The result of this decrease in body mass is that drugs and alcohol remain in the bloodstream for a longer time. The prolonged effect of drugs and alcohol magnifies the risk of weakness, falls, and fractures.

Blood Components and the Immune System

Long-term alcohol abuse impairs the immune response, making the body much more susceptible to infection and cancer. Severe alcohol ingestion may also cause low blood sugar, or **hypoglycemia**. Vitamin stores, including vitamin B_{12}, folate, and iron, are significantly depleted. Without these substances, essential nutrients are not absorbed, contributing to overall malnutrition. In addition, alcohol suppresses the functioning of the bone marrow, where most blood cells are made. These elements are essential in creating blood cells vital to oxygen transport. Lowered ability to transport oxygen can lead to confusion, falls, memory loss, or fatigue.

Screening for Substance Abuse or Misuse

Screening for substance misuse or abuse by the EMS provider is a critical element of the patient

> **Medication Tip**
>
> Alcohol and medications unable to be metabolized by the liver or excreted in the kidneys can build to toxic levels and may even be life threatening in the older adult.

encounter. The tools in the following tables may be useful to identify older patients at risk. The CAGE questionnaire (▶ **Table 11-6**) is extremely useful in identifying older patients at risk for alcoholism. Two questions answered with a "yes" should prompt the EMS provider to consider that the patient is abusing alcohol, and

CASE STUDY 2

You are dispatched back to the home of the 78-year-old Army officer two weeks after having responded to a call for the same patient. This time, the patient is unresponsive and the respiration rate is 10 breaths/min and shallow. A neighbor who came to check on the man states that the patient was evaluated by a doctor two days ago for depression. Upon observing the home, you find an empty bottle of amitriptyline (Elavil) and an empty bottle of whiskey.

What should you consider as your first priority?

What is significant about the medication amitriptyline?

What must you consider, given the amount of amitriptyline taken by the patient?

make appropriate referrals. If substance abuse or even possible overdose is suspected, the questions suggested in (▶ **Table 11-7**) can be used to guide your focused history.

The EMS provider may also pose the questions in (▶ **Table 11-8**) to detect harmful drinking.

Approaching the Older Patient

A few key strategies can make the evaluation of the older adult easier. Gain the patient's and family's trust by identifying yourself in a calm and re-

TABLE 11-7   Focused History Questions Pertaining to Substance Abuse or Possible Overdose

1. How much did you ingest?

2. What substance did you take?

3. What actions have been taken?

4. When did you take it?

5. If any injury resulted, when did it occur?

Source: American Academy of Orthopaedic Surgeons. *Emergency Care and Transportation of the Sick and Injured.* 8th ed. Sudbury, MA: Jones and Bartlett; 2002:434.

TABLE 11-6   CAGE Questionnaire for Alcoholism

1. Ever felt the need to cut down on your drinking?	Yes/No
2. Ever felt annoyed by criticism of your drinking?	Yes/No
3. Ever felt guilty about drinking?	Yes/No
4. Ever take a morning drink (eye-opener)?	Yes/No

Source: Ewing JA. Detecting alcoholism: The CAGE questionnaire. *JAMA.* 1984; 252:1905–1907.

TABLE 11-8   Detecting Harmful Drinking

How many days per week do you drink?

How many drinks do you have on those days?

Maximum intake on any one day?

What type (ie, beer, wine, or liquor)?

What is in "a drink"?

Note: Greater than or equal to 2 drinks/day for women, or greater than or equal to 3 drinks for men, is potentially harmful.

Source: Reuben DB, Herr K, Pacala JT, et al. *Geriatrics at Your Fingertips: 2002 Edition.* Malden, MA: Blackwell Science for the American Geriatrics Society; 2002.

assuring manner (▶ **Figure 11-12**). Be honest and direct with the patient, describing every intervention you want to perform. Communicate clearly and slowly; some older adults may have hearing impairments. Remain totally nonjudgmental and refrain from imposing your values or ideas on the patient or family. Remember that it may take additional time to thoroughly listen to and answer any question posed by the older adult. Be ready to commit additional time on scene.

Assessment Goals

Using the GEMS diamond, the EMS provider has the tools to properly assess environmental, medical, and social aspects of the older adult. Your objective is twofold: (1) recognize any major life-threatening condition, and (2) reduce any factors that may be contributing to unnecessary stress for both the patient and family.

History

It is imperative to gather an accurate history. Avoid asking any questions in an accusatory or threatening way. The interview is less likely to produce good information if you lose the patient's trust. Gather data from family members, friends, or caretakers, including questions about signs of substance abuse. Use the questions suggested in Table 11-7 to guide your focused history when substance abuse is a possibility.

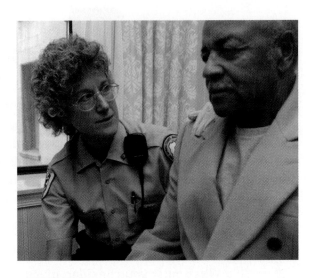

Figure 11-12 Identify yourself and communicate with the patient in a calm and reassuring manner.

Environmental Observations

Perform a scene size-up and ensure that the environment is safe for both the patient and EMS provider. Carefully assess the older adult's surroundings (▶ **Figure 11-13**). Remember that many older adults at risk of substance abuse live alone, with limited financial resources. Look for unsanitary or dangerous home conditions that may place the patient at risk. This may include the presence of a gun or other weapon. Carefully document any finding that may support substance abuse. Particular attention

---

CASE STUDY 3

You are on the scene with an 85-year-old woman who is complaining of vomiting bright red blood. Family members deny any previous medical history. Your review of medications notes an antihypertensive, a cholesterol-reducing agent, and nonsteroidal anti-inflammatories (NSAIDs). A family member comments during your review, "She likes to take her Advil, Ibuprofen, and Motrin all at once."

What about the family member's comment alerts you to potential misunderstanding of the patient's current medication regimen?

How should you handle this situation?

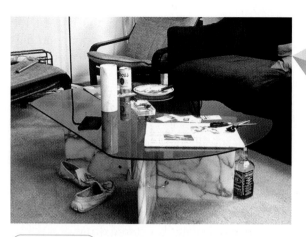

Figure 11-13 Carefully observe the patient's surroundings for dangerous conditions or signs of substance abuse.

Attitude Tip

Observations you make of the older patient's home environment, along with your assessment of psychosocial status, may provide valuable clues to a history of depression, alcoholism, or other substance abuse. When such observations are reported to the emergency department (or other receiving facility) staff, they will likely improve the patient's long-term outcome, reducing any associated risk of serious decline when the patient returns home.

Medication Tip

Older adults commonly self-medicate with similar classes of OTC drugs. Failing to understand that the drugs are the same type of medication increases the potential for overdose or adverse effects.

---

should be paid to the presence of alcoholic beverages, whether they are empty or full, and the presence of prescription or OTC medication bottles. Note the date of the initial prescription and the number of pills remaining in any of the bottles. This may be useful in determining if an overdose has occurred.

Medical Examination and Care

If the scene is safe, perform an initial assessment of the older adult, as outlined in Chapter 5, and give appropriate medical care where indicated. Clear, maintain, and protect the airway if the level of consciousness is altered from either drug or alcohol ingestion. Be prepared to provide additional oxygenation and possibly ventilatory support in anyone who shows signs of **cyanosis** (bluish skin color) or **dyspnea** (shortness of breath). Consider the need to mechanically clear or suction the airway if the patient vomits.

Evaluation of pupillary size may assist the emergency department professional in identifying potential drug overdose. The most common example is the class of opiate narcotics (eg, codeine, demerol, morphine) that cause pinpoint pupils. Several drug types can also produce pupillary dilation.

Assess for any signs of physical trauma, such as altered mental status, fractures, or bruising, because many older patients are at risk for falls, especially when compromised by alcohol or medication abuse. Older patients are also at higher-than-normal risk of **subdural hematoma** (intracranial bleeding between the dural layer and the brain). This risk rises generally with age, and increases further in heavy alcohol users.

Also assess hydration status, because alcohol and certain medications including diuretics remove fluids, thus dehydrating the patient. Evidence of self-neglect, a decline in personal hygiene, disheveled clothing, poor grooming, and weight loss are red flags indicating possible alcohol or medication misuse or abuse. In addition, findings of fatigue, difficulty concentrating, unexplainable confusion, incontinence, or insomnia may also be physical clues suggesting substance abuse.

Consider that the older adult who is withdrawing from chronic alcohol abuse may be suffering from a condition known as **delirium tremens** (DTs). Delirium tremens may occur 24 hours to 1 week following the cessation of alcohol ingestion, or when alcohol consumption stops abruptly. Objective findings on examination include fine tremors, sweating, agitation, hallucinations, and confusion. Delirium tremens is a life-threatening condition and is much more severe in the older adult than in younger patients.

These patients require prompt evaluation and medical transport. In addition, an older adult experiencing DTs has the potential of experiencing seizure activity. Every attempt should be made to protect the airway and prevent accidental injury. Administer oxygen immediately following the episode, because the patient was likely deprived during the seizure. At no point should any type of physical restraint be used in an attempt to prevent physical harm.

Short-acting benzodiazepines such as lorazepam (Ativan) and oxazepam (Serax) can safely be used to treat DTs. They are not oxidized in the liver, which may be damaged due to long-term alcohol abuse.

Look for several additional emotional factors that may point to substance abuse. During assessment, older adults may ask for a tranquilizer or an antianxiety medication. In addition, the patient may be withdrawn; exhibit feelings of hopelessness, worthlessness, or guilt; or demonstrate paranoid tendencies or thoughts of suicide.

Social Setting

Continuously observe interactions between the patient and family. The EMS provider may notice **enabling behavior** demonstrated by family members that can indicate substance abuse. Enabling behavior is defined as actions by someone who promotes continued self-destructive behavior of another individual. An example is a spouse who continues to makes excuses for continued alcohol ingestion, stating, "He needs his beer daily to keep him happy."

It is also important that the EMS provider observe for behavioral signs of neglect or abuse. A complete discussion of self-neglect and neglect can be found in Chapter 14.

Management Considerations

The episodic, short-term nature of most EMS responses to older adults makes it difficult for providers to significantly affect the psychological well-being of older patients. As an EMS provider and patient advocate, you can intervene in a variety of ways to help the older adult afflicted with any psychological issue. Continuously treat the older patient with respect, compassion, and dignity. Many have lost the independence or autonomy they have enjoyed for years, becoming totally dependent on others for care.

Consider these points:

1. Review all medication regimens with both the patient and family, clarifying drug, dose, and time of day the medication is to be taken. This practice may reveal accidental multiple dosing or missed doses. It may also identify expired drugs or medications that have been discontinued by the doctor, but remain in the patient's medicine cabinet.

2. Ensure that your ambulance carries a current list of phone numbers and e-mail addresses of helpful community contacts, including social service agencies, companion groups, drug and alcohol rehabilitation programs, and crisis intervention hot lines that can be provided on request to the patient or family. Appendix A lists national examples of such resources.

3. For individuals whom you suspect want help, but are reluctant to seek it, consider initiating that first telephone contact for the patient while on scene ▶ **Figure 11-14** . Your empathetic support and assistance through the interaction may be what the patient emotionally needs to seek treatment. The key to success in medically treating an older adult afflicted with substance abuse is their (and your) recognition that a problem does in fact exist. Studies have shown remarkable treatment success in older adults who began to abuse alcohol late in life.

4. The attention of a caring and competent professional can be enough reassurance to get a depressed or suicidal person through the acute crisis, while other agencies are marshaled for more aggressive intervention. It is of paramount importance that EMS providers report—verbally and in writing—their impressions or perceptions of potentially suicidal older adults. One explanation for the high suicide completions-to-attempts ratio is the fact that

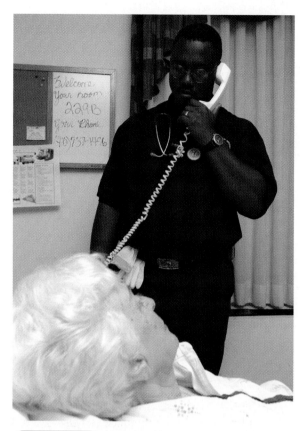

Figure 11-14 Offer to make the first telephone contact for a patient who you think wants help but is reluctant to seek it.

many suicidal older adults never cry for help, make repeated attempts, or otherwise seek help. The EMS provider who is astute enough to recognize the warning signs for suicide is in a position to initiate referrals and assure that emergency department personnel are aware of the potential for self-harm.

5. Objective data gathered on the scene indicating substance abuse or medication problems should be conveyed to the patient's family physician or the emergency department. Substance abuse and medication problems are often unrecognized among this population group. Your "eyes and ears" assessment data give other health care providers an accurate picture of what is truly occurring in the patient's environment.

6. Patients experiencing altered levels of consciousness secondary to drug or alcohol abuse or lack of oxygen (hypoxia), or even depression, may be mentally incapacitated. These patients—although they require medical attention—may refuse your assistance, and could become violent. They should never be left unattended. Doing so endangers the patient and may constitute patient abandonment, thus placing the EMS provider in legal jeopardy.

Summary

Fortunately, EMS providers should not be faced too frequently with older adults suffering from substance abuse or serious suicidal intentions. When these patients are encountered, it is vital that all members of the health care team be aware of the issues and take appropriate steps to ensure patient safety and initiate effective treatment. On the other hand, older adults suffering from depression will be frequent clients for almost all EMS providers. The challenge facing any professional concerned with care of the older adult is to recognize the signs of depression and aggressively intervene to prevent the ultimate care failure—suicide.

Case Study Summaries

CASE STUDY 1 SUMMARY

All the serious risk factors for suicide in the older adult appear to be present with this patient. Recent loss of a spouse, no nearby family support systems, evidence of alcohol use, personal experience with firearms (military background), loss of interest in personal hygiene/surroundings, and frequent non-urgent EMS calls should all alert the EMS provider to the risk of suicide. Comments like "You probably shouldn't bother taking care of me" are often overlooked; how-ever, they are very important signs that a patient may be contemplating suicide, and should be taken seriously. The loss of self-esteem and sense of self-worth associated with the older adult faced with living alone and not "contributing" to family or society (this patient spent more than 20 years in service to his country) are often potent feelings leading to suicidal ideation. Given the danger of suicide, transport to the emergency department is advised.

CASE STUDY 2 SUMMARY

Given the empty bottles of medication and alcohol, this patient is probably experiencing an overdose. Given the history conveyed in Case Study 1, this overdose may have been intentional with the intent of killing himself. Amitriptyline, also known as Elavil, is a tricyclic antidepressant. Taken in large quantities, this drug is extremely dangerous and has the potential of causing a wide range of signs or symptoms, including delirium, coma, seizure activity, dilated pupils, dry membranes, and even cardiac arrhythmias.

The patient's altered mental status and decreased and shallow respiratory status mandate the EMS provider to protect the airway while delivering necessary oxygen. The patient should have an IV established, as well as his ECG monitored. In cases of tricyclic antidepressant overdose, sodium bicarbonate administration (50 mEq) IV push should be considered. However, check your local protocol regarding specific medications and dosages.

CASE STUDY 3 SUMMARY

The most important priority for the EMS provider at this time is protection of the patient's airway. A history of vomiting bright red blood should prompt the EMS provider to assess hemodynamic status to ensure that the patient is not experiencing hypovolemic shock from blood loss. The EMS provider, after hearing the medication history of the patient, should recognize that all the medications mentioned by the family member are classified as nonsteroidal anti-inflammatory drugs (NSAIDs). These medications taken incorrectly, either without food or in large amounts, can cause gastric irritation, erosion, and subsequent bleeding. In this case, the patient is misusing the medications. This is an optimal time for the EMS provider to educate regarding the proper use of NSAIDs.

Endnotes

1. National Institutes of Health.

2. American Psychological Association. *Diagnostic and Statistical Manual of Mental Disorders (DSM-IV)*. Washington, DC: Author; 1994.

3. Conwell Y. Suicide in Elderly Patients. In: Schneider LS, Reynolds CF III, Lebowitz BD, Friedhoff AJ, eds. *Diagnosis and Treatment of Depression in Late Life*. Washington, DC: American Psychiatric Press; 1994:397–418.

4. National Institutes of Health.

5. American Academy of Orthopaedic Surgeons. *Emergency Care and Transportation of the Sick and Injured*. 8th ed. Sudbury, MA: Jones and Bartlett; 2002:439.

6. Adams WL, Cox NS. Epidemiology of problem drinking among elderly people. *International Journal of Addiction*. 1995;30(13–14):1693–1716.

7. Adams WL, Yuan Z, Barboriak JJ, Rim AA. Alcohol-related hospitalizations of elderly people: Prevalence and geographic variation in the United States. *JAMA*. 1993;270(10):1222–1225.

8. Barry PP, Ackerman K. Chemical Dependency in the Elderly. In: Hazzard WR, Blass JP, Ettinger WH, Halter JB, Ouslander JG, eds: *Principles of Geriatric Medicine and Gerontology*. 4th ed. New York: McGraw-Hill; 1999:1358.

9. Florida Alcohol and Drug Abuse Program. *Chemical Dependency in the Elderly*. Florida Department of Health and Rehabilitative Services. Available at: http://www.fadaa.org/resource/justfact/elderly.html. Accessed July 2, 2002.

10. National Clearinghouse for Alcohol and Drug Information. *Use and Abuse of Psychoactive Prescription and Over the Counter Medications*. Available at: http://www.health.org/govpubsBKD250/26t.htm. Accessed July 2, 2002.

11. American Academy of Orthopaedic Surgeons. *Emergency Care and Transportation of the Sick and Injured*. 8th ed. Sudbury, MA: Jones and Bartlett; 2002:440.

Other Medical Emergencies

1 Discuss abnormal changes of the gastrointestinal system with age, as well as epidemiology, pathophysiology, assessment, intervention, and transport of gastrointestinal emergencies in the older patient, including GI bleeding, peptic ulcer disease, bowel obstruction, diarrhea, diverticulitis, gallbladder disease, and problems with elimination.

2 Discuss abnormal changes of the endocrine system with age, as well as epidemiology, pathophysiology, assessment, intervention, and transport of endocrine emergencies in the older patient, including diabetes and thyroid disorders.

3 Discuss abnormal changes of the integumentary system with age, as well as epidemiology, pathophysiology, assessment, intervention, and transport of older patients with integumentary emergencies, including pressure ulcers.

4 Discuss the epidemiology, pathophysiology, assessment, intervention, and transport of older patients with nutritional emergencies, including malnutrition and dehydration.

5 Discuss the epidemiology, pathophysiology, assessment, intervention, and transport of older patients with environmental emergencies, including hypothermia, hyperthermia, and their predisposing factors.

6 Discuss the epidemiology, pathophysiology, assessment, intervention, and transport of older patients with sepsis and infectious diseases.

CHAPTER 12

Luis F. Amador, MD

Colleen Christmas, MD

Teresita M. Hogan, MD, FACEP

David E. Milkes, MD

Robert C. Salinas, MD, CAQ (G)

William H. Seifarth, MS, NREMT-P

George Triadafilopoulos, MD

Andy Trohanis, MA, EMT-B

CASE STUDY 1

You are dispatched to the home of a 70-year-old man who reports vomiting 2 to 3 cups of red blood and having frequent black, tarry stools for 2 days. He has a history of a recent heart attack. His current medications include aspirin for his heart disease and ibuprofen for his arthritis.

On exam, the patient looks pale and diaphoretic, with beads of sweat on his forehead. His vital signs reveal a blood pressure of 84/40 mm Hg and a heart rate of 120 beats/min. Otherwise, examination of the patient's heart, lungs, and abdomen is normal.

What is this patient's current medical problem, and how severe is it?

What other symptoms should you ask the patient about?

How will you transport and manage this patient?

Other Medical Emergencies

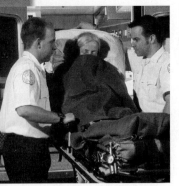

Gastrointestinal Emergencies

Age-related Changes in the Gastrointestinal System

The changes in the gastrointestinal (GI) system that occur in older patients are attributable either to the age of the patient or to diseases that tend to occur with increased age. The changes attributable to age alone are increased stomach acid production and decreased saliva production, sense of taste, liver size, and liver blood flow. These changes in body functions can lead to problems. For example, decreased taste contributes to reduced food intake in older patients, thereby increasing their risk of malnutrition. And, as liver size and liver blood flow decrease, the ability of the liver to metabolize or break down drugs also diminishes. So, the same dose of a drug consumed by an older person may result in higher blood levels than it would in a younger person. This difference in metabolism contributes to the more frequent medication side effects in older patients.

Medication Tip

Decreased liver blood flow and size reduce its metabolic function. This contributes to the more frequent medication side effects experienced by older patients.

Certain gastrointestinal diseases are more common in older patients. Most GI cancers occur in older patients. __Diverticulosis__ (many small pouches protruding from the inner lumen of the colon) is primarily a disease of older age. About 30% of persons over age 50 and 66% of those over age 80 have diverticulosis.[1] Older patients are also more likely to develop difficulty swallowing due to common illnesses such as stroke, medication side effects, or other rarer diseases. The presence of a swallowing disorder is important to recognize because it may increase the risk of aspiration pneumonia, in which contents from the mouth or stomach enter the lungs and cause infection.

Upper GI Bleeding

Upper gastrointestinal hemorrhage occurs when there is bleeding from the esophagus, stomach, or __duodenum__ (▼ Figure 12-1). When severe, this condition is a true medical emergency that must be recognized and assessed quickly. Not only are older patients more prone to having upper GI bleeding, they are also at greater risk of complications, urgent surgery, and death. In severe cases, the death rate in patients over 80 years old approaches 25%.[1]

It is not possible to determine the cause of upper GI bleeding without an __endoscopic examination__ (inspection of the inside of a hollow organ or body cavity) of the esophagus, stomach, and duodenum. However, the patient history can offer some clues as to the cause. Regular use of __nonsteroidal anti-inflammatory drugs (NSAIDs)__ or alcohol may result in bleeding from irritation of the lining of the stomach (gastritis) or from __ulcers__ (a hollowing out or disintegration of tis-

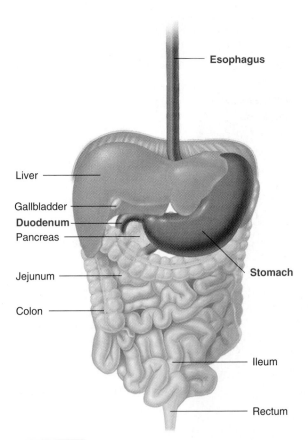

Figure 12-1 Upper GI bleeding occurs in the stomach, esophagus, and duodenum.

sue) in the stomach or duodenum. Forceful vomiting can cause tears in the esophagus that may bleed. Cirrhosis of the liver from chronic alcohol use or chronic infectious hepatitis may cause large veins (varices) to form in the esophagus. These veins can rupture and result in massive bleeding. Stomach cancer or esophageal cancer can also produce upper GI bleeding. Recent weight loss or difficulty swallowing would raise the suspicion of an underlying cancer as the source of bleeding.

Upon arrival at the scene, even more important than knowing the cause of bleeding is being able to assess its severity. Slower bleeding is characterized by emesis that has the appearance of coffee grounds. With minor bleeding, the heart rate and systolic blood pressure are normal. Brisk bleeding presents with **hematemesis** (vomiting red blood) or **melena** (black, tarlike stools). The most severe cases of upper GI bleeding have abnormal vital signs with tachycardia (heart rate greater than 100 beats/min), hypotension (systolic blood pressure less than 90 mm Hg), or both. These abnormal vital signs indicate that the patient has lost at least 10% of his or her total blood volume. The loss of so much blood can make patients appear pale, with cool or cyanotic extremities, as well as feel agitated and dizzy.

An important difference between older patients with GI bleeding and younger ones is that older patients are more likely to have other medical conditions that can be worsened by the bleeding. Hypotension and tachycardia cause increased stress on the heart and are harder for the older patient to tolerate. An older patient with coronary artery disease is at high risk for heart attack in the setting of active GI bleeding. Hypotension can also result in decreased blood flow to the brain, which could cause a stroke in an older patient. Furthermore, older patients are more likely to take blood-thinning medications such as warfarin (Coumadin), which can make the bleeding more severe.

In assessing older patients with upper GI bleeding, note any underlying risk factors such as NSAID or alcohol use. Then determine the severity of bleeding based on the history and vital signs. Remember that tachycardia or hypotension in an older patient with hematemesis or melena represents severe upper GI bleeding, a true medical emergency. These patients require general steps to treat shock (supine position with feet up,

maintenance of body temperature, oxygen, and reassurance) and immediate transport. En route, start a large-bore IV (16-gauge, if possible) because the patient will require fluid resuscitation and blood transfusion. Patients should be monitored with a cardiac monitor when these services are available, to watch for arrhythmias and changes suggestive of cardiac ischemia. Determine any history of heart disease or stroke. Ask patients with a history of heart attack or coronary artery disease if they are experiencing any chest pain.

> **Medication Tip**
>
> Medications can be major contributors to GI bleeding problems. NSAIDs and alcohol often cause GI bleeding, and blood thinners such as warfarin may make it more severe.

Peptic Ulcer Disease

Older patients are more likely than younger ones to develop ulcers in the stomach or duodenum (peptic ulcer disease). The main risk factors for developing peptic ulcers are regular use of NSAIDs and infection with *H. pylori* (an ulcer-associated bacteria of the stomach), both of which are more common in older patients. Some other medications have also been implicated in ulcer formation. Up to 15% of patients over age 60 regularly use NSAIDs, such as aspirin or ibuprofen.[1] Older patients taking both NSAIDs and corticosteroids, such as prednisone, are at even greater risk for developing ulcers than those taking NSAIDs alone.

> **Medication Tip**
>
> Patients taking NSAIDs are at even greater risk of GI bleeding when they are also taking steroids such as prednisone.

The main symptom of peptic ulcer disease is **dyspepsia** (a gnawing, burning pain in the upper abdomen), which usually improves immediately after eating but returns several hours later. Other causes of dyspepsia include acid reflux, gastritis, and gastric cancer.

It is important to realize that older patients with peptic ulcer disease are less likely than younger patients to complain of dyspepsia. Another important difference is that older patients are more likely to present initially with a complication of peptic ulcer disease such as anemia, GI bleeding, or **bowel perforation** (a hole or opening in the tissue of the bowel).

A perforated peptic ulcer is a medical emergency. Typical symptoms include abdominal pain and fever. Physical exam findings include **peritoneal signs** such as a rigid abdomen and few bowel sounds. However, older patients with a perforated peptic ulcer often deny any symptoms or history of peptic ulcer disease, and are less likely than younger patients to have peritoneal signs.

In assessing older patients who complain of dyspepsia, be sure to ask if they take NSAIDs, aspirin, or steroids. Be aware that not all older patients with peptic ulcer disease will complain of dyspepsia. For example, an older patient taking NSAIDs who only complains of weakness and looks pale may actually have peptic ulcer disease that has caused anemia. In a patient with signs of a bowel perforation (rigid, silent abdomen), immediate transportation to an emergency department is warranted.

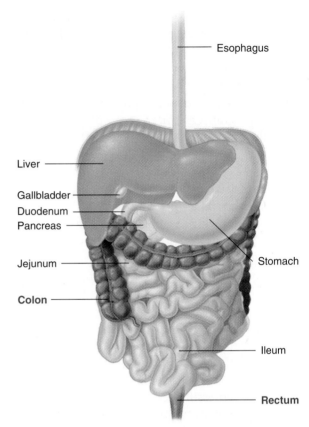

Figure 12-2 Lower GI bleeding takes place primarily in the colon and rectum.

Lower GI Bleeding

Lower GI hemorrhage primarily describes bleeding from the colon and rectum ▶ **Figure 12-2** . It is often less brisk than upper GI bleeding, and in 80% of cases the bleeding stops spontaneously.[2] However, in the older population, even minor lower GI bleeding needs to be fully investigated. It should never simply be attributed to hemorrhoids, because colon polyps and colon cancer are also possible, among other causes. Only after all other causes have been excluded by hospital personnel can lower GI bleeding be attributed to hemorrhoids.

As with upper GI bleeding, it is not possible to determine the cause of lower GI bleeding accurately without a medical work-up, usually a colonoscopy. However, certain features of the history may suggest the cause. In the older population, severe lower GI hemorrhaging is usually from diverticular bleeding or abnormal blood vessels in the colon wall, known as arteriovenous malformations (AVM). Colon polyps and colon

cancer usually cause slow GI bleeding, but in rare cases may present with severe bleeding.

Minor lower GI bleeding is characterized by small amounts of red blood covering formed brown stools, or scant amounts of red blood noticed on the toilet paper. Patients with minor lower GI bleeding will have normal vital signs and usually do not require admission to the hospital, though they should be examined there. Severe lower GI bleeding is characterized by passing significant amounts of red blood or maroon colored stools from the rectum. Patients may describe the whole toilet bowl as appearing full of red blood. In the most severe cases, tachycardia and hypotension will be present. These findings indicate a true medical emergency.

Assessment should begin with identifying any risk factors such as a history of previous lower GI bleed, symptoms or signs suggestive of colon cancer, recent constipation or diarrhea, and use of medications such as blood thinners. Next, determine the severity of bleeding based on the

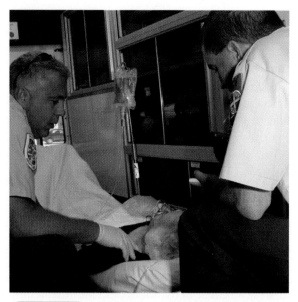

Figure 12-3   Treat any patient who has GI bleeding and altered vital signs with general measures for shock.

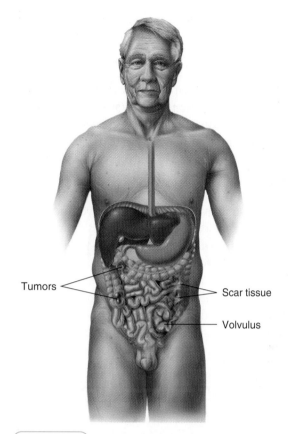

Tumors

Scar tissue

Volvulus

Figure 12-4   Bowel obstruction can be caused by scar tissue from surgery, twisting of the intestine (volvulus), or tumors inside or outside of the intestine.

history and vital signs. Tachycardia or hypotension in a patient passing red blood or maroon colored colon stools indicates a severe lower GI bleed. Treat for shock as described above for severe upper GI bleeding (▲ **Figure 12-3**). Severe lower GI bleeding requires immediate transportation to the nearest emergency department.

Bowel Obstruction

Older patients who complain of an acute onset of nausea, vomiting, and abdominal pain may have a bowel obstruction. They may also report constipation, but this is a later finding. The vomitus is typically **bilious**, with a dark yellow-greenish color that produces a bitter taste.

The most common cause of bowel obstruction is from scar tissues called adhesions that form after previous abdominal surgery (▶ **Figure 12-4**). Other causes of bowel obstruction include twisting of the intestines around themselves (volvulus) and tumors growing inside the bowel that block the intestine. Cancers in the abdominal cavity can also cause bowel obstruction by compressing the outside of the intestines.

A careful history may suggest other causes for nausea and vomiting. GI infections usually present with nausea and vomiting, but patients will also complain of diarrhea and fever. Older pa-

tients take more medications than younger patients, and are more likely to have side effects. Therefore, an older patient who develops nausea and vomiting after starting a new prescription may be experiencing a side effect of the medication.

Medication Tip

In your history of an older patient with nausea and vomiting, be sure to ask if the patient has recently started a new medication. Side effects such as nausea and vomiting are more likely in older patients than in young people.

When evaluating an older patient with symptoms suggestive of bowel obstruction, be sure to ask about any history of abdominal surgery or cancer. Also ask about fever, diarrhea, or new medications that may suggest other causes of nausea, vomiting, and abdominal pain. On abdominal exam, the typical findings of bowel obstruction include diffuse abdominal tenderness, abdominal distension, and high-pitched rushing sounds heard on auscultation with a stethoscope. Older patients with frequent vomiting are more prone to dehydration than younger patients. Significant dehydration is suggested by dry lips and mouth, a heart rate greater than 100 beats/min, a systolic blood pressure less than 90 mm Hg, or a significant decrease in the blood pressure with standing (orthostatic hypotension). Fever also increases the risk of dehydration.

Older patients with signs and symptoms suggestive of bowel obstruction or dehydration require emergency transportation. Start an IV line in patients you suspect are dehydrated. Patients who are vomiting should be transported with their heads raised at least 45 degrees; have oral suctioning ready to help prevent aspiration pneumonia.

Nausea, Vomiting, and Diarrhea

Most of us are personally familiar with the experience of nausea, vomiting, and diarrhea. Nausea is the queasy sensation warning you that vomiting may be near at hand and vomiting (emesis) is the uncontrolled eruption of stomach contents up the esophagus and out the mouth. Diarrhea is defined as a change in the frequency and consistency of the bowel movement (more runny, more often).

Diarrhea can be a severe problem in older patients. Approximately 1,000 older patients die each year due to diarrheal illnesses.[1] Older patients who live in nursing homes are at greater risk than others for developing diarrhea. Feeding tubes contribute to diarrhea both because of the effects of the solutions put in the tubes and because they are a risk factor for gastrointestinal infections. Diabetes is also a risk factor, and may cause chronic diarrhea by damaging the function of the intestines. Those persons who are not active enough to provide themselves with water have a particularly high risk of dehydration with diarrhea.

There are many causes of diarrhea, but certain clues may help distinguish the cause. Fever, bloody diarrhea, and a history of eating undercooked food are suggestive of an infectious diarrhea. Bloody diarrhea may also suggest **inflam-**

matory bowel disease, a chronic inflammation of the gastrointestinal tract. Ulcerative colitis and Crohn's disease are two examples of inflammatory bowel disease. Recent antibiotic use can cause diarrhea by changing the bacterial composition of the bowel. Diarrhea may represent a side effect of newly started medication. Patients with diabetes can develop diarrhea as a complication of the diabetes itself. Older patients who abuse laxatives may also present with diarrhea, and patients who have undergone radiation therapy for abdominal or pelvic cancers can develop diarrhea secondary to radiation damage of the bowel.

Nausea, vomiting, and diarrhea are common complaints among older people, often with potentially serious consequences. Vomiting and diarrhea can cause dehydration and life-threatening **electrolyte** imbalances. In assessing older patients with diarrhea, the key issue is to determine if they are dehydrated (▼ Figure 12-5). Check for findings of significant dehydration (dry lips and mouth, tachycardia, hypotension). Those patients suffering from bloody diarrhea who appear cold, clammy, and pale may have severe anemia and will likely require blood transfusion. Maintain appropriate body substance isolation; many of the causes of nausea, vomiting, and diarrhea are infectious. Dehydration should be recognized and treated appropriately.

Start an IV line in patients with diarrhea who are dehydrated or appear anemic. Use a large-bore IV such as 14- or 16-gauge if possible. A

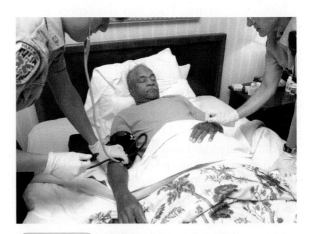

(**Figure 12-5**)   Patients not active enough to drink water are at high risk of dehydration when they have diarrhea. Ask about water intake and check for signs of dehydration.

crystalloid bolus of 10 mL/kg may be indicated. Recognize and treat significant underlying medical problems such as cardiac ischemia or increased intracranial pressure. If cardiac monitoring is available, peaked T waves suggest too much potassium (hyperkalemia) (▼ **Figure 12-6A**) and flattened T waves suggest a low potassium level (hypokalemia) (▼ **Figure 12-6B**). Anti-emetic (anti-vomiting) medication such as promethazine (Phenergan) or prochlorperazine (Compazine) may be appropriate, depending on local protocols or standing orders.

Older patients with diarrhea may lose control of their bowel movements (fecal incontinence). When available, provide patients with clean, dry clothing if they have soiled their clothes. They may also be anxious or embarrassed about having "an accident" en route. It is important to reassure these patients that they are not responsible for any incontinence and need not be embarrassed.

Diverticulitis

The presence of diverticula (pouchlike protrusions from the bowel), or diverticulosis, is primarily a condition found in older patients (▶ **Figure 12-7**). Approximately 10% to 20% of patients with diverticulosis will develop an infection within a diverticulum, a condition known as **diverticulitis**.

The typical symptoms of diverticulitis are left lower quadrant abdominal pain and fever. Rarely, the pain will be in the right lower quadrant. Diarrhea may also be reported. A fistula (abnormal connection) may develop between the colon and

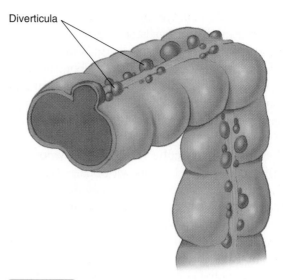

Figure 12-7 Approximately 10% to 20% of patients with diverticula will develop an infection in one of them (diverticulitis).

surrounding organs. For example, patients who describe the release of fecal material when they urinate have developed a fistula between the colon and bladder. Diverticulitis can also result in perforation of the colon and spillage of fecal material into the abdominal cavity.

In assessing patients who complain of left lower quadrant pain, ask if there is a known history of diverticulosis. Many older patients have undergone colon cancer screening with flexible sigmoidoscopy or colonoscopy; when asked, they may recall being told they have diverticulosis. Next, it is extremely important to assess for the presence of fever. Those patients without fever can usually be treated as outpatients with oral antibiotics if they are able to consume liquids without vomiting, but those with fever will likely require a computed tomography (CT) scan and hospitalization for IV antibiotics. On abdominal exam, a palpable mass in the lower abdomen may represent a large abscess that has formed from a perforated diverticulum. The development of peritoneal signs represents a surgical emergency that requires immediate attention.

Gallbladder Disease

The prevalence of gallstones is higher in the older population. Up to 33% of patients over 70 years old have gallstones.[1] Older patients are also at

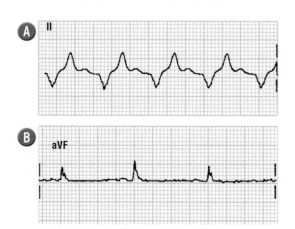

Figure 12-6 Electrolyte imbalances that can cause nausea, vomiting, and diarrhea may also show on the EKG strip as hyperkalemia **(A)** or hypokalemia **(B)**.

greater risk than younger ones of developing complications from gallstones. The risk of death during surgery to remove the gallbladder (cholecystectomy) increases with age. For the older population, the risk of death during minimally invasive cholecystectomy is 3%; during emergency cholecystectomy, it is 20%.[1]

Pain from the gallbladder, or biliary pain (also known as **biliary colic**), is the classic symptom of gallstone disease. Patients with biliary colic typically complain of sharp right upper quadrant pain (**▼ Figure 12-8**). The pain may radiate to the back and the right shoulder. Episodes of biliary colic are usually separated by several weeks or months. Biliary colic may also cause nausea and vomiting. A commonly held belief is that biliary colic worsens after eating fatty or greasy meals, but this association is nonspecific and controversial.

Controversy

It is commonly believed that eating fatty or greasy meals worsens biliary colic, but this is not a proven or universally accepted medical fact.

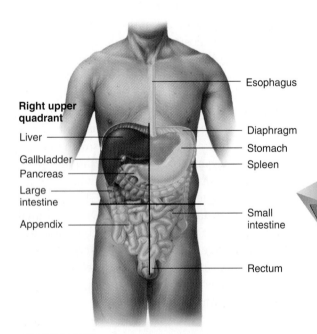

Right upper quadrant

Liver
Gallbladder
Pancreas
Large intestine
Appendix

Esophagus
Diaphragm
Stomach
Spleen
Small intestine
Rectum

Figure 12-8   Older patients with sharp right upper quadrant pain for more than 1 hour may have biliary colic, which indicates gallbladder disease. Right upper quadrant pain with fever can be a sign of infection of the gallbladder or biliary system.

Right upper quadrant pain with fever is a worrisome combination that could signify an infection of the gallbladder (**cholecystitis**) or the biliary system. Older patients with right upper quadrant pain, fever, and jaundice (yellow appearance of the eyes and skin) represent a true medical emergency because they are very susceptible to having the biliary infection spread to the blood, causing overwhelming sepsis and shock.

In assessing older patients with complaints of biliary colic, it is most important to determine the presence of fever and jaundice. The presence of fever, jaundice, and right upper quadrant abdominal pain likely represents a complication of gallstones, and these patients need immediate medical evaluation. Physical examination of the abdomen should focus on localizing tenderness to the right upper quadrant. Patients with a systolic blood pressure less than 90 mm Hg may have dehydration, sepsis, or shock from overwhelming infection. Start a large-bore IV line and begin fluid administration if you see these signs.

Attitude Tip

Remember that complaints from older patients, such as bloody stools, bowel obstruction, vomiting, diarrhea, flulike symptoms, and fever may sound trivial, but may signal a serious or life-threatening condition worthy of an ED evaluation.

Problems with Elimination: Fecal Incontinence and Constipation

Incontinence

Older patients frequently report problems with elimination. Up to 7% of older patients suffer from fecal incontinence.[3] This condition may have a negative impact on quality of life by causing social isolation. It is important to encourage these patients to have a medical evaluation because certain causes of fecal incontinence are treatable, including diarrhea and **fecal impaction**, which is hardened feces lodged or collected in the rectum or sigmoid. Often, simply increasing dietary fiber, taking bulking agents such as psyllium seed, and using antidiarrheal medications can significantly improve quality of life. Sudden onset of fecal incontinence and back pain in a patient with cancer necessitates emergency evaluation because this may be the first evidence of a tumor compressing the nerves of the spinal cord.

Constipation

Constipation is defined as having less than one bowel movement every 3 days. Constipation is an extremely common symptom, affecting 30% of patients over 65 years old.[3] Patients should be encouraged to have a medical evaluation, because nearly all causes of constipation are treatable and patient well-being is usually improved. Although rarely indicated for younger patients, a colonoscopy may be warranted in an older patient with constipation to rule out colon polyps or colon cancer. Adequate hydration, sufficient dietary fiber, exercise, and the use of bulking agents are frequently the only interventions needed to treat constipation (▼ **Figure 12-9**). Nursing home patients, inactive persons, and those with Parkinson's disease are at higher risk for serious causes of constipation such as fecal impaction and massive dilation of the colon. Although rare, these severe types of constipation can cause abdominal pain, nausea, and vomiting; if not treated urgently, they can also result in bowel perforation in rare cases.

Prevention

As a member of the health care team, you have a unique opportunity to help educate and advise patients about prevention. A small amount of time and thought focused on prevention can help to avert some gastrointestinal emergencies in older patients. Ask patients who take NSAIDs for joint pain and arthritis to speak to their doctor about alternative medications. Some patients can achieve the same symptom relief from acetaminophen, and thereby reduce their risk of peptic ulcer disease and upper GI hemorrhage. Encourage an older patient on NSAIDs who complains of dyspepsia to discuss this with the doctor, because early detection of peptic ulcer disease leads to earlier treatment and prevents complications such as perforation or bleeding. Reinforcing the importance of regular exercise, adequate hydration, and sufficient dietary fiber can reduce the incidence of constipation. Also, a high-fiber diet will minimize the development of diverticulosis and may decrease the incidence of diverticulitis and lower GI hemorrhage from diverticular bleeding. All patients over 50 years old should ask their doctors about colon cancer screening, because routine screening may detect cancer at a treatable stage and avert complications such as bowel obstruction and anemia.

Malnutrition and Dehydration in the Older Patient

Age-related Effects

To understand nutrition and hydration in older people, remember that certain age-related changes can affect fluid and nutrient needs and utilization. First, with aging, total body water content decreases; because of lower muscle mass, energy requirements also drop (▶ **Figure 12-10**). Sedentary behavior can worsen muscle loss, so that even less energy is used. The senses of taste and smell both diminish with age, and there is some evidence that the perception of thirst when dehydrated may lessen. Thus, there are several reasons that the "drives" to eat and drink are weaker in older people.

Compromised ability to sense changes in temperature can contribute to failure to seek a cooler environment and increase fluid intake during a heat wave. Finally, changes in kidney function can result in the inability to concentrate urine and

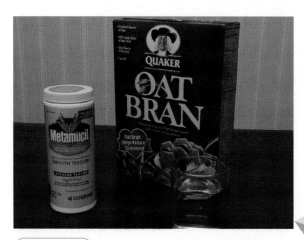

Figure 12-9   Adequate hydration, sufficient dietary fiber, exercise, and the use of bulking agents are frequently the only interventions needed to treat constipation.

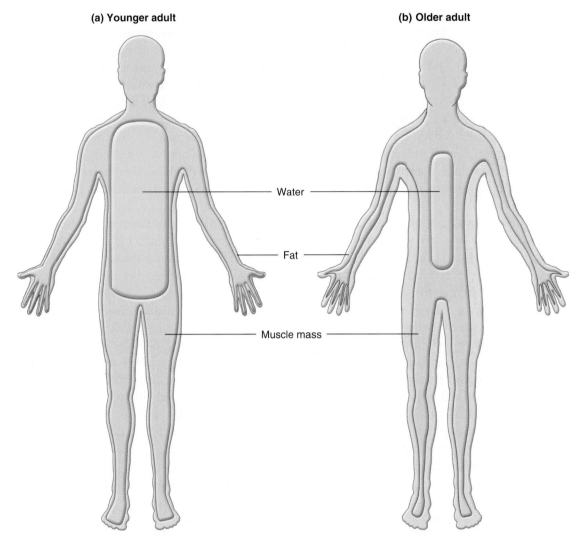

(a) Younger adult   **(b) Older adult**

Water

Fat

Muscle mass

Figure 12-10   Muscle mass and total water content in the body decrease with age. Fat normally increases.

conserve water even with significant dehydration. These age-related changes in body composition, senses, and water handling predispose an older person to undernutrition and dehydration, particularly when the effects of illnesses on the ability to eat and drink are also present. For example, illness, injury, or medications that limit mobility or cause fever, diarrhea, sweating, swallowing disorders, or confusion may all adversely affect oral intake of food and fluids.

Identifying Malnutrition and Dehydration

We often refer to patients as *malnourished,* but there is no uniform definition of malnutrition. Obesity is the most common form of malnutri-

tion in the United States, though this is generally not how the term is used. More often, it describes a person who is very thin (low weight) or losing weight, is losing or has low muscle or fat mass, is eating poorly, or has abnormal blood "markers" of nutritional status such as cholesterol, albumin, and prealbumin. Though many of these body composition and blood markers are strongly associated with high risk for adverse outcomes and death, they also can all be affected by diseases not related to nutrient intake, adding to the complexity in defining who is malnourished. What is important for the EMS provider to determine is whether or not the individual may be *undernourished*—suffering from a condition in which providing extra nutrients would result in some benefit ▶ **Figure 12-11**. This section explains how to

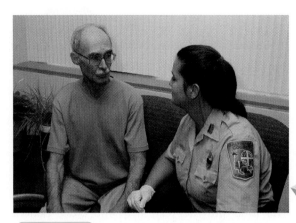

Figure 12-11   It is very important for the EMS provider to determine if an older patient may be undernourished.

make the determination. Fortunately, hydration problems have been more extensively studied, and there is less debate over what constitutes volume depletion (dehydration).

Though there is no accepted definition of malnutrition, it is well known that very high and very low body weight are associated with higher morbidity and mortality in older—just as in younger—populations, though it appears that the ideal body weight is somewhat higher in older individuals. Similarly, dehydration is associated with a high morbidity and mortality in the older population; hospitalized older patients with dehydration have seven times the mortality rate of patients of the same age with normal water balance.[4] Thus, although malnutrition or dehydration is not generally the main reason EMS is called for an older patient, these conditions are probably common and may be important to address to prevent later illness.

Assessment

History

Determination of when a food or fluid problem exists in an older patient can represent a significant challenge for health care providers. First, when malnutrition or dehydration is suspected, it is useful to ask the patient or caregiver about symptoms of illness such as weight loss, poor appetite, fever, confusion, or diarrhea; about chewing or swallowing problems; about the presence of illnesses that may affect oral intake such as depression, dementia, or stroke; and about the use of alcohol and medications that affect eating and

body water. One of the most common reasons for undernutrition in the community-dwelling older person is a social one: Don't forget to ask if this person has difficulty getting groceries, preparing meals, and paying for food, or frequently eats alone. Finally, ask if the patient is hungry or thirsty, and has been passing a normal amount of urine.

Physical Examination

On examination, you may note poor condition of teeth, or loose-fitting dentures, that can contribute to weight loss. Examine the patient and the environment for signs of abuse or neglect (see also Chapter 14, Elder Abuse), and document the presence of any medications or alcohol bottles. Look in the refrigerator to see that the patient actually has food. You may see evidence of chronic illnesses, such as a barrel chest in a patient with severe pulmonary disease, or red palms (**palmar erythema**) and fluid in the abdomen (**ascites**) in a patient with liver cirrhosis. Note evidence of self-neglect and general poor self-care, such as torn or soiled clothes and an unclean living environment.

The clinical assessment for dehydration is challenging; older people may have some signs of dehydration simply because of age and may not manifest other common signs until dehydration is very severe. Thus, determination of dehydration requires quite a bit of detective work; at times it may be unclear until laboratory values are available (▼ **Figure 12-12**). Possible signs to look for are dry

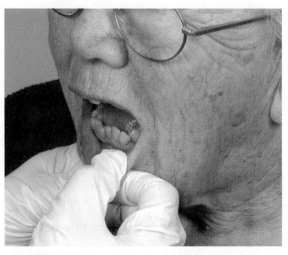

Figure 12-12   Clinical assessment for dehydration and malnutrition can be challenging. Dry mucous membranes are among the signs to look for.

mucous membranes, flat neck veins, increased heart rate or low blood pressure, absence of urine output, and a weight that is significantly less than the patient's usual. Evaluation of skin turgor ("tenting"), though useful in children and younger adults, is very unreliable in older patients.

Treatment and Transport

Remember that dehydration is not well tolerated by the older patient; treat abnormal vital signs as soon as possible. If the patient is not mentating well and blood pressure is low, IV fluid will be required until the patient is stabilized. Early transport is particularly urgent if your training level does not enable you to give IV fluid therapy. At times, starting an IV can be very difficult in an older person whose veins tend to roll and may be collapsed because of low blood volume. Because of concern for underlying cardiac, pulmonary, and renal diseases in the older patient, monitor IV fluid administration closely to avoid overhydration. The patient's ECG should be monitored as well. If glucose monitoring is available, the patient's blood glucose level should be checked. If hypoglycemic, consider the administration of D_{50} intravenously, according to local protocol. Pay special attention to skin condition in an undernourished or dehydrated person, who often has very thin skin that is easily subject to tears and pressure ulcers. Treat the skin gently when preparing the patient for transport.

> ### Attitude Tip
>
> **Pay special attention to gentle handling of the skin in an older patient who may be undernourished or dehydrated; the skin will be particularly vulnerable to tears and pressure ulcers.**

Prevention

The EMS provider can help the older patient avoid significant health problems by educating the patient about nutritional and fluid needs, and by making appropriate referrals for services when the need is discovered. In patients with difficulty affording, getting to, preparing, or eating food, it may be helpful to make a referral for financial services, personal care aides, or food delivered by in-home services. Contact your local Meals on Wheels agency or senior center. Senior centers often provide meals at a nominal fee. Or call your state unit on aging, listed in the government pages of the phone book, for additional resources.

For patients with difficulty chewing or swallowing, poor appetite or other signs of depression, or indications of a medical reason for poor consumption of food and fluids, referral for a medical evaluation may be warranted. Further, when there is evidence of increased need for oral hydration, such as in a patient with diarrhea or

CASE STUDY 2

You are dispatched to a 68-year-old woman with a chief complaint of flulike symptoms. The patient is sitting on her couch and complains that she has been feeling progressively weak and has had no energy. She says that she's lost some weight over the past few weeks and is constantly thirsty.

Her vital signs are: blood pressure, 98/62 mm Hg; pulse, 104 beats/min; and respirations, 16 breaths/min. Her skin is warm and dry, and her mouth appears dry. She has no allergies and takes one multivitamin daily.

What condition is this patient likely experiencing?

What additional assessment should be done on this patient?

What prehospital treatment should this patient receive?

when the environment is very hot, education to promote proper hydration is in order.

Endocrine System

The endocrine system, like the nervous system, functions as a control center for the body. The endocrine system uses hormones (chemicals that affect bodily functions) to control numerous physiological processes including growth, metabolism, "fight or flight" responses to stress, salt and fluid balance, sexual maturation, cellular uptake of glucose, and others. Through these processes, the endocrine system assists the body in maintaining homeostasis, or internal normalcy. Among the numerous endocrine disorders that affect older patients, diabetes and thyroid disorders are particularly important.

Diabetes

Diabetes is the most common endocrine disorder in older patients. Over 18% of the US population, or 6.3 million people age 65 and older, have diabetes.[5] The incidence of diabetes increases with age.

Diabetes is divided into two categories: type I and type II. **Type I diabetes**, also known as *insulin-dependent diabetes*, is managed with daily injections of insulin, exercise, and proper diet. Type I diabetes results from the destruction of the pancreas' insulin-producing cells and evokes a quick onset of signs and symptoms, usually over a few days (▶ **Figure 12-13A**). Type I diabetes usually starts at a young age. **Type II diabetes** is commonly referred to as *non–insulin-dependent diabetes,* though often patients with this type of diabetes will also use insulin when oral medications are inadequate. It is usually managed with oral medications, exercise, and proper diet (▶ **Figure 12-13B**). Type II diabetes usually has a slower onset (weeks to months) than type I because the pancreas is still producing insulin. Type II diabetes is commonly associated with an inadequate amount of insulin production, or a resistance by the body to its own insulin. Most, but not all, type II diabetics are overweight. Treatment of type II diabetes with oral medications is usually adequate to stabilize the condition and normalize blood glucose levels, but sometimes insulin injections may also be required.

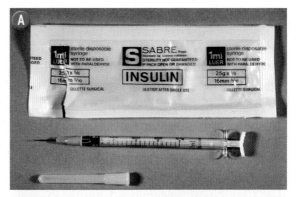

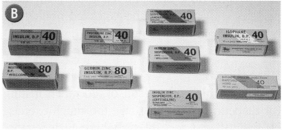

Figure 12-13   Type I diabetes is managed with daily insulin injections **(A)**. Type II diabetes care usually involves oral medications **(B)**. Exercise and proper diet are important parts of self-care for both types.

Ideally, diabetics maintain good control of their disease and have access to knowledgeable diabetes care practitioners. Maintaining good blood sugar control probably decreases complications from the disease, such as heart disease and stroke, blindness, kidney disease, and amputations. Older patients with diabetes are even more affected by complications than younger people:

♦ Evidence of heart disease is present in up to 20% of people with diabetes over the age of 45, and the incidence increases with age.

♦ Diabetes is the leading contributor to new cases of blindness for adults up to age 74.

♦ Diabetes is one of the leading causes for renal failure requiring dialysis in the United States.

♦ Diabetic patients over age 65 are twice as likely to be hospitalized for kidney infections as those without diabetes.[6]

Managing diabetes in older patients is even more difficult than in younger patient groups. Diabetes management requires precise dosing, especially for patients using insulin. Older patients are at a disadvantage in regard to precise dosing because insulin syringes have small markings that can be difficult to see for patients with vision problems. Some commercial devices are available to assist patients in dosing their insulin (▼ **Figure 12-14**).

Types of Diabetic Emergencies

Both types of diabetes have the potential to create a diabetic emergency. The two most common emergencies are hypoglycemia (low blood glucose levels) and diabetic ketoacidosis. There is also a condition, encountered mostly in older persons with type II diabetes, called nonketotic hyperglycemic-hyperosmolar coma.

Hypoglycemia

Hypoglycemia is the result of too much insulin (or diabetic oral medication), too much exercise or activity, or a lack of carbohydrate ingestion. Any combination of these three hastens development of a hypoglycemic state. Onset of hypoglycemia is generally quick, but the condition is reversible if treated promptly. If left untreated, hypoglycemia can be fatal. Signs and symptoms of hypoglycemia include:

- Altered level of responsiveness, with a history of diabetes
- Odd or bizarre behavior
- Increased hunger
- Diaphoresis
- Anxiety
- Tremors
- Fast heart rate

Note that older patients are frequently taking medications that can alter the signs and symptoms of hypoglycemia. For example, patients tak-

ing beta-blocker heart medications may not feel shaky or have an increased heart rate even when their blood glucose levels are very low. Treatment for an older hypoglycemic patient includes:

- Airway maintenance
- Oral glucose between the gum and cheeks (follow local protocols) (▼ **Figure 12-15A**)
- Blood glucose monitoring, an IV of an isotonic fluid, and IV injection of 50% dextrose (follow local protocols) (▼ **Figure 12-15B**)

Diabetic Ketoacidosis

Diabetic ketoacidosis (DKA) occurs when a patient has **hyperglycemia** but the cells resort to burning fat for energy. The lack of insulin in the body prevents proper amounts of glucose from entering the cells, where it is used for energy. The cells are then forced to burn fat for energy, which creates ketone bodies and ketoacids as byproducts. The ketone bodies and

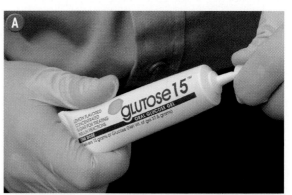

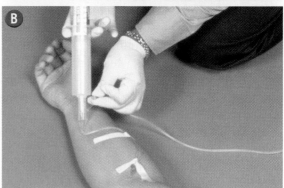

(**Figure 12-15**)   Administering glucose is appropriate in diabetic emergencies unless you have a reliable blood glucose measurement indicating hyperglycemia. Available forms include oral glucose paste **(A)** and 50% glucose solution for IV administration **(B)**.

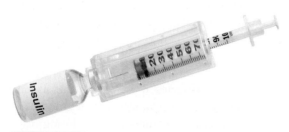

(**Figure 12-14**)   Devices such as syringe magnifiers are available to assist patients in dosing their insulin.

acids cause an acidotic state within the body. The onset of diabetic ketoacidosis is usually slow, but the effects can be fatal. Common signs and symptoms associated with diabetic ketoacidosis include:

♦ Increased thirst

♦ Increased urination

♦ Kussmaul (rapid and deep) respirations

♦ Unexplained rapid weight loss

♦ Dehydration

♦ Blurred vision

♦ Altered level of responsiveness

♦ Sweet, pungent odor to the breath

Treatment for an older patient with diabetic ketoacidosis includes:

♦ Airway maintenance

♦ Oral glucose between the gum and cheeks (follow local protocols)

♦ Blood glucose monitoring; an IV with an isotonic fluid; and consider a fluid bolus of 10 mL/kg if rales, wheezing, renal failure, and respiratory distress are not present (follow local protocols)

Nonketotic Hyperglycemic-Hyperosmolar Coma

Nonketotic hyperglycemic-hyperosmolar coma (NKHHC), a complication of type II diabetes that is commonly seen in older patients, has a high mortality rate. It frequently occurs because of an infection or trauma. The complication is caused by inadequate fluid intake during a period of elevated blood glucose levels. The high glucose levels lead to increased urination, as the body tries to "dump" glucose in the urine. The low fluid intake and increased urination result in dehydration. Patients with NKHHC most often present with blood glucose levels greater than 500 mg/dL, decreased level of consciousness (usually unresponsive), and possibly seizures.

Treatment involves maintenance of airway, breathing, and circulation (ABCs) and immediate transport. Administer IV fluid therapy following local protocols.

Prevention of Diabetic Emergencies

Good blood sugar control reduces complications and emergencies associated with diabetes. To im-

prove older patients' awareness and help them maintain good control, EMS providers can offer these supportive actions:

♦ Provide diabetes screening and awareness for communities. This will provide for early detection of type II diabetes in some persons, and cut back the potential for complications. *Approximately 50% of persons with type II diabetes are not aware of their disease until after the onset of a complication!*[7]

♦ Offer diabetes workshops for older patients in the community to promote and encourage proper diabetes management. Use diabetes health professionals in local communities to facilitate the workshops. *Proper control, complying with medication regimens, exercise, and proper diet can cut back diabetes complications by up to 60% in those with type I diabetes!*[8]

♦ Provide education (or make a referral for education) to patients about the signs and symptoms of hyperglycemia and hypoglycemia so that they may seek early treatment when these occur.

♦ All persons with diabetes should be taught to contact their health care provider right away for instructions if they are unable to eat or drink, to make adjustments in their medications to avoid hypoglycemia.

Thyroid Disorders

The thyroid gland undergoes changes in both its structure and function with aging (▶ **Figure 12-16**).

Hypothyroidism

Up to 5% of patients older than 65 have low levels of thyroid hormones, a condition known as **hypothyroidism**.[9] The prevalence of hypothyroidism rises with age, is higher in women, and is higher in institutionalized older patients than in those living in the community.[9] Unfortunately, less than a third of the older patients with hypothyroidism present with typical signs and symptoms, so many patients attribute the changes to normal aging. Signs and symptoms of hypothyroidism include:

♦ Feeling cold

♦ Fatigue/low energy

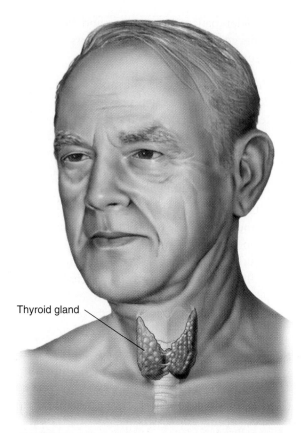

Figure 12-16 The thyroid gland undergoes changes in both its structure and function with aging.

- Constipation
- Thinning of hair or eyebrows
- Confusion
- Increased occurrence of falls
- Bradycardia
- Decreased appetite
- "Puffy" face
- Unexplained weight gain

Hyperthyroidism

Hyperthyroidism, an overabundance of thyroid hormones, is less common in older patients and is usually the result of overmedication with thyroid medications. The rate of hyperthyroidism, up to 2% of the older population, is no different than in other age groups.[9] In contrast to younger populations where the condition is more common in women, in the older age groups, men and women are equally affected. Older patients more commonly do not present with the classic signs

and symptoms of hyperthyroidism that are listed below. More often, they present with weakness or lack of interest in anything (apathy), and commonly present with cardiac symptoms such as new or worsened congestive heart failure, new atrial fibrillation, or angina. Classic signs and symptoms of hyperthyroidism include:

- Feeling hot
- Inability to sleep
- Fatigue
- Palpitations
- Tachycardia
- Diarrhea
- Feeling anxious or "fidgety"
- Unexplained weight loss

The most common complication in older patients with hyperthyroidism is atrial fibrillation, occurring in 27% of older patients with hyperthyroidism.[9] The likelihood of developing heart failure and death are greater if a normal heart rhythm is not restored. Additionally, the diagnosis of hyperthyroidism in an older patient carries an increased likelihood of depression, myopathy, and osteoporosis.

A **thyroid storm** is a rare, life-threatening condition that may occur in patients with hyperthyroidism. The condition is usually triggered by a stressful event or increased volume of thyroid hormones in the circulation. In addition to the normal signs and symptoms of hyperthyroidism, the following are usually present: fever, severe tachycardia, nausea, vomiting, altered mental status, and possibly heart failure.

Medication Tip

Most older patients with hyperthyroidism actually have a hypothyroid condition and have taken too much medication, or are consuming medications that interact with their thyroid medicine.

Treatment for both hypothyroidism and hyperthyroidism is usually deferred to the hospital. In the event that a patient is unstable (tachycardic or bradycardic with serious signs and symptoms), treat the patient for the instability with appropriate cardiac or other therapies.

Prevention of Thyroid-related Emergencies

Prehospital providers can assist in avoiding emergencies related to thyroid disorders by taking two actions:

♦ Encourage patients with symptoms to seek medical attention. Thyroid disorders may be easily diagnosed with blood tests.

♦ Remind or encourage older patients with thyroid disorders to comply with their medication plans (▼ Figure 12-17). Common medications for thyroid conditions are listed in (▼ Table 12-1).

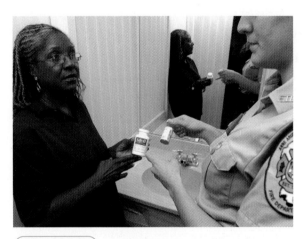

Figure 12-17 Remind or encourage older patients with thyroid disorders to comply with their medication plans and check with their health care provider before consuming any over-the-counter medications that may interact.

TABLE 12-1 Common Medications for Thyroid Conditions
Levothyroxine (Synthroid, Levothroid, Levoxine)
Dextrothyroxine (Choloxin)
Liothyronine (Cytomel)
Thyroglobulin (Proloid)
Liotrix (Euthroid)

Integumentary System Emergencies

Integument means a natural outer coat, such as the skin. The skin, hair, and nails make up the integumentary system. It is the largest organ or system in the human body and like any other, it changes over time. These changes could be physiologic as part of normal aging, or pathologic due to disease. This section discusses skin structure, function, and aging, and common skin diseases among older patients.

Structure and Physiology of the Aging Skin

Skin Layers

The skin has two main layers. The **epidermis** is the outer, protective layer; the inner, living layer is the **dermis** (▼ Figure 12-18). These layers stretch over the body, protect it from losing fluid, and provide a barrier against harmful external substances.

Medication Tip

Proper use of a device such as a blood pressure cuff at diastolic measure is an excellent alternative to a constricting band, which could damage an older person's skin during IV therapy.

The epidermis is only a few cells (0.07 to 1.4 mm) thick. It contains pores, pigments, and ducts. The surface of the epidermis consists of dead cells that shed constantly. The epidermis changes with age. One of these changes is flattening

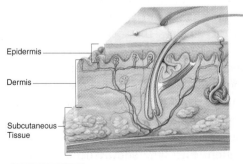

Figure 12-18 The skin has two main layers, the epidermis and dermis, which are connected by the dermal-epidermal junction.

CASE STUDY 3

Mrs. Smith is a 90-year-old woman with a history of dementia and left hip fracture. Her daughter, who visits daily, found her on the floor of the house, lethargic and confused. She called 9-1-1 for help. An EMS crew arrived 8 minutes later and found her unable to follow commands and with a temperature of 103°F. Blood pressure and pulse were within normal limits and respiratory rate was 24 breaths/min.

They transported Mrs. Smith to the nearest emergency department for evaluation. After 4 hours, she was transferred to an acute-care hospital bed for treatment of sepsis and a urinary tract infection. In the acute care unit, the nurse noticed an area of tissue redness about 2 inches square in the sacral region that would not blanch (turn white when pressed).

At which stage is Mrs. Smith's pressure ulcer?

What caused Mrs. Smith's pressure ulcer?

of the dermalepidermal junction. The dermal-epidermal junction is the connection between the two layers. This junction has several connecting structures that help with communication and nutrient transfer between the layers. Flattening of the junction increases the tendency of the skin to tear or blister. In addition, the epidermis is continually losing and gaining new cells, a process called epidermal turnover. This process declines with age, to around 30% in a person in their 70s of what it was in their 20s. This slowing affects the healing time of a wound. These are some of the normal changes that occur with age and affect the functions of the epidermis.

The dermis has many functions, but the main ones are mechanical protection and thermoregulation. The dermis protects the body against trauma and changes in external temperatures. Some of the changes that occur in the dermis with age are decreases in its thickness (atrophy) and blood flow. Deterioration of the ability to regulate blood flow, combined with other changes in the dermis, also has an impact on wound healing.

Subcutaneous fat is the layer beneath the dermis. Its major purposes are protection and thermoregulation. First, the subcutaneous fat layer protects the body against trauma and pressure of the dermis. Second, the layer limits conductive heat loss and helps the body control temperature.

The thickness of the subcutaneous fat layer decreases with age, affecting these functions. (Subcutaneous fat is different from total body fat, which increases with age. Total body fat lies mainly around muscles and other organs.) ▼ Table 12-2 presents skin changes with age.

Pressure Ulcers

A **pressure ulcer** (▶ Figure 12-19) is caused by pressure that compromises the blood supply to an area of tissue. This area of tissue then dies (infarcts). Other names that describe this process are decubitus ulcer, pressure sore, and bedsore.

TABLE 12-2 Functional Skin Changes with Aging

Elasticity declines.

Body loses heat more easily.

Skin bruises and tears more easily.

Sweat production declines.

Wound healing declines.

Cell replacement declines.

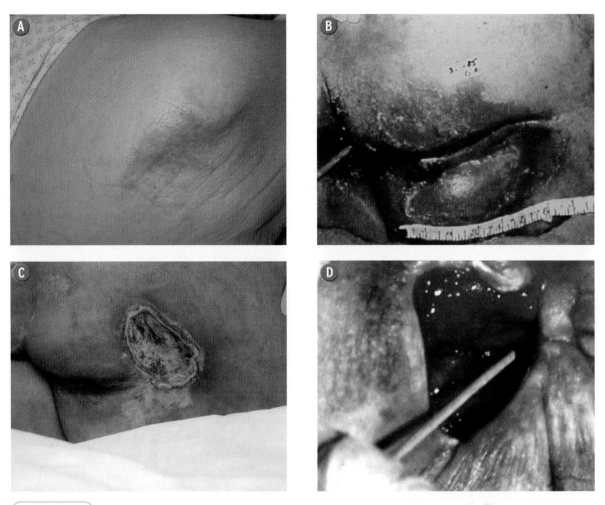

Figure 12-19   A pressure ulcer, or decubitus ulcer, develops when pressure compromises blood supply and thus oxygenation to an area of tissue. **(A)** Stage 1. **(B)** Stage 2. **(C)** Stage 3. **(D)** Stage 4.

Occurrence

Pressure ulcers occur mainly in immobile or debilitated patients. Currently, an estimated 1.5 million or more Americans are affected. At least 57% of all pressure ulcers are thought to develop in the hospital.[10] Pressure ulcers in long-term care facilities have been reported to occur in 2.4% to 23% of patients at time of admission.[11,12] They are a frequent problem in older adults, and can cause pain and distress for the patient and family.

Pathophysiology

Pressure ulcers are usually localized in areas close to a bony prominence (**hard site**). Pressure affects blood flow and oxygenation of the tissues between bony prominences and the skin. It first causes failure to oxygenate and deliver nutrients in the area, then accumulation of waste products, and finally tissue damage or death (necrosis). Time is an important factor in this process, as well as pressure. The damage also depends on the person's general health and the type of tissue affected. For example, muscle tissue damage can occur after applying enough pressure to affect the blood flow for approximately 2 hours. But with higher pressure, the time required to cause damage decreases. Muscle and subcutaneous tissues are more susceptible to pressure and hypoxia than epidermal tissues. Therefore, damage usually occurs in the underlying tissues first and will not be clearly visible in the epidermis.

Pressure ulcers commonly occur in areas around the sacrum, greater trochanter, ischial tuberosity, heel, scapula, and fibular head (▼ **Figure 12-20**). Approximately 95% of pressure ulcers occur in the lower part of the body.[13] Three key factors in addition to pressure contribute to development of pressure ulcers: friction, moisture, and shearing forces (forces sliding past each other in opposite directions). For example, shearing forces and friction occur when the patient slides down in bed, stretching subcutaneous tissues and compromising blood supply. Moisture, often from incontinence or perspiration, is another important factor. This can lead to tissue maceration that makes the skin more susceptible to pressure, friction, or shearing forces.

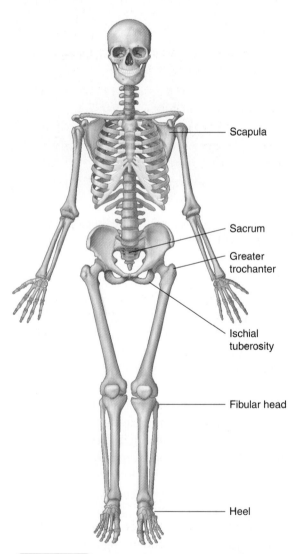

Scapula

Sacrum

Greater trochanter

Ischial tuberosity

Fibular head

Heel

Figure 12-20 Pressure ulcers commonly occur in areas around the scapula, sacrum, greater trochanter, ischial tuberosity, fibular head, and heel.

Risk Factors

Any factor that increases exposure to pressure in the hard sites of the body increases the risk for pressure ulcers. Conditions that affect mobility, such as spinal cord injury, brain injury, or neuromuscular disorder, or any acute illness that makes the patient less active, increase the risk for a pressure ulcer. Problems with nutrition, fecal or urinary incontinence, and neuropathies also can significantly increase the risk for pressure ulcers.

Clinical Stages

Pressure ulcers can be classified in four different stages, describing the severity of the sore (▼ **Table 12-3**). Stage I is **nonblanching erythema**. To evaluate this stage, gently apply pressure to the area of tissue redness with a finger; this will not produce a blanching (whiteness) as a rash does. It is important to note that, in stage I, the damage occurs under the skin, which will be intact. In stage II, the damage extends through the epidermis and dermis. This could appear as a superficial ulcer or blister. In stage III the epidermis, dermis, and subcutaneous tissues are affected. Fat is visible at the base of the ulcer. In Stage IV, the ulcer extends into muscle, tendons, or bone. On occasion, ulcers cannot be classified because of scar tissue formation or a covering of black dead tissue (**eschar**), which makes it difficult to know how deep the ulcer is. In all cases, in addition to the stage of the ulcer, it is important to describe the surrounding structure, location, appearance, and size. This will help in treating the sore, following its progress, and communicating with other health care professionals.

TABLE 12-3 Pressure Ulcer Stages	
Stages	**Description**
I	Nonblanching erythema; damage beneath the skin
II	Blister or ulcer affecting the epidermis and dermis
III	Ulcer exposing the fat down to the fascia
IV	Ulcer exposing muscle or bone

Complications

Pressure ulcers can cause pain and discomfort in the affected area. Patients with pressure ulcers have increased mortality rates, either because of underlying clinical problems that lead to ulcers, or as a complication of the ulcers themselves. Complications that can occur with pressure ulcers include bleeding, cellulitis, sepsis, and **osteomyelitis**. Osteomyelitis is inflammation of the bone caused by infection and is a frequent complication of pressure ulcers that can affect ulcer healing if the infection is not appropriately treated. These complications occur more commonly in stages III and IV. Any nonhealing ulcer has to be evaluated for infection, especially osteomyelitis.

Prevention and Care

Prevention should be targeted at persons with risk factors for pressure ulcers, but because nearly all older patients will have thinning of their skin, it is prudent to practice good preventive skin care management on all older patients. Most importantly, decrease pressure—especially on hard sites. This can be done with careful positioning to spread the maximal areas of pressure over a large region, with frequent changes of position to promote mobility, and with use of pillows to package the patient so that areas of high risk, such as the sacrum and heels, are cushioned from hard surfaces (▼ **Figure 12-21**). Also, it is important to inspect the skin regularly and avoid friction or tearing forces, excessive moisture, and skin irritants.

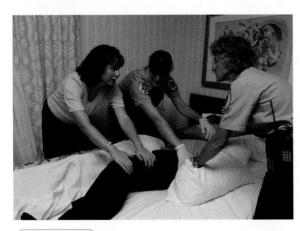

Figure 12-21 To help prevent pressure ulcers, encourage or help the patient to decrease pressure on hard sites by changing position frequently.

Treatment

Aside from assessment and pressure relief, specific pressure ulcer treatment is beyond the scope of the EMS provider. However, by knowing what these treatments are, the EMS provider is better able to educate patients, family members, and caregivers.

All the preventive measures also need to be followed during treatment of pressure ulcers, in addition to specific treatment measures (▼ **Table 12-4**). The primary treatment is to relieve pressure from the area of skin damage to allow the growth of new skin. In addition, treat any infection. Dressing will depend on the stage and characteristics of the ulcer.

Attitude Tip

Pressure ulcers can develop after lying on a hard surface for 2 hours. With any immobile patient in your care for 2 hours or more, especially on a hard backboard, relieve discomfort and reduce pressure ulcer risk by finding safe ways to reposition the patient. When possible, avoid hard surfaces and package the patient with pillows to relieve pressure, particularly on bony areas of the body.

Infection in the Aging Skin

Herpes Zoster

Herpes zoster (shingles) is caused by the reactivation of a varicella virus on nerve roots. This condition is more common in the older population. Most people that develop herpes zoster are in good health, but those with cancer or im-

TABLE 12-4 Pressure Ulcer Treatment

Assess the stage of the ulcer.

Relieve pressure.

Assess and manage nutritional status.

Cleanse ulcer at each dressing change.

Select ulcer dressing.

Provide pain relief.

munosuppression are at higher risk. This condition affects any nerve in the body, but the thoracic nerves and the ophthalmic division of the trigeminal nerve are most common. The disease usually starts with pain in the affected area. Subsequently, a cluster of tiny blisters (**vesicles**) erupts on reddened skin in the same area. The rash is typically unilateral; it rarely crosses the midline.

One of the most common complications of herpes zoster is pain, or postherpetic neuralgia. This condition affects up to half of those 60 and older, and can last longer than a year.[14] During the acute phase of the infection, the person may suffer severe pain and require narcotic pain relievers. Antiviral medications such as acyclovir or famciclovir can be used, preferably within 48 hours of the activation of the disease. These medications decrease healing time, new lesion formation, and pain.

Candida

Candida is a fungal organism that usually grows in moist areas like the groin and other skin folds. Those who are obese, diabetic, and have recently been treated with antibiotic or steroid therapies are at risk for overgrowth with *Candida*. The skin develops a reddish rash with small red spots (**papules**). Treatments include strategies to decrease moisture, topical antifungal medication, and on occasion, systemic antifungal therapy.

Cellulitis

Cellulitis is an acute inflammation within the skin caused by a bacterial infection (**▼ Figure 12-22**).

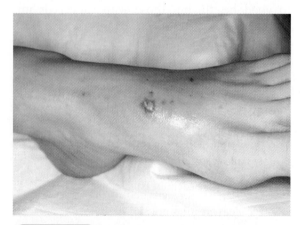

Figure 12-22) Cellulitis is a diffuse, acute inflammation within the skin caused by a bacterial infection.

This condition usually affects the lower extremities. Symptoms can include fever, chills, and general malaise. Cellulitis can cause warmth, swelling, redness (**erythema**), tenderness, and enlarged lymph nodes in the affected area. Blood tests may show elevation of the white blood cell counts and bacteria. Treatments include antibiotic therapy, assuring adequate fluid intake, and local dressings if there is an open sore.

Rashes

A rash is a temporary eruption or inflammation in the skin. It can be caused by exposure to a toxic substance, or an allergic reaction. Exposure to the poison ivy plant causes a type of rash called **contact dermatitis**. Symptoms include redness and swelling, which can sometimes be severe. Treatment is similar to any other contact dermatitis. Avoid exposure to the irritating agent, and use topical steroid creams and antihistamine medication.

Drugs or medications can also cause many dermatological problems. Older patients are particularly at risk because they often use multiple medications. The skin can react in different ways to a new medication. In addition, some medications make the skin more sensitive to sunlight. When a patient complains of a rash, obtaining a medication list is very important.

Medication Tip

Rashes and other skin problems can be medication reactions. Because older patients often use multiple medications, this is yet another condition for which they are at higher risk than the younger population.

Vascular Ulceration

In addition to pressure sores or ulcers, a group of vascular conditions can cause ulcers. Examples include **venous ulceration** and **arterial ulceration**. Venous ulceration is caused by an increase of the venous pressure in the lower extremities. Some factors predispose people to venous ulcers, including obesity, multiple pregnancies, and family history. Initially, the person will complain of edema and discomfort in the ankle. If untreated, an ulcer can develop in the affected area. The venous ulcer, usually located on the medial aspect of the ankle, can become infected. Treatment is to relieve the edema and treat any infection. Arterial ulcers are caused by a decrease in oxygen supply to an area of tissue, secondary to atherosclerosis. They are usually located in the toe or anterior tibial area. The treatment consists of improvement in the blood flow with medication, and sometimes surgery. The patient should avoid tobacco use, which can worsen the disease by further decreasing blood flow.

Sepsis and Infectious Disease

Infections in older persons can be severe and dangerous. **Sepsis** is the disease state that results from the presence of microorganisms or their toxic products in the bloodstream. Sepsis is the 13th most common cause of death in the United States. Of all older patients who become septic, 37% to 50% will die[15] (▼ **Figure 12-23**). Therefore, this is a serious problem that every EMS provider should know how to recognize and to treat. Think of sepsis whenever you see a hot, flushed patient who is also tachycardic and tachypnic. Think septic shock when hypotension is also present.

The term "sepsis" is used loosely, and often interchangeably with septicemia and bacteremia. The following definitions outline the differences:

♦ *Sepsis:* the presence of two or more of these criteria in response to any infection:

♦ Oral temperature greater than 38°C or less than 36°C

♦ Respiratory rate over 20 or $PaCO_2$ less than 32 mm Hg

♦ Heart rate of greater than 90 beats/min

♦ Leukocyte count over 12,000 or less than 4,000

♦ *Septic shock:* Sepsis with hypotension that is unresponsive to fluid resuscitation, plus any of these:

♦ Organ dysfunction

♦ Acute mental status changes

♦ Other conditions that would be determined in the hospital (metabolic acidosis, low urine output, acute respiratory distress syndrome)

♦ *Bacteremia (fungicemia):* The presence of viable bacteria (fungi) in the bloodstream as evidenced by positive blood cultures.

While bacteremia must have a bacterial cause, sepsis can occur due to bacteria, fungi, or viruses.

Alterations in Immune Function with Age

Almost every aspect of immune function is affected by aging. Older persons are therefore more prone to infection and secondary complications than the young. Chronic conditions such as diabetes, dementia, malnutrition, cardiovascular disease, chronic pulmonary disease, and cancer all place older individuals at greater risk of serious infection (▶ **Table 12-5**).

Older persons manifest infections differently. Although fever is often present with minor illness in the young, fever in older persons usually indicates serious infection. However, as many as 30% of older persons with serious infection may not have a fever at all (▶ **Figure 12-24**). This is due to the inability of older persons to mount a fever. In fact, these patients may even have hypothermia! Therefore, when the temperature is either too high or too low, think infection. In many cases, the temperature will be normal; the only sign of underlying infection may be an acute decline in baseline functional status. Anorexia, fatigue, weight loss, falls, or change in mental status may be the primary symptoms of infection in these patients.

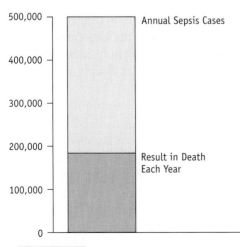

(**Figure 12-23**) Of all patients who become septic, at least 37% will die.

TABLE 12-5   Age-related Risk Factors for Infection

Decreased pulmonary function and cough reflex

Decreased gastric acidity and GI motility (activity)

Heart disease

Thin, easily traumatized skin; skin ulcers

Impaired immune mechanisms

Inadequate nutrition and hydration

Chronic use of medications

Chronic diseases

Urinary retention or incontinence

Institutional living

Need for invasive medical devices (eg, catheters and tubes)

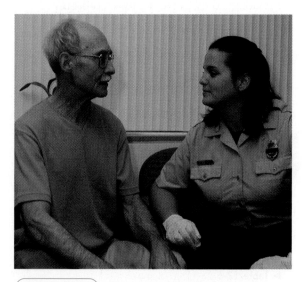

Figure 12-24   As many as 30% of older persons with serious infection may not have a fever at all. Check for less obvious signs and symptoms such as anorexia, fatigue, weight loss, falls, or change in mental status.

Infection in Community-Dwelling Versus Nursing Home Patients

Infections in independent, community-dwelling older people differ from those of institutionalized (usually nursing home) residents. Nursing home residents often get more serious infections because they are exposed to antibiotic-resistant bacteria that live in nursing home patients. It is also easy to pass infection from person to person in the close confines of a nursing home. Health care providers with poor handwashing techniques and lack of universal precautions may cause infections by carrying bacteria from one patient to the next. Also, patients who reside in a nursing home are usually sicker than those who live in the community, and therefore cannot fight off an infection as well.

Attitude Tip

Your compliance with handwashing and other universal precautions procedures will help protect your older patients from the transmission of infections between patients. Nursing home residents are at particular risk.

Causes

Pneumonia is the leading cause of death from infection in Americans older than 65 (▸ **Figure 12-25**). Atypical presentations are common. Approximately one third present without sputum production or fever, and half present without cough. In these patients, tachypnea is the most common presenting sign. However, you must still always check for history of cough, fever, chills, and upper respiratory infection symptoms. Ask about sore throat, sinus symptoms, and ear pain. Look for signs of respiratory congestion, shortness of breath, and crackles (rales) on lung auscultation.

The GI system is a common trigger for sepsis. Common symptoms signaling this cause are abdominal pain, nausea, vomiting, and diarrhea. Ask for history of gallbladder disease, or diverticulitis and colitis.

The urinary system also contributes to sepsis. Discomfort urinating, frequent need to urinate, and urgency are common symptoms of a urinary tract infection (UTI). Patients with indwelling Foley catheters are at high risk. People with any difficulty urinating or with incontinence are also prone to UTI.

Finally, the skin and joints may be a source of infection and sepsis. Look for red, hot, and tender areas of skin, especially at points of skin appropriate IV antibiotics as soon as possible. Just as EMS providers may put heart attack patients on the track for nitroglycerin, clot-dissolving therapy such as tPA, or catheter lab intervention, you should put the septic patient on the fast track for fluids and antibiotics—whether you provide them yourself or deliver the patient promptly to the hospital.

Be sure you get a thorough history of medications, especially antibiotics: what kind and when taken. Also get a good history of immunizations. Has the patient received a flu shot or a pneumonia vaccination? Ask about their exposure to disease: What illnesses is he or she in contact with? Especially know about infections in a nursing home patient's roommate and others from that floor (▼ Figure 12-26).

It is essential for EMS providers to maintain universal precautions for the protection of all older people. Also be sure to disinfect equipment such as your stethoscope so it does not serve to spread bacteria.

Use respiratory precautions on any patient with cough or congestion. When you personally have a cold or flu, ensure that you wear a mask to stop the spread of respiratory droplets. What is a minor nuisance to you may cause sepsis in an older person. Also protect yourself from infection. Congested, coughing patients usually will benefit from supplemental oxygen. Note that an oxygen mask, fitted well to the patient's face, can serve as respiratory isolation to protect you from droplet spread.

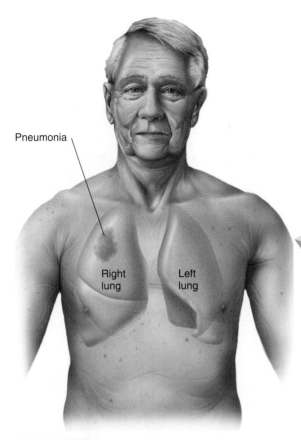

Pneumonia

Right lung

Left lung

Figure 12-25 Pneumonia is the leading cause of death from infection in Americans older than 65.

breakdown or ulcers. This often means lifting or rolling the bedridden patient to see hard sites at the back and sacrum. Diapers may also hide areas of skin infection. Because an older person's skin is less of a barrier, be careful to adequately prep the skin before starting IV lines. Don't be the cause of a skin infection from a contaminated IV site.

Treatment and Prevention

Have a high level of suspicion for these life-threatening disease states. Know the subtle findings compatible with sepsis and treat abnormal vital signs. Administer high-flow oxygen for respiratory complaints, especially if accompanied by tachypnea. When patients are hypotensive, give a fluid bolus. If the patient is hot, flushed, and hypotensive, the circulation is being shunted peripherally and is not reaching the vital organs. In these cases, give more fluid.

The most important life-saving intervention, after ensuring the ABCs, is to get these patients

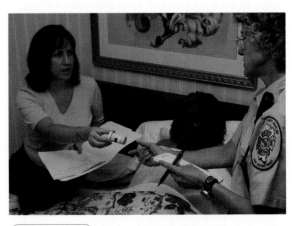

Figure 12-26 For a septic patient, get a thorough history: medications (especially antibiotics), immunizations, and illnesses the patient has been in contact with.

As an EMS provider, make sure that you also receive all your immunizations, including a flu shot every year. This is more to protect the frail older person than yourself, but you will benefit, too. Never use an oxygen mask solely for respiratory isolation. Also provide the correct liter flow for the device being used.

Attitude Tip

Every older patient, regardless of symptoms, has either pneumonia or a UTI until proven otherwise!

Environmental Emergencies

The term "environmental emergencies" is used broadly to include numerous medical conditions resulting from exposure to weather, abnormal conditions, terrain, differing pressures, or a variety of other conditions. The environmental emergencies that most commonly affect older patients include heat disorders (heat cramps, heat exhaustion, and heatstroke) and hypothermia.

Temperature Regulation

Heat and cold emergencies are commonly the result of exposure to extreme temperatures. Even in the harshest of conditions and temperatures, the body attempts to maintain a state of normalcy and balance. To achieve a constant temperature, the **hypothalamus** acts as the control center. Located at the base of the brain, the hypothalamus works in conjunction with **thermoreceptors** throughout the body to help minimize changes in body temperature and determine what corrective actions need to be taken to do so (▶ **Figure 12-27**). If the hypothalamus detects that the body temperature is low, it triggers shivering in an attempt to increase the core temperature. On the other hand, if the hypothalamus detects that temperature is too high, it triggers sweating in an effort to lower the temperature.

In varying temperatures and conditions, a normal body is constantly generating or losing heat to maintain a normal temperature. The body generates heat (thermogenesis) through several processes, including:

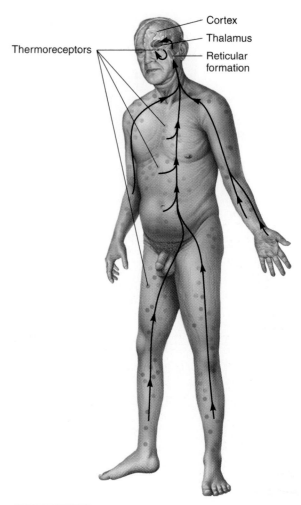

Figure 12-27   The hypothalamus works in conjunction with thermoreceptors throughout the body to minimize changes in body temperature.

♦ Shivering—The movement of muscles generates heat as a byproduct.

♦ Endocrine response—Endocrine glands react by releasing catecholamines (hormones such as epinephrine) to increase the rate of metabolism, create a fever, and ultimately generate heat.

♦ Digestion and metabolism—The process of digesting and metabolizing food creates heat as a byproduct.

The body loses heat through these processes:

♦ Evaporation of sweat

♦ Dilation of blood vessels near the skin to cool the blood

♦ Respiration—Exhaling warm air

CASE STUDY 4

You are dispatched for a 67-year-old man who fell approximately 1 hour ago. The patient is outside and the temperature is approximately 71°F. The patient complains that he is very cold and that his left ankle hurts. His vital signs are within normal limits, but his skin is cool to touch.

In addition to treating his ankle, what else should be treated, and how?

What makes this older patient more susceptible to hypothermia?

Various predisposing factors make older patients more susceptible to environmental emergencies. The temperature regulation mechanisms are not as effective in older persons as they are in younger adults. Due to decreased density and sensitivity of the thermoreceptors, responses to regulate temperatures in both cold and hot environments are frequently delayed. Additionally, *older* patients on fixed incomes are not always financially able to set home thermostats to meet their "comfort needs." Some may therefore live in cooler or warmer environments than their bodies can adjust for (▼ **Figure 12-28**).

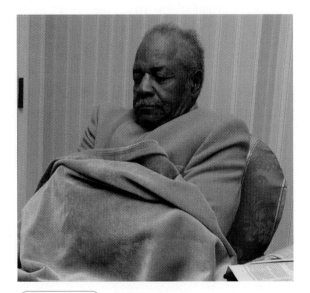

Figure 12-28 Older patients on fixed incomes are not always financially able to set home thermostats to maintain living environments that their bodies can adjust for.

Hypothermia

In colder conditions, older patients are susceptible to hypothermia as a result of normal aging processes and other factors. A normal compensatory mechanism to generate heat is shivering. By the age of 70, 30% of muscle mass is lost, decreasing the amount available for potential heat generation through shivering.[16] The lack of heat-generating ability is compounded by the fact that older patients have less insulation (thinner skin, less hair, and less subcutaneous fat). Another source of heat generation, the release of catecholamines, is also diminished in older patients due to the steady decline in normal metabolism.

Chronic medical conditions also affect the older person's ability to cope with colder environments. Diabetic patients are six times more likely to suffer from hypothermia, in part due to vascular disease that alters thermoregulatory mechanisms.[17] Patients with impaired heart function are also more susceptible to hypothermia emergencies because of common medications used to control their disease (beta blockers). Patients with mobility problems may not be able to seek appropriate shelter from the cold, and patients with dementia may be unable to figure out how to make themselves warmer when they are cold.

Little data are available to pinpoint the exact number of deaths from hypothermia, but the mortality rate of identified cases is 50%. Persons with hypothermia who are older than 75 are five times more likely to die than those younger than 75.[17]

Assessment

Assessment of hypothermic patients centers on the use of thermometers that accurately measure core temperature. To obtain an accurate core temperature in the patient with hypothermia, use a special low-reading rectal thermometer, placed into the rectum for 5 to 8 minutes ▼ **Figure 12-29**.

The signs and symptoms of hypothermia vary. Normal body temperature is 98.6°F (37°C). Mildly hypothermic patients, between 95°F and 97°F (35°C to 36.1°C), typically complain of feeling cold, whereas patients with lower body temperatures may not complain of any coldness at all. Assessment findings are typically not specific and can suggest other conditions, including metabolic disorders and stroke. Patients may present with confusion, weakness, tachycardia (early sign), hypertension (early sign), lower core body tempera-

ture, and shivering (may not be present due to normal aging processes described earlier). Hypothermia is subdivided into four categories of severity according to core temperature ▼ **Table 12-6**.

Treatment

Treatment of older hypothermic patients is the same as other age groups. Stabilization of the ABCs and removal from the cold environment are crucial. Move the patient to a warm environment, such as a heated ambulance, and remove all wet clothes. Provide warmed and humidified oxygen, if available. Avoid rough handling of the patient to minimize the chance of triggering abnormal heart rhythms. When resuscitating cold patients, remember that a patient is not dead until warm and dead. Follow local protocols for resuscitation of hypothermic patients.

Controversy

Especially in moderate to severe cases of hypothermia, treatment steps are less agreed upon than for many other types of medical emergencies. Know and follow local protocols.

Hyperthermia

Hyperthermia is quantified as a high core temperature (greater than 101°F or 38.3°C). In warmer conditions, older patients have a de-

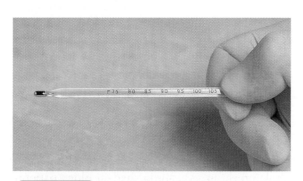

Figure 12-29 To assess core temperature accurately in hypothermia patients, use a special low-reading rectal thermometer.

TABLE 12-6	Characteristics of Systemic Hypothermia			
Core Temperature	90°F to 95°F (32°C to 35°C)	89°F to 92°F (32°C to 33°C)	80°F to 88°F (27°C to 31°C)	< 80°F (< 27°C)
Signs and Symptoms	Shivering, foot stamping	Loss of coordination, muscle stiffness	Coma	Apparent death
Cardiorespiratory Response	Constricted blood vessels, rapid breathing	Slowing respirations, slow pulse	Weak pulse, arrhythmias, very slow respirations	Cardiac arrest
Level of Consciousness	Withdrawn	Confused, lethargic, sleepy	Unresponsive	Unresponsive

Source: American Academy of Orthopaedic Surgeons. Table 18-1. *Emergency Care and Transportation of the Sick and Injured.* 8th ed. Sudbury, MA: Jones and Bartlett; 2002:455.

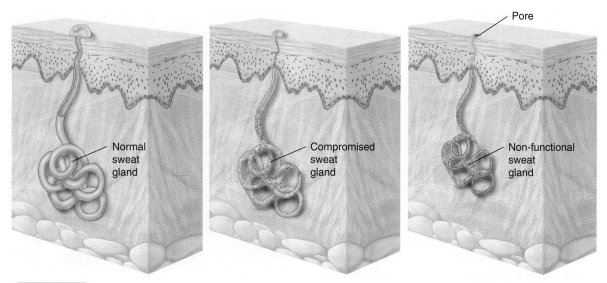

Figure 12-30 Because some sweat glands function poorly with age and others do not work at all, the older body has a decreased ability to cool itself by perspiring.

creased ability to perspire than a younger adult. Some sweat glands function poorly with age, and others do not function at all (▲ **Figure 12-30**). This diminishes the body's ability to cool itself. Additionally, older patients with a history of heart disease are at increased risk of heat emergencies. Reduced heart function makes the patient less able to cope with higher environmental temperatures, and increased heat and humidity also worsen heart failure. As with hypothermia, patients with mobility problems or with dementia may be unable to remove themselves from a hot environment. Heat emergencies tend to worsen other chronic medical conditions, as well. Deaths caused by lung disease (eg, chronic obstructive pulmonary disease), diabetes, and hypertension increase by more than 50% during heat waves.[17]

Many medications predispose older patients to heatstroke. Anticholinergics, phenothiazines, tricyclic antidepressants, and antihistamines tend to decrease the function of the hypothalamus, reduce peripheral sweat output, and cause a decreased mental ability to respond to heated environments. Medications such as opioids, sedatives, and alcohol also alter the patient's ability to respond to heat stress. Amphetamines have a tendency to raise the body temperature by interacting with the hypothalamus. Beta blockers impair the cardiovascular response and ultimately decrease the ability of the

compensatory mechanisms for heatstroke. Diuretics, through fluid loss, exacerbate heat emergencies by depleting the body of needed fluids.

Types of Heat Emergencies

Heat emergencies are traditionally classified into three categories: heat cramps, abnormal redness of the skin due to capillary congestion (as in inflammation), and heatstroke.

Heat cramps (muscle cramps) commonly occur during intense physical activity in a hot, humid environment and are the result of salt and electrolyte imbalance. The cramps are usually preceded by intense sweating, increased thirst, and then an increase in the core body temperature. Treatment for these patients involves removal from the warm environment, oral fluid replacement (including electrolyte drinks), and IV therapy if permitted. Follow local protocols.

Heat exhaustion, more severe than heat cramps, is characterized by nausea, vomiting, increased thirst, dizziness, confusion, and hypotension. Heat exhaustion is the result of fluid depletion. The patient may present with cramping and the core body temperature may be elevated. Oral fluid replacement may be tried if the patient's symptoms are mild. IV fluid replacement is the most effective treatment. ECG monitoring should also be considered. Follow local protocols for specific treatment.

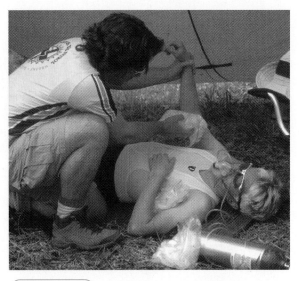

▶ Figure 12-31

<u>Heatstroke</u> is the most life threatening of heat disorders. People over the age of 50 account for 80% of all deaths from heatstroke. Heatstrokes are 12 to13 times more common in people 65 years and older than in younger adults.[17] Heatstroke is characterized by a very high temperature—usually over 106°F (41°C). Typically, there may be headache and dizziness early on, followed by altered mental status (unresponsiveness) and an absence of sweating. The pulse rate of older patients with heatstroke is most often very slow and thready, and the heatstroke patient usually presents with hypovolemia. Treatment should include removal from the warm environment, management of the ABCs, and active cooling—with care not to cool the patient too much. Stop slightly above normal temperature 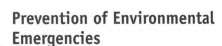. Initiate IV fluid therapy and ECG monitoring. Some patients present with ECG changes in ST segments and T waves, premature ventricular contractions, or supraventricular tachycardia. Follow local protocols for specific guidance.

Figure 12-31 Treatment for heatstroke includes active cooling, with care not to cool the patient too much. Stop slightly above normal core temperature.

Prevention of Environmental Emergencies

EMS providers can help to minimize environmental emergencies in older patients by doing the following:

♦ Provide access information to shelters, both in cold and hot seasons.

♦ Initiate "well-being checks" for known older people living by themselves during hot and cold seasons.

♦ Provide public information to older patients on how to minimize exposure to the elements and ultimately reduce the chances of suffering an environmental emergency.

♦ When time permits on a call to an older patient's residence, check to see that home heating or cooling systems are working.

Summary

Older people tend to have less body reserves. They may not tolerate medical emergencies as well as patients of younger age would, and these emergencies can result in life-threatening conditions for the older patient. Recognition and early EMS intervention will have a positive impact on outcome. Be aware of the differences in this population so you can provide them with lifesaving care.

Chapter Resources

Case Study Summaries

CASE STUDY 1 SUMMARY

Vomiting red blood (hematemesis) and passing black, tarlike stools (melena) are indicators of active upper GI bleeding. The abnormal vital signs, tachycardia, and hypotension characterize the bleeding as severe. Because this patient uses NSAIDs on a regular basis, he is at increased risk for developing upper GI bleeding from peptic ulcers. The patient's medical history includes a recent heart attack. Therefore, be sure to ask the patient if he is having any chest pain that could signify myocardial ischemia or a heart attack. This situation represents a true medical emergency, and the patient should be transported to the nearest emergency department immediately. En route, give standard shock treatment, including supplemental oxygen. Start a large-bore IV for fluid resuscitation, and place the patient on a cardiac monitor.

CASE STUDY 2 SUMMARY

The patient is likely suffering from type II diabetes. Her onset was slow, over several weeks, and her signs and symptoms of presentation are classic. In the field, this patient should have her blood glucose levels taken if you are trained and equipped to do so. Treatment in the field should include oxygen, and glucose or dextrose administration unless you have an accurate glucose measurement that indicates hyperglycemia. Start an IV and give a fluid challenge, per local protocols.

CASE STUDY 3 SUMMARY

Mrs. Smith's pressure sore measures 2 inches wide and 2 inches long. Due to the depth and characteristics of the tissue, Mrs. Smith's pressure ulcer can be categorized as stage 1. Immobility caused pressure, which in turn resulted in decreased blood flow and tissue damage.

The goals of treatment are to treat the current pressure sore and to prevent new ones from developing. First, relieve pressure from the affected area and rotate the person every 2 hours while the patient is in your care. There are several ways to relieve pressure from the bony prominences, for example, an air mattress. In addition, the pressure ulcer has to be assessed. Nutrition status should also be assessed, and pain relief may be called for.

Chapter Resources

253

Due to the patient's decreased abilities to preserve and generate heat, he is predisposed to hypothermia. The decreased muscle tone, loss of body fat, and less than optimal thermoregulatory abilities make this older patient more susceptible to hypothermia. Even in the 70°F weather, the patient should be made and kept warm by removing any wet clothing, providing additional blankets, and keeping the ambulance warm.

Bibliography

Barzilai N. Disorders of Carbohydrate Metabolism. In: Abrams W, Beers M, Berkow R, eds. The Merck Manual of Geriatrics. Rahway, NJ: Merck & Co. Available at: www.merck.com/pubs/mm_geriatrics/sec8/ch64.

Bledsoe B, et al. *Paramedic Care: Principles and Practice, Medical Emergencies*. Upper Saddle River, NJ: Prentice Hall; Medical Emergencies: 2001.

Defloor T. The risk of pressure sores: A conceptual scheme. *Journal of Clinical Nursing*. 1999;8(2): 206–216.

Guralnik JM, Harris TB, White LR, et al. Occurrence and predictors of pressure ulcers in the National Health and Nutrition Examination Survey follow up. *J Am Geriatr Soc*. 1998;36:807–812.

Knies R. Geriatric Thermoregulation. Available at: www.enw.org/Research-GeriTherm.htm.

Maklebust J. Pressure ulcers: Decreasing the risk for older adults: Body positioning and good skin care are two of the preventive steps geriatric nurses can take to reduce the risk of pressure ulcers in their elderly patients. *Geriatric Nursing*. 1997;18(6): 250–254.

Merck Research Laboratories. *The Merck Manual of Geriatrics*. 3rd ed. Abrams W, Beers M, Berkow R, eds. Rahway, NJ: Merck & Co.; 2000:1231–1238, 1261–1276.

Morrison S. Monitoring decubitus ulcers: A monthly survey method. *Q Rev Bull*. 1984;10:112–117.

Thomas D. *Geriatric Medicine*. 3rd ed. New York: Springer Verlag, 1997:767–785.

Endnotes

1. Quirk DM, Friedman LS. Approach to Gastrointestinal Problems in the Elderly. In: Yamada T, et al., eds. *Handbook of Gastroenterology*. Philadelphia: Lippincott Williams and Wilkins; 1999:1015–1033.

2. Elta GH. Approach to the Patient with Gross Gastrointestinal Bleeding. In: Yamada T, et al., eds. *Handbook of Gastroenterology*. Philadelphia: Lippincott Williams and Wilkins; 1999: 714–743.

3. Bree Johnston C, Goldstein MK, Triadafilopoulos G. Constipation, Diarrhea, and Fecal Incontinence. In: Osterweil D, et al., eds. *Comprehensive Geriatric Assessment*. New York: McGraw-Hill; 2000:421–441.

4. Molaschi M, Ponzetto M, Massaia M, Villa L, Scarafiotti C, Ferrario E. Hypernatriemic dehydration in the elderly on admission to hospital. *J Nutr Health Aging*. 1997;1(3):156–160.

5. Bledsoe B, et al. *Paramedic Care: Principles and Practice. Volume 5: Special Considerations/Operations*. Upper Saddle River, NJ: Prentice Hall; 2001:179.

6. American Diabetes Association. Available at: http://www.diabetes.org:80/main/application/commercewf?origin=*.jsp&event=link(B4_4). Accessed on April 23, 2002.

7. American Diabetes Association. Available at: http://www.diabetes.org:80/main/application/commercewf?origin=*.jsp&event=link(B1_1). Accessed on April 23, 2002.

8. Diabetes Control and Complications Trial. Available at: http://www.niddk.nih.gov/health/diabetes/pubs/dcct1/dcct.htm. Accessed on April 23, 2002.

9. Merck Research Laboratories. Thyroid Disorders. In: Abrams W, Beers M, Berkow R., eds. The Merck Manual of Geriatrics. 3rd ed. Rahway NJ: Merck & Co.; 2000. Available at: http://www.merck.com/pubs/mm_geriatrics/sec8/ch65.htm.

10. Peterson NC, Bittman S. The epidemiology of pressure sores. *Scand J Plast Reconstr Surg Hand Surg.* 1971;5:62–66.

11. Langemo DK, Olson B, Hunter S, et al. Incidence of pressure sores in acute care, rehabilitation, extended care, home health, and hospice in one locale. *Decubitus.* 1989;2:42.

12. Young L. Pressure ulcer prevalence and associated patient characteristics in one long-term care facility. *Decubitus.* 1989;2:52.

13. Vasconez LO, Schneider WJ, Jurkiewicz MJ. Pressure sores. *Curr Probl Surg.* 1977;62:83-89.

14. Goldfarb MT, Ellis CN, Voorhees JJ. *Geriatric Medicine.* 3rd ed. New York: Springer-Verlag; 1997; 50:667–681.

15. Smith RL, Meixler SM, Simberkoff MS. Excess mortality in critically ill patients with nosocomial bloodstream infections. *Chest.* 1991;100(1): 164–167.

16. Knies, RC. Geriatric Thermoregulation. Available at Emergency Nursing World web site: www.enw.org/Research-GeriTherm.htm.

17. Merck Research Laboratories. Hyperthermia and Hypothermia. In: Abrams W, Beers M, Berkow R., eds. The Merck Manual of Geriatrics. 3rd ed. Rahway NJ: Merck & Co.; 2000. Available at: http://www.merck.com/pubs/mm_geriatrics/sec8/ch67.htm.

Pharmacology and Medication Toxicity Emergencies

LEARNING OBJECTIVES

1 Discuss physiological changes in older people with regard to the effects of medication on the body in terms of drug distribution, metabolism, and excretion.

2 Describe the epidemiology in the older population of polypharmacy, drug toxicity, medication noncompliance, dosing errors, and drug sensitivity.

3 Discuss the use and effects of commonly prescribed medications for older people.

4 Discuss the use of vitamins, herbal medications, and over-the-counter medications and their effects on the older patient, including drug interactions.

5 Discuss the assessment, intervention, treatment, and transport of the older patient with complaints related to medication toxicity or medication nonadherence.

6 Discuss ways EMS providers can help prevent medication misuse in older people.

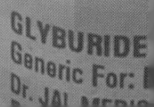

CHAPTER 13

Susan K. Bowles, PharmD

Robert L. Maher, Jr, PharmD

Kevin Spelman, AHG

CASE STUDY 1

You arrive at the scene to find a 72-year-old man who says he has experienced chest pain over the past several hours. You note that he is slightly obese, is in moderate distress, and has an enlarged right leg that is tender to the touch. Chest auscultation is clear. Blood pressure is 140/90 mm Hg, pulse is 102 beats/min and regular, and respirations are 30 breaths/min and regular.

The patient's wife indicates that the patient has been treated for a "blood clot" in his right leg over the past eight weeks.

What questions should you ask regarding the patient's medication use?

(continued on page 265)

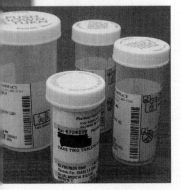

Age-related Changes in the Body's Processing of Drugs

The introduction of new medications over the past 60 years has provided health care practitioners with important tools to cure some diseases and relieve the symptoms of many chronic illnesses. Despite the benefits of such medicines, drug-related adverse effects can and do occur. These adverse effects occur 2 to 3 times more frequently in the aging population than in individuals under 30.[1]

Older people represent only 12% of the total population,[2] but consume the greatest proportion of medications, in the range of 3.1 to 7.9 prescription and nonprescription medications at one time.[3] Older age itself is not an independent risk factor for drug-related adverse events, but the number of medications used may significantly increase the risk of drug-related complications.

Further, older people do not always respond to drug therapy in the same manner as younger persons. The aging process involves several physiologic changes in **pharmacokinetics** (absorption, distribution, metabolism, and elimination of medicines). Those changes may alter the way in which an older person responds to a particular medication. Older patients, who experience more chronic illness and generally use more medications, often also lack the compensatory mechanisms that protect younger individuals from experiencing medication side effects. In combination, these factors increase the risk of drug-related adverse events in older persons.

Adverse drug events in the older population are recognized as a serious public health problem, because of the high potential for morbidity and mortality. Up to 40% of hospitalizations among older persons have been estimated to be related to adverse drug events.[4] Because EMS providers are often an older person's first contact with the medical system once an adverse drug event has occurred, it is important that EMS providers become familiar with the age-related changes in function and composition of the body in relation to medications (▶ **Figure 13-1**).

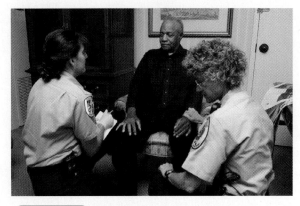

Figure 13-1   EMS providers are often an older person's first contact with the medical system once an adverse drug event has occurred.

Passage of Drugs Through the Body

Absorption

Several age-related changes occur in the gastrointestinal tract. Gastric acidity decreases, gastric emptying slows, and the absorptive surface of the intestine is diminished. However, there is little evidence that drug absorption changes significantly in most older people. Thus, absorption of orally administered medications is generally not a major part of altered drug response in older patients. Due to the greater number of medications taken by older individuals, it is important to look for drug–drug interactions that could decrease the absorption of medications such as calcium with levothyroxine (Synthroid) or ciprofloxacin (Cipro).

Distribution

Several age-related changes in body composition can alter the distribution of medications throughout the body. Lean body mass and total body water decrease by 10% to 20%, while fat tissue increases 20% to 40%.[5] These changes have the potential to alter the distribution of both water-soluble and fat-soluble medications.

In general, the drop in total body water results in higher blood levels of the more water-soluble drugs. Thus, initial doses of water-soluble drugs such as aminoglycosides (eg, gentamicin), digoxin, or lithium should be lower in older persons. In contrast, fat-soluble drugs tend to have lower blood levels. Because fat tissue acts as a reservoir for fat-soluble medications, the increase in fat tissue means these medications are eliminated more slowly, potentially prolonging the pharmacologic effect. Thus, lower doses of some fat-soluble drugs may also be warranted, and others are best avoided altogether. For example, blood levels of diazepam (Valium) may be lower in older patients following a single dose, but the sedative effect may be prolonged due to a decrease in elimination or metabolism. Because of this, diazepam is generally not recommended for older people.

Some drugs, such as phenytoin (Dilantin) and warfarin (Coumadin), are carried in the bloodstream attached to proteins ▼ Figure 13-2. Older people who have a low level of blood proteins because of liver diseases, malnutrition, or other chronic diseases require lower doses of these drugs. In some cases, blood tests can be used to monitor the levels of the drug.

Drug Metabolism and Elimination

The primary routes of drug elimination are through the kidney and the liver. The liver is the main site of drug metabolism. Both routes are subject to age-related changes.

Kidneys

The kidneys undergo two age-related physiologic changes—a decline in renal blood flow and a reduction in both the size and number of **nephrons** (the kidneys' basic filtering units)—which can affect the elimination of medications by the kidney in older people. The resulting slowdown in renal filtration decreases the elimination of medications that are predominately excreted by the kidney. As a result, it is often necessary to decrease the dose of these drugs, or make the doses less frequent. Examples include cimetidine, digoxin, lithium, amantadine, and aminoglycoside antibiotics (eg, gentamicin and tobramycin).

> **Medication Tip**
>
> The kidneys and the liver are the primary routes of drug elimination. Age-related changes in the function of these organs can have a major impact on drug effects, and may require changes in dosages and frequency.

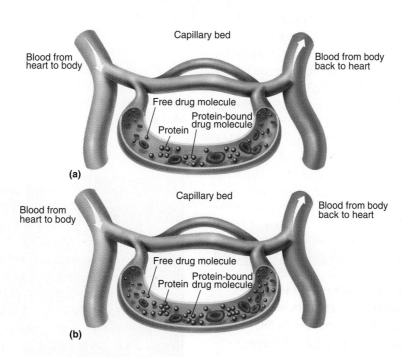

Figure 13-2 Some medications "bind" to proteins in the blood, a process called plasma-protein binding **(A)**. When drug elimination is significantly decreased by renal or hepatic disease, changes in protein binding can be important **(B)**.

Another factor is the accumulation of **active metabolites** that are eliminated by the kidneys. Active metabolites are byproducts of a drug, after it has been partially or fully metabolized, that have active drug effects on the body. For example, meperidine (Demerol) undergoes metabolism by the liver into the active compound, normeperidine, which is eliminated renally. Because of the risk of central nervous system side effects, meperidine should generally be avoided in older patients.

Changes in kidney function can also alter the effect of diuretics on electrolyte balance. For example, the use of potassium-sparing diuretics such as triamterene and spironolactone increases the risk of hyperkalemia (excessive blood levels of potassium). Thiazide (hydrochlorothiazide) or loop diuretics (furosemide) raise the risk of hyponatremia (low sodium levels). Although these effects can occur in younger persons who use these medications, older persons are especially at risk.

Liver

The primary site of drug metabolism in the body is the liver, although some occurs at other sites (▶ **Figure 13-3**). Age-related pharmacologic changes that can alter drug metabolism include a reduction in liver mass and decreased liver blood flow. However, disease states, nutrition status, other drugs, consumption of tobacco or alcohol, and genetics are also important factors in drug metabolism.

The clinical effects of age-related changes on hepatic elimination depend on the degree to which medications undergo metabolism. Because nearly all older people have declines in kidney and liver function with aging, as a rule it is best to "start low, go slow" with medications in this age group. That is, a new medication should be started at the lowest possible dose, and only changed slowly to allow any build-up of the medication from sluggish metabolism or elimination, to occur.

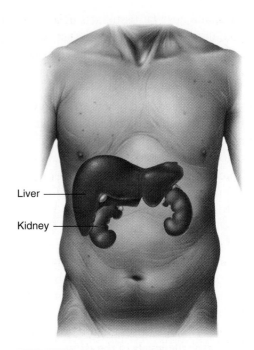

Figure 13-3   The primary site of drug metabolism in the body is the liver. The kidneys and the liver are the main routes of drug elimination.

Liver
Kidney

Therapeutic (Pharmacodynamic) Changes

The term **pharmacodynamics** refers to the pharmacologic or therapeutic effect of a medication or combination of medications. Pharmacodynamic changes associated with aging have not been well studied in older populations, and are therefore poorly understood. Generally, older patients are considered to have an enhanced response to most medications. In other words, many drugs appear

Attitude Tip

You and your EMS agency can support community education and assistance programs to help the older population establish and maintain EMS-accessible medical information and medication containers and storage devices, such as the "OK MedCard/MedFile," "Vial-of-Life," "U.S. MedGear," and others (▶ **Figure 13-4**).

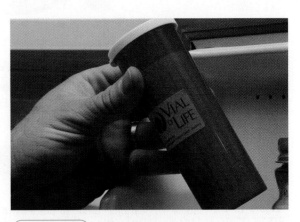

Figure 13-4   Medication containers such as the Vial of Life can be distributed to older patients at risk for medication-related emergencies.

to have an increased potency in older people. Examples include warfarin (Coumadin), opioids, oxycodone/acetaminophen (Percocet), and benzodiazepines such as lorazepam (Ativan).

Attitude Tip

Remember that older patients frequently need reductions in the dose or strength of medications as they mature.

Drug Interactions

A drug interaction occurs when the combination of a medication with other medications (drug-drug interaction), a food or nutrient (drug-nutrient interaction), or a disease state (drug-disease interaction) results in a change in the pharmacologic effect or toxicity of the drug. Drug interactions occur more frequently as the number of drugs used increases; therefore, since older patients are the largest consumers of medications, they are at increased risk of drug interactions. Other risk factors associated with drug interactions in older patients include mixing alcohol or over-the-counter medications with prescription drugs, having drugs prescribed by multiple physicians, and purchasing medications from more than one pharmacy (▼ Figure 13-5). Of

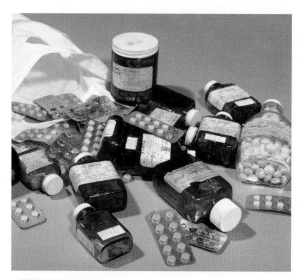

Figure 13-5 Risk factors for harmful drug interactions include use of multiple medications, combination of alcohol and medications, and prescriptions from more than one physician or pharmacy.

particular concern to older people is the association between drug interactions and the increased risk of adverse drug events. Older people don't tolerate adverse effects of drugs as well as their younger counterparts. When older patients present to EMS providers, it is important to take a thorough medication history—and at times to transport medication (both prescription and non-prescription) with the patient, to ensure that all potential drug interactions are identified.

Drug–Drug Interactions

Drug-drug interactions occur when two drugs administered together alter the pharmacokinetics or pharmacodynamics of at least one of the medications. When one drug interferes with another in this way, the result can be either the magnification or reduction of the pharmacologic action of the affected drug. Some common drug-drug interactions are listed in (▶ Table 13-1).

Antacids and vitamins containing aluminum, calcium, iron, magnesium, and zinc can decrease the oral absorption of tetracycline, bisphosphonate bone medications (eg, alendronate or risedronate), and the quinolone antibiotics. Decreased absorption can result in therapeutic failure. Patients taking these medications do not need to avoid antacids and vitamins, however, because the interaction usually can be avoided by separating administration of the interacting drugs by 2 hours.

Interactions affecting elimination usually involve drug metabolism, when one drug either enhances or decreases the metabolism of another one. Increased drug metabolism can result in failure of a medication to exert its therapeutic effect, whereas inhibition of metabolism can result in greater pharmacologic effect or drug toxicity. Patients are at highest risk of complications from metabolic drug interactions when an interacting drug is stopped or started. Even if patients or caregivers provide a list of medications, EMS providers should specifically ask if any new medicines have been started recently or if the dose of any medications has changed.

Pharmacodynamic interactions between two or more drugs occur when one medication directly enhances or inhibits the action of another drug, usually in the same system. For example, alcohol combined with central nervous system depressants such as tricyclic antidepressants,

TABLE 13-1   Common Drug Interactions in Older Patients

Drug	Interacting	Drug Effect
Antacids (Rolaids, Tums)	Bisphosphonates, quinolone antibiotics, tetracycline	Impaired absorption
Anticholinergics (benztropine)	Older antihistamines, neuroleptics, opioids, tricyclic antidepressants	Additive anticholinergic effects (confusion, constipation, urinary retention)
Antidiabetic agents (oral anti-hyperglycemics, insulin, glyburide)	Beta-blocking drugs	Inhibition of usual symptoms (except sweating) during hypoglycemic episodes
Benzodiazepines (Valium, Xanax)	Alcohol, tricyclic antidepressants, opioids	Increased sedation
Digoxin (Lanoxin)	Quinidine	Reduced elimination, resulting in increased digoxin concentrations
	Potassium-wasting diuretics	Increased effect of digoxin on the heart
Potassium-sparing diuretics (Aldactone, Dyrenium, Midamor)	Potassium supplements Angiotensin-converting enzyme inhibitors	**Hyperkalemia** (high potassium)
Phenytoin (Dilantin)	Cimetidine, quinolone antibiotics, erythromycin	Inhibit phenytoin metabolism, resulting in elevated blood levels
	Phenobarbital, rifampin	Trigger phenytoin metabolism, resulting in decreased blood levels and potential loss of seizure control
	Enteral feeding products	Reduce phenytoin absorption, resulting in decreased blood levels and potential loss of seizure control

(continued)

sedating antihistamines, or benzodiazepines can increase CNS depression. The additive effects of various drugs of this type can also produce effects such as confusion, constipation, and urinary retention.

Drug–Nutrient Interactions

Many clinically important drug–nutrient interactions are related to the absorption process. As mentioned, the body will not absorb some antibiotics properly if they are taken with vitamins or supplements that contain calcium, magnesium,

or iron. It is therefore important that these medications not be taken with dairy products or other foods containing high levels of these minerals (▶ Figure 13-6).

Nutritional supplements or **enteral** products (used for people with feeding tubes) may also contain minerals that can interfere with drug absorption. For example, tube feedings can impair the absorption of phenytoin, which may result in poor seizure control.

The administration of some medications with grapefruit juice can produce clinically important drug–nutrient interactions. Components of grape-

TABLE 13-1   Common Drug Interactions in Older Patients (*continued*)

Drug	Interacting	Drug Effect
Theophylline (Elixophyllin, Theodur)	Cimetidine, quinolone antibiotics, erythromycin	Inhibit theophylline metabolism, resulting in elevated blood levels and potential toxicity
	Phenobarbital, rifampin	Trigger theophylline metabolism, resulting in decreased blood levels and potentially decreased therapeutic effect
Warfarin (Coumadin)	Amiodarone, cimetidine, erythromycin, clarithromycin, levofloxacin	Inhibit warfarin metabolism, resulting in increased anticlotting (anticoagulant) effect
	Phenobarbital, rifampin	Trigger warfarin metabolism, resulting in decreased anticoagulant effect
	Nonsteroidal anti-inflammatory drugs (NSAIDs)	Exaggerate warfarin's anticoagulant activity, increasing the risk of bleeding
	Nutritional supplements and enteral feeding products with high vitamin K content	May interfere with anticoagulant effect

Note: This table is not meant to be a complete list of drug interactions.

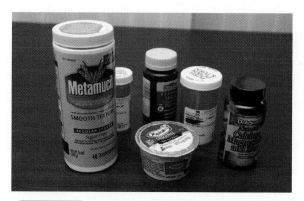

Figure 13-6   The body will not absorb some antibiotics properly if they are taken with vitamins or supplements that contain calcium, magnesium, or iron, or with dairy products or other foods containing high levels of these minerals.

fruit juice interfere with the phase of metabolism that occurs in the intestinal wall. This results in higher blood levels of the drug and an overall increase in pharmacologic effect and risk of drug tox-

icity. Drugs affected include some calcium channel blockers (nifedipine, felodipine, verapamil), cyclosporine, triazolam, lovastatin, and astemizole.

Medication Tip

Grapefruit juice can interfere with metabolism of some drugs, and several minerals can affect absorption of a number of antibiotics. Vitamin K alters the anticoagulant effect of warfarin.

There are some circumstances in which drug–nutrient interactions are pharmacodynamic in nature. For example, if the dietary intake of vitamin K increases significantly from food, nutritional supplements, or enteral products, it can interfere with the anticlotting (anticoagulant) effect of warfarin. If vitamin K intake decreases significantly, patients may experience an increase in anticoagulant effect, and therefore an increased risk of bleeding. Patients taking warfarin who present either with possible clotting events or with bleeding complications should be questioned about any recent changes in their diet, and the use of nutritional supplements or enteral nutrition.

Drug–Disease Interactions

A drug–disease interaction occurs when one or more medications act to worsen an existing disease. For example, the effect of nonsteroidal anti-inflammatory drugs (NSAIDs) on the kidney can interfere with blood pressure control or place some patients at risk of developing congestive heart failure.[6] Of particular concern for older people is the potential for medications to compromise mental function and physical mobility.

Drug-induced mental impairment can occur in older patients as a direct result of medications on the central nervous system, or secondary to metabolic imbalances caused by drugs. Patients with pre-existing cognitive problems are at the greatest risk, but drug-induced confusion can occur in any older patient. (▼ Table 13-2) lists several drugs that can produce confusion. In many instances, confusion is not due to a single agent, but to the additive effects of two or more drugs used together. Drug toxicity may also manifest atypically in some older patients, initially presenting as confusion (▼ Figure 13-7).

Attitude Tip

Drug-induced confusion can occur in any older patient. Do not assume dementia or psychiatric problems: Assess the patient for medication problems and other medical causes.

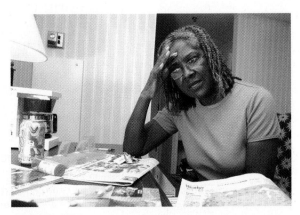

Figure 13-7 Though it is not the typical presentation, drug toxicity may initially show itself in the form of confusion.

TABLE 13-2 Some Drugs Associated with Confusion in Older People	
Drug	**Mechanism**
Antidiabetic agents (oral antihyperglycemics, insulin, glyburide)	Hypoglycemia presenting as confusion
Anticholinergics (benztropine)	Anticholinergic effect on CNS
Antiparkinson agents (bromocriptine, levodopa/carbidopa [Sinemet])	Direct effect on CNS
Benzodiazepines (Valium, Xanax)	Direct effect on CNS
Digoxin (Lanoxin)	Anticholinergic effect on CNS
Diuretics (Lasix, hydrochlorothiazide)	Electrolyte imbalance presenting as confusion
Opioids (Demerol, Percodan, codeine)	Direct effects on CNS; excessive sedation
Phenytoin (Dilantin)	Drug toxicity presenting as confusion
Tricyclic antidepressants (Elavil, Vivactil)	Anticholinergic effect on CNS; excessive sedation

Note: This table is not meant to provide a complete list of agents causing confusion in older people.

CASE STUDY 1 (continued)

In Case Study 1, you encountered a 72-year-old man who had experienced chest pain over several hours and who had been treated for a blood clot in his right leg for the past 8 weeks. After questioning the patient, you learn the following:

♦ He is currently taking warfarin 3 mg daily.

♦ He had his blood tested when leaving the hospital, and twice since his discharge. He was told that his blood was in the right range. His last blood test was taken one month ago, as he found it difficult to go to the lab for his blood test.

♦ He is taking a "water pill" (hydrochlorothiazide 12.5 mg once daily) for his blood pressure, pills for his "sugar" (metformin 500 mg three times a day), "arthritis pills" (acetaminophen 500 mg four times a day) and "pills for my thyroid" (levothyroxine 75 µg once daily).

♦ The patient indicates that the dose of his "thyroid pills" were decreased about a month ago from 100 µg daily to his current dose of 88 µg daily.

♦ The patient's wife indicates that she gives him all of his medications. He takes his "water pill," "thyroid pill," one "arthritis pill," and one "sugar pill" with breakfast each morning, one "sugar pill" and one "arthritis pill" at lunch, one "sugar pill," one "arthritis pill" and his "blood thinner" at dinner, and one "arthritis pill" just before bedtime.

♦ The patient reports taking a single multi-vitamin with iron daily. He has not been using any other OTC medications. He states that he is not taking any herbal medications.

♦ The patient indicates that he is trying to lose weight so he started to eat more salad.

What is your assessment and treatment of this patient?

Impaired physical mobility secondary to medications can occur as a result of several different mechanisms (see Table 13-4). Drugs can trigger movement disorders or affect balance through a variety of mechanisms. Drugs such as benzodiazepines, neuroleptics, selective serotonin-reuptake inhibitors (eg, Paxil, Zoloft), and tricyclic antidepressants can cause movement disorders and altered balance that increase the risk of falls.

Drug–Herb Interactions

The available information on pharmacokinetics is largely dominated by drug–drug interactions, with little data on drug–herb interactions. In one study of 108 suspected interactions identified, 68.5% were unable to be linked to the herb due to poor reporting.[7] This raises two questions when there is a problem: (1) Is the adverse effect being caused by an agent other than the herb, such as another pharmaceutical or food substance? (2) Is the suspected herbal preparation actually consistent with its label?

Though frequently discussed, the occurrence of drug–herb interactions is relatively rare. Nevertheless, it is prudent to include questions about the use of supplements and herbal medicines in your history. Many people do not think of herbs as supplements, so it is necessary to specify both

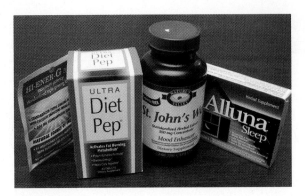

Figure 13-8   Herbal supplements are popular for a variety of purported health effects.

categories in history taking. Among the most popular herbal remedies the provider is likely to encounter are Echinacea (*Echinacea* spp.), Ma Huang (*Ephedra* spp.), Ginkgo (*Ginkgo biloba*), and St. John's Wort (*Hypericum* spp.) (▲ **Figure 13-8**).

When you suspect a drug–herb interaction, determine and record the following:

◆ Patient diseases and conditions

◆ Medications being taken: name, dose, timing

◆ Herb(s) involved:

  ◆ Brand name, label information

  ◆ Dosage and timing, including timing relative to medications

  ◆ Transport a sample, in case lab analysis is needed

Because drug–herb interactions are not common, ensure that your assessment covers other possible causes of existing signs and symptoms. Do not let the patient's "diagnosis" prevent a thorough assessment.

Echinacea

Echinacea, used to treat colds and flus, is not toxic to the liver as was once thought. However, its use with immunosuppressive drugs such as cyclosporine, corticosteroids, and chemotherapy drugs may be inappropriate, and long-term use may alter immune function.

Ephedra

Ephedra, also known as Ma Huang and Mormon Tea, is used to treat asthma and other lower respiratory conditions, as well as upper respiratory conditions. It is effective because it contains substances such as ephedrine and pseudoephedrine,

which stimulate the sympathetic nervous system to cause bronchodilation. Ephedra also causes CNS stimulation.

Most recently, the natural-products industry has marketed ephedra in "fat burning" (thermogenic) products. These products can cause agitation, tremors, and insomnia when combined with the category of drugs that includes theophylline, aminophylline, and caffeine. (Many of the thermogenic products contain caffeine.) Thermogenic products can also cause blood pressure elevation when combined with monoamine oxidase inhibitors (phenelzine, tranylcypromine), and they may speed the elimination of corticosteroids such as dexamethasone. In addition, although interactions are not as great a concern with selective (type A) monoamine oxidase inhibitors, the dosage is. If your patient has taken such a medication, record the dosage of it and any other medications taken. Moclobemide is an example of a selective monoamine oxidase inhibitor.

> **Medication Tip**
>
> The use of herbal medications by older patients is growing in popularity despite the lack of adequate medical research describing their benefits, risks, and potential interactions with other medications.

Ginkgo

Ginkgo, used for pulmonary conditions in traditional Chinese medicine, is currently used for cerebrovascular dysfunctions and memory enhancement. Ginkgo is contraindicated in patients using anticoagulants and NSAIDs because the combination inhibits platelet function, and thus may cause bleeding problems.

St. John's Wort

St. John's Wort, mentioned by Hippocrates, Dioscorides, and Galen in their writings, was used traditionally both topically and internally. The herb is a popular treatment for mild to moderate depression; it also is used to treat anxiety, seasonal affective disorder, sleep disorders, and as an antiviral medication. St. John's Wort is one of the best selling herbs in Germany, outselling Prozac 20 to 1.[8] St. John's Wort is contraindicated in patients taking selective serotonin-reuptake inhibitors (SSRIs) such as Paxil and Zoloft, as well as monoamine oxidase inhibitors (▼ **Figure 13-9**). In addition, this medication causes photosensitivity and has led to reports of severe sunburn.

In lab research, extracts of St. John's Wort have been shown to inhibit binding of naloxone (Narcan) to opioid receptors. This raises the concern that naloxone may be less effective than usual in counteracting narcotic overdoses when St. John's Wort is present.

> ## Attitude Tip
>
> **Don't forget to gather related vitamin and mineral supplements, and herbal or other over-the-counter (OTC) remedies being taken by the patient, which could contribute to adverse drug reactions or other polypharmacy complications.**

Assessing Problems Related to Medication Toxicity or Adverse Effects

Two goals for the clinical care of an older patient are to enhance the patient's health-related quality of life and to maintain function. Prescribing medication in older persons can play a role in achieving this goal by curing a disease, reducing or eliminating symptoms of a disease, slowing a disease process, or preventing a disease.

However, the benefits of medications in the older patient can often be outweighed by the occurrence of drug-related problems such as medication toxicities (adverse drug reactions) and therapeutic failure, which can lead to reoccurrence or worsening of disease symptoms. The patient's health beliefs, physical and mental impairments, and economic situation may contribute to alteration of the medication plan, which can cause either underdosing or overdosing. Drug-related problems in the older person are common reasons for hospitalization; the two main reasons are adverse drug reactions and intentional nonadherence.[4] Other factors that can contribute to drug-related problems include biological changes of aging, drug interactions, and withdrawal reactions from stopping a medication abruptly.

History

A vital initial step in identifying drug-related problems is obtaining a comprehensive medication history from the patient or a caregiver. Several difficulties can prevent you from getting an accurate and complete medication history. In communicating with the older patient, make an initial assessment of any possible barriers such as hearing or vision impairment. Additional problems in history taking and communication include cognitive impairment and underreporting. When barriers do exist, it becomes important to identify family members or caregivers who can help with the history (▼ **Figure 13-10**).

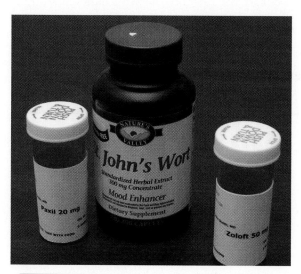

Figure 13-9 St. John's Wort, a popular herbal treatment for mild to moderate depression, is contraindicated in patients taking SSRI-type antidepressants, such as Paxil and Zoloft.

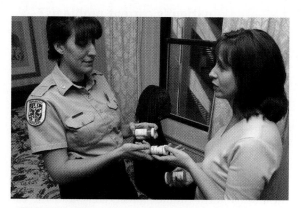

Figure 13-10 When there are barriers to communicating with the patient, involve family members or caregivers who can help with the history.

CASE STUDY 2

You are dispatched to the home of an 86-year-old man who is in acute respiratory distress. He appears confused and is wheezing. He is requesting a nebulizer treatment. You notice that the patient's elbow is bruised. When you ask about it, he can't remember how it happened. The patient comments that he thinks he got dizzy earlier and may have fallen. On the patient's kitchen table you notice about 15 to 20 medication bottles and several breathing inhalers. You collect a list of the medications on the table and find the following:

1. Guaifenesin 600 mg PO bid
2. Cimetidine 400 mg PO qid
3. Wellbutrin (bupropion) 75 mg PO bid
4. Zyban (bupropion) 150 mg PO qd— currently taking samples from general practitioner
5. Amitriptyline 75 mg PO qam
6. Digoxin 0.25 mg PO qd
7. NTG 0.4 mg/h patch, topically, qam and off at night
8. Clonidine 0.1 mg PO bid
9. Furosemide 60 mg PO qd
10. ASA EC 325 mg PO qd

11. Albuterol inhaler 2 puffs PO qid
12. Ipratropium 2 puffs PO qid
13. Albuterol nebs prn
14. Smx/tmp DS 1 tablet PO bid
15. Tylenol 3 one or two tablets every 4 hours as needed for pain—use average 2 tablets per day
16. Pericolace 1 capsule PO bid
17. OTC Correctol prn—use average 1 per week
18. OTC Zantac prn—use average one or two per day
19. Mupirocin ointment to nares qd, alternate nostrils every 5 days

What important questions do you need to try to ask this patient with regard to a medication history?

In terms of adverse drug reactions, what concerns do you have for this patient?

Are there any medications that potentially may be contributing to the patient's current problems?

Key Questions

In reviewing the medication history, assess the patient's or caregiver's knowledge of current medications. (▶ Table 13-3) lists common questions to ask. In collecting a detailed history, gather information such as the name of the medication (both brand and generic names if available), its strength, the dosage form (liquid, tablet, etc.), and the directions about how the patient is to take the medication. Documenting printed directions is impor-

tant, but remember that the patient may not follow the directions because of problems with the medication (side effects), financial difficulties, or health beliefs. Information about actual use is very important because additional adverse drug events can occur if hospital personnel are not aware of the patient's nonadherence to instructions.

In collecting information on the medication dosage, be sure to determine the measurement of strength that is being used (eg, mg or mcg); the

TABLE 13-3   Key Questions in a Medication History of an Older Patient
1. What medications you are taking?
2. What is the purpose of these medications?
3. Do you currently take any medications that you can purchase without a doctor's prescription for any medical condition? Herbal products? Vitamins and nutritional supplements?
4. Have you ever had an allergic reaction to a medication, such as hives or difficulty breathing?
5. Have you ever had a bad reaction to a medication that made you have to stop taking that medication and/or report it to your doctor?
6. Do you use more than one pharmacy and physician?
7. Do you carry a medication list so your pharmacy and physician can review a current list of what you are taking?
8. Have you stopped taking any medication recently?
9. Have you added any new medications recently?
10. How do you remember to take your medications on a daily basis?
11. Do you smoke or drink alcohol? If so, how often?
12. Do you use any other drugs? If so, how often?

risk of medication error rises if there are errors in the unit of measurement. The patient or caregiver's understanding of the medication's purpose is another important point to explore and record. For instance, consider the case of an older male patient with asthma who has frequent breathing attacks. Upon interview, the patient reports that when he uses his inhaled corticosteroids (Flovent), he finds no acute relief. Confusion about what his medications are for has prevented the patient from picking the right inhaler for immediate relief. If properly informed, he would use the inhaled corticosteroids on a daily basis for pre-

vention of asthma attacks, and a bronchodilating inhaler (beta-agonist, such as albuterol) for acute relief. This could help prevent emergency department (ED) or hospital admissions in the future.

Over-the-Counter Medications

Also ask if the patient uses any medications purchased over-the-counter (OTC), without requiring a physician's order. Another method to get an accurate report of OTC medicine use is to conduct a review of symptoms, going from head to toe through various organ systems and inquiring about medication use. For instance: What medication do you take for a headache? To help with your bowels? For an upset stomach? Beside OTC medication use, ask if the patient is taking any medication that was not prescribed specifically for him or her. Older persons may use family members' medications on a trial basis to see if they help.

Adherence

Determine whether the patient is adherent with medication directions. Methods for evaluating adherence include direct patient reporting, and counting the number of pills in the bottle to see if the number remaining matches up with the interval since the last time the prescription was refilled (▼ Figure 13-11).

Poor adherence is often associated with underuse of a medication; however, there are certain

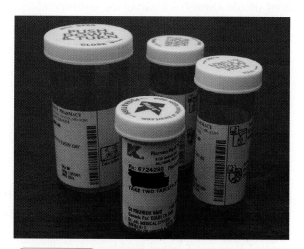

Figure 13-11 You may be able to evaluate medication adherence generally by comparing information on the container label (total number of pills dispensed, date dispensed, and number of pills to be taken per day) with the number of pills remaining in the container.

medication classes such as narcotics and benzodiazepines that have been associated with overuse (abuse). Reporting of medication adherence is a valuable aid to the ED physician in determining future treatment for the patient's disease, and can help reduce adverse drug reactions in hospital. Other factors to learn and report that may help with future adherence include impaired hearing, vision, cognition, ability to open safety caps, financial ability to obtain medications, and ability to swallow or apply medications appropriately.

Multiple Sources

Assessing the older person's use of multiple pharmacies and physicians helps identify risk factors for drug-drug interactions and adverse drug interactions, which are more likely when the patient does not share medication information with the different service providers. Additional information for the prevention of prescribing problems includes recording any history of allergies to medications, history of adverse drug events, and smoking or alcohol use.

Common Adverse Drug Events

Adverse drug events are often hard to detect in older patients. Medication toxicities can mimic signs and symptoms associated with various disease states or conditions. When trying to determine reasons for functional impairment in the older person, medications should always be a part of the assessment.

The three most common organ systems involved in drug-related side effects are the cardiovascular, central nervous, and gastrointestinal systems.[9]

Cardiovascular Problems

The most frequent adverse effects on the cardiovascular system are orthostatic hypotension and dizziness that can contribute to falls and syncope. Medicines used to treat high blood pressure are the usual causes of these problems. ▶ **Table 13-4** lists common medication classes associated with these side effects.

Central Nervous System Problems

The common CNS effects triggered by medications are confusion and psychiatric symptoms. Many medications can contribute to these side effects ▶ **Table 13-5**. Most medications associated with mental confusion or psychiatric symptoms have anticholinergic or fat-soluble properties.

TABLE 13-4 Drug Classes Associated with Syncope and Falls

Class of Medication	Example
Antihypertensives	propranolol (Inderal)
Vasodilators	hydralazine (Apresoline)
Antiarrhythmics	procainamide (Procan SR, Pronestyl)
CNS agents and sleeping and anxiety medications, especially antipsychotics, antidepressants, and benzodiazepines	diazepam (Valium)
Antiparkinsonian	levodopa/carbidopa (Sinemet)
NSAIDs	indomethacin (Indocin)
Antidiabetic	glyburide (Micronase)

Adapted from: Owens NJ, Silliman RA, Fretwell MD. The relationship between comprehensive functional assessment and optimal pharmacotherapy in the older patient. *DICP ANN Pharmacother.* 1989;23:847–854.

TABLE 13-5 Drug Classes Associated with Psychiatric Disorders

Class of Medication	Example
Anticholinergics	amitriptyline (Elavil)
Anticonvulsants	phenobarbital (Luminal)
Antihistamines	diphenhydramine (Benadryl)
Antiparkinsons	pergolide (Permax)
Cardiovascular	clonidine (Catapres)
Gastrointestinal	cimetidine (Tagamet)
NSAIDs	indomethacin (Indocin)
Antipsychotics	haloperidol (Haldol)

Medications that are fat soluble are more easily absorbed into the brain and therefore increase the risk of these adverse effects in the brain. Medications with anticholinergic properties are most likely to cause confusion (delirium). Most drug information handbooks can help EMS providers determine if a medication has one of these properties ▶ **Figure 13-12**.

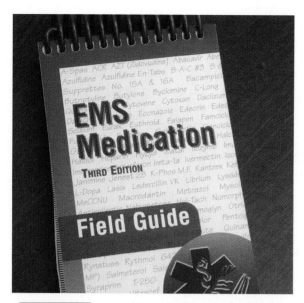

Figure 13-12 A drug handbook will help determine whether a medication has anticholinergic or fat-soluble properties, and thus could be causing confusion or psychiatric symptoms.

Medication Tip

The cause-effect relationships between medications and a patient's signs and symptoms can be complex. When in doubt, treat ABCs, gather as much information as possible about medications, and report thoroughly to receiving personnel.

Gastrointestinal Problems

Gastrointestinal side effects, such as nausea and vomiting, can contribute to nutrition problems when the patient does not eat well as a result. The situation can often be dealt with by administering the medication with food, switching to a medication less likely to cause nausea and vomiting, or reducing the dosage. In assessing this side effect, ask when the patient takes the medication and whether it is taken on a full or empty stomach. Because absorption may be decreased when administered with food, the recommendation to take it with food should come from the pharmacist or physician. Constipation is another gastrointestinal problem that is common in older patients. Anticholinergic medications and narcotics often cause constipation. Evaluate the patient's food and water intake and bowel history, along with other medication information.

Other Common Categories of Adverse Events

Anticholinergic Effects

Medications with anticholinergic properties can cause problems in the older person besides mental confusion: dry eyes, dry mouth, constipation, and urinary retention. Traditional over-the-counter antihistamines are the main anticholinergics that cause these problems. For example, diphenhydramine (Benadryl), found in cough and cold preparations and sleeping aids such as Tylenol PM, has anticholinergic effects strong enough to cause delirium in some cases.

Metabolic Disturbances

Another common adverse drug event is metabolic disturbance, such as low potassium (hypokalemia), low sodium (hyponatremia), or low bicarbonate. All of these conditions can contribute to possible cardiovascular side effects (arrhythmias), mental confusion, and acid-base imbalances. Diuretics such as hydrochlorothiazide and furosemide (Lasix) can cause these conditions (▼ **Figure 13-13**). High potassium (hyperkalemia) can be produced by potassium-sparing diuretics such as spironolactone, which is often used in congestive heart failure. The class of medications known as angiotensin-converting enzyme (ACE) inhibitors, used for conditions such as high blood pressure, diabetes, and congestive heart failure, may also contribute to hyperkalemia; impairment of renal function makes this more likely. Another major metabolic disturbance that can be attributed to medications is

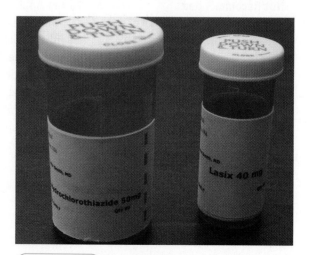

Figure 13-13 Common diuretics such as hydrochlorothiazide and furosemide (Lasix) can cause metabolic disturbances that may lead to arrhythmias, confusion, or acid-base imbalances.

hypoglycemia, caused either by insulin products or medications used in type 2 diabetes such as glyburide (in the category of *sulfonylureas*). In assessing problems with hypoglycemia, get a good history of the patient's eating patterns and the time of administration of these medications.

Information Resources

A current drug information handbook with a section listing common adverse reactions is an important tool for an EMS provider to carry at all times. Making a thorough list of drugs with high potential to cause adverse effect in older patients is a difficult task. Research attempts to determine which drugs pose higher risks have led to the list in (▼ Table 13-6). Being familiar with these medications—and carrying a copy of the list—may help you spot medication problems in older patients. Most of these medications have either anticholinergic or fat-soluble properties.

Controversy

Exactly which medications pose the highest risks to older patients is not well established. However, carrying drug information resources may help you spot medication-related problems.

An additional reason for the difficulty in determining adverse drug events is the exclusion of older people from clinical trials of medications. There are usually a small number of patients above the age of 65, and patients with more than one medical condition or above the age of 85 are almost always excluded. There is very limited data about dosing or adverse events in patients older than 85. In frail older persons, adverse drug events should always be considered a possible emergency. Your local poison control center is another resource for information on toxicity emergencies.

Identifying Drug Withdrawal Problems

A common objective in the management of older patients is eliminating unwanted medications. Many patients intentionally stop a medication on their own, a practice that can lead to an **adverse drug withdrawal event (ADWE)**. An ADWE is a set of clinical signs or symptoms caused by discontinuing use of a drug. Cardiovascular and CNS drugs most frequently cause ADWEs. Hospitalizations, or ED or urgent care clinic visits, often result. Two key points about ADWEs are that some may actually be a worsening of a

TABLE 13-6   Medications That May Cause Adverse Effects in Older Patients

Not Recommended	Rarely Appropriate	Moderate Risk
barbiturates (Phenobarbital)	carsiprodol (Soma)	amitriptyline (Elavil)
belladonna alkaloids (Donnatal)	chlordiazepoxide (Librium)	chlorpheniramine (Chlor-Trimeton)
chlorpropamide (Diabinese)	chlorzoxazone (Parafon Forte)	cyproheptadine (Periactin)
dicyclomine (Bentyl)	cyclobenzaprine (Flexeril)	diphenhydramine (Benadryl)
flurazepam (Dalmane)	diazepam (Valium)	disopyramide (Norpace)
hyoscyamine (Levisin)	metaxalone (Skelaxin)	doxepin (Sinequan, Zonalon)
meperidine (Demerol)	methocarbamol (Robaxin)	hydroxyzine (Atarax, Vistaril)
meprobamate (Equagesic)	propoxyphene (Darvon)	indomethacin (Indocin)
pentazocine (Talwin)		methyldopa (Aldomet)
propantheline (Pro-Banthine)		oxybutynin (Ditropan)
trimethobenzamide (Tigan)		promethazine (Phenergan)
		reserpine
		ticlopidine (Ticlid)

Adapted from: Zhan C, Sangl J, Bierman AS, Miller MR, et al. Potentially inappropriate medication use in the community-dwelling elderly: findings from the 1996 medical expenditure. JAMA 2001;28(22):2823–2829.

patient's underlying disease, and that withdrawal events can occur as long as 4 months after discontinuing a medication.

One type of physiological withdrawal reaction is the development of a new set of clinical symptoms. For example, abrupt cessation of SSRIs (Paxil, Zoloft) can produce dizziness, nausea, vomiting, anxiety, agitation, and flu-like symptoms (lethargy and sleepiness). Withdrawal events that worsen an underlying disease can occur even if a patient's medication is slowly tapered. An example is diuretic withdrawal, which may aggravate a patient's heart failure. When assessing a patient whose condition or disease is worsening, ask if the patient has recently stopped taking a medication (▶ **Figure 13-14**). (▼ **Table 13-7**) reviews common examples of physiological ADWEs in older persons.

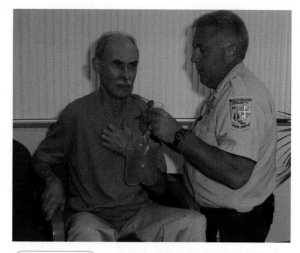

Figure 13-14   When assessing a patient whose condition or disease is worsening, ask if the patient has recently stopped taking a medication.

TABLE 13-7 Drugs Associated with Physiological Medication Withdrawal Syndromes	
Medications	**Physiological Withdrawal Syndrome**
Alpha-antagonist [Clonidine (Catapres)]/antihypertensives	Hypertension, palpitations, headache, agitation
Angiotensin-converting enzyme (ACE) inhibitors (Captopril, Lotensin, Zestril)	Hypertension, heart failure
Anticonvulsants (Dilantin)	Seizures
Antidepressants (Elavil, Zoloft, Paxil)	Anxiety, irritability, gastrointestinal distress, fatigue, muscle pain, headache, chills, insomnia, recurrence of depression
Antiparkinsonian agents (Sinemet, Eldepryl, Mirapex)	Rigidity, tremor, pulmonary embolism, psychosis, hypotension
Antipsychotics (Clozaril, Serentil, Haldol)	Nausea, restlessness, insomnia, movement disorder
Benzodiazepines (Valium, Xanax)	Agitation, confusion, seizures, insomnia
Beta-blockers (Tenormin, Toprol, Lopressor)	Angina, myocardial infarction, anxiety, tachycardia, hypertension
Corticosteroids (prednisone, Medrol, Prelone)	Weakness, anorexia, nausea, hypotension
Muscle relaxers (Baclofen, Lioresal)	Hallucinations, paranoia, nightmares, mania, depression, anxiety, confusion
NSAIDs (ibuprofen, indomethacin, Celebrex)	Recurrence of arthritis and gout symptoms
Narcotic analgesics (oxycodone, Percocet, Methadone)	Restlessness, anxiety, anger, insomnia, chills, abdominal cramping, diarrhea, diaphoresis
Sedative/hypnotics (barbiturates)	Anxiety, muscle twitches, tremor, dizziness

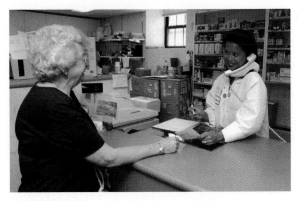

Figure 13-15 Having the patient, pharmacist, and physician work together can help improve adherence by ensuring that dosing schedules fit the patient's lifestyle, and that the patient can afford the prescriptions.

Nonadherence and Its Risks

Nonadherence can increase morbidity and mortality in the older patient, and may also increase overall health care costs. With an increasing older population and a rising number of prescriptions being written for older patients, there has been an increase in the rate of nonadherence, as well. Many factors can contribute to this:

♦ Forgetting to take medications on time.

♦ Not remembering the correct amount or dose.

♦ Poor technique with medicine administration devices [eg, metered-dose inhalers (MDIs), insulin syringes].

♦ Difficulty understanding the label or other directions.

♦ Difficulty opening containers.

♦ Financial problems (cannot afford medications).

Nonadherent behavior is generally thought of as causing a decline in health, but the opposite can also be true: nausea and vomiting, for instance, can convince a patient to stop taking medications. The patient may also believe that he or she is taking too many medications, and decide to take a "drug holiday" to see if they are all really necessary. The number of doses that need to be taken in a day can also lead to nonadherence. Medications that require dosing three or four times daily can contribute to confusion about the drug plan, especially if the patient has any cognitive impairment. The following may help improve adherence:

♦ Have the physician modify medication schedules to fit the patient's lifestyle.

♦ Have the physician and pharmacist work with the patient in selecting medications that are more affordable (▲ **Figure 13-15**).

♦ Have the pharmacy dispense easy-to-open containers.

♦ Switch to dosage forms that are easier to swallow.

♦ If vision impairment is a problem, have the pharmacy provide labels and directions with larger type.

♦ Provide adherence-enhancing aids such as special blister packaging, pillboxes of various sizes, drug calendars, insulin pens, or dosage-measuring devices.

As the list above suggests, it is important to determine the causes of nonadherence before selecting a strategy to address it. Identification of family members to become caregivers may assist in improving adherence, especially if the patient is cognitively impaired. Additional topics to assess are medication storage and the risk of sharing medications with family members. If the patient has reasons for intentional nonadherence, inform the patient's primary care physician of the situation.

Intervention, Management, and Transport

Depending on the adverse drug event, administration of reversal drugs may be required. In this situation, it is usually standard to stop the medication and administer the reversal medication, which can cause new side effects. For example, diphenhydramine is often used to reverse allergic reactions to medications. High doses of diphenhydramine may contribute to delirium, constipation, and urinary retention in the older person. Patients having an anaphylactic reaction to a medication may require high doses of IV corticosteroids, such as methylprednisolone, which can cause psychiatric symptoms. When treating a side effect from a medication, use caution about the medication you are administering.

Prevention

Throughout this chapter, many methods to reduce adverse drug events and improve adherence have been mentioned. The most important contribution an EMS provider can make is to get a complete medication history that includes medication adherence, OTC medication use, nutritional supplements, and herbal medication use.

Other specific ways to prevent adverse medication-related events in older patients include:

♦ Collecting all of the patient's medications, including OTC drugs, and bringing them to the ED when time does not allow for a detailed medication history.

♦ Assessing whether a patient is taking the medication in exactly the way indicated on the prescription container (▼ Figure 13-16).

♦ Calling the patient's pharmacy to get a better report on medication adherence.

♦ Assessing any problems with body systems that may be associated with drug side effects.

♦ Encouraging the patient to develop a complete medication list to carry at all times, and to have it updated regularly by the physician or pharmacist.

Drug-related problems and side effects can contribute to the functional decline of an older person, and to an increase in ED visits. Successful treatment of older patients has relied for years on the multidisciplinary team approach; by making themselves part of that team, EMS providers can help improve the care of the older patient.

Summary

Older people are at increased risk of experiencing adverse drug events because of several factors, including age-related physiologic changes that can affect the distribution and elimination of drugs. In addition, older patients consume the largest proportion of medications. As the number of drugs increases, the risk of drug interactions also rises. It is important that EMS providers obtain a thorough medication history, and possibly transport medication with the patient, to identify adverse drug events.

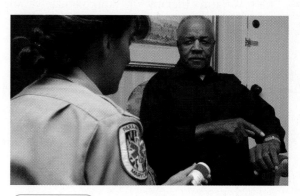

Figure 13-16 Assess whether a patient is taking the medication in exactly the way indicated on the prescription container.

Case Study Summaries

Based on the patient's presentation, you should ask the following questions:

- What medications is he taking for his "blood clot" and in what dose?
- When was the last time he had his blood tested for his "blood thinner" medication?
- What other medications is he taking?

- Have there been any changes to his prescription medications in the past few weeks?
- Does he have any difficulty in remembering to take his medications?
- Is he taking any over-the-counter or herbal medications?
- Has he made any changes to his diet lately?

CASE STUDY 1 SUMMARY (continued)

This patient is potentially experiencing a pulmonary embolism due to not receiving adequate anticoagulation with his warfarin therapy. The signs and symptoms that the patient is experiencing are consistent with a pulmonary embolism in light of his recent history of deep vein thrombosis (blood clot in his leg). The most likely source of a pulmonary embolism is his deep vein thrombosis given his swollen and tender right leg.

There are several clues to suggest his blood thinner medication may not be at sufficient levels. First, the patient has not had a blood test for his warfarin therapy in approximately one month. While his levels were reportedly adequate a month ago, several factors have since occurred that may result in warfarin having a decreased effect. Most importantly is the dose reduction in the patient's thyroid medication (levothyroxine). Thyroid hormones, such as levothyroxine, increase the breakdown of clotting factors that antagonize the anticoagulation

(anti-clotting) effect of warfarin but may also increase the metabolism of warfarin itself. When the dose of levothyroxine is changed, the patient should have his blood tested to be sure he does not have to have his dose of warfarin adjusted as well.

The patient also states that he has changed his diet recently, indicating that he is "eating more salad" in an effort to lose weight. Leafy green vegetables, such as lettuce, have a high vitamin K content, which also serves to decrease the effect of warfarin. Again, this could have been detected by the blood test, but this drug-dietary interaction was not identified as the patient has not followed-up with regular blood tests.

Both drug interactions contributed to warfarin having a decreased effect, which were not identified due to the patient's not following up with regular blood tests. Therefore, the patient did not receive adequate treatment for his deep vein thrombosis, possibly resulting in a pulmonary embolism.

Upon interviewing this patient you find that he is confused, and unsure about his medications. You may write down the list of medications to bring into the ED, with the correct name, strength, directions, and the last time the patient had it refilled, to verify adherence. Note when checking for adherence that you may want to check the number of pills in the bottle and compare it to the refill dates and directions.

You may also want to ask the patient if he uses the inhalers on the table and check to see if the patient understands the proper technique for using the breathing inhalers. Improper technique may be leading to difficulty in receiving the proper amount of drug to control his breathing problem. You may also recommend that the patient use a spacer to aid with the breathing inhalers.

Evaluate if any medications may have been stopped suddenly to assess if there is any risk of the patient developing adverse drug withdrawal symptoms. Upon arrival at the ED, notify the physician on call of any suspicion of an adverse drug withdrawal. Also, have the ED check a digoxin level. Digoxin toxicity could contribute to the patient's mental confusion.

Note that the patient is taking the same medication in different forms: Cessation Zyban (buproprion) 150 mg for smoking, and Wellbutrin (buproprion) for depression. It appears the patient is seeing different doctors for the two prescriptions. This could be leading to an increase in the risk of side effects that may be contributing to his current problems of confusion and potential risk for falls.

In addition, the patient appears to have fallen recently. Consider evaluating the patient's blood pressures and check if he has orthostatic vital signs. Several medications (eg, clonidine, amitriptyline) on the patient's list may be contributing to his orthostatic condition and to risk of falls.

It appears that the patient has a case of polypharmacy. You may be able to prevent future adverse medication effects by providing the patient with a list of his medications and encouraging him to bring that list to every physician visit for evaluation (see Appendix B: Medication Diary for a list that can be filled out and distributed to patients). Encouraging use of a pill box or other organized system may help with adherence to the prescribed regimen and may help avoid overdosing and withdrawal. Reporting to the ED observed evidence of the inability to safely self-administer medications may result in initiating a plan to have medication administration supervised. See if there is anybody who could provide caregiver support.

Endnotes

1. Turnheim K. Drug dosage in the elderly. Is it rational? *Drugs Aging.* 1998;13:357–379.

2. US Bureau of Census. *Demographic and Socio-economic Aspects of Aging in the United States.* Current Population Reports, ser P-23, no. 138. Washington DC: Government Printing Office; 1984.

3. Beers MH, Baran RW, Frenia K. Drugs and the elderly, part I: the problems facing managed care. *Am J Manag Care.* 2000;6:1313–1320.

4. Grymonpre RE, Mikenko PA, Sitar DS, Aoki FY, Montgomery PR. Drug-associated hospital admissions in older medical patients. *J Am Geriatr Soc.* 1988;36:1092–1098.

5. Parker BM, Cusack BJ, Vestal RE. Pharmacokinetic optimization of drug therapy in elderly patients. *Drugs Aging.* 1995;7:10–18.

6. Field TS, Gurwitz JH, Glynn RJ, et al. The renal effects of nonsteroidal anti-inflammatory drugs in older people: findings from the Established Populations for Epidemiologic Studies of the Elderly. *J Am Geriatr Soc.* 1999;47:507–511.

7. Fugh-Berman A, Ernst E. Herb-drug interactions: review and assessment of report reliability. *Br J Clin Pharmacol.* 2001;52:587–595.

8. Murray M. Common questions about St. John's Wort extract. *American Journal of Natural Medicine.* 1997;4(7):14–19.

9. Graves T, Hanlon JT, Schmader KE, et al. Adverse events after discontinuing medications in elderly outpatients. *Arch Intern Med.* 1997;157:2205–2210.

Bibliography

Ament PW, Bertolino JG, Liszewski JL. Clinically significant drug interactions. *Am Fam Phys.* 2000;61(6):1745–1754.

American Herbal Pharmacopoeia and Therapeutic Compendium. St. John's Wort (*Hypericum perforatum*) monograph. *Herbalgram. The Journal of the American Botanical Council and the Herb Research Foundation.* 1997;(40):1–16.

Bailey DG, Malcolm J, Arnold O, Spence JD. Grapefruit juice-drug interactions. *Br J Clin Pharmacol.* 1998;46:101–110.

Blum MR, Riegelman S, Becker CE. Altered protein binding of diphenylhydantoin in uremic plasma. *New Engl J Med.* 1972;286:109.

Blumenthal M (ed). *The Complete German Commission E Monographs.* Boston: Integrative Medicine Communications; 1998.

Breidenbach T, Kliem V, Burg M, Radermacher J, Hoffmann MW, Klempnauer J. Profound drop of cyclosporin A whole blood trough levels caused by St. John's wort (*Hypericum perforatum*) [letter]. *Transplantation.* 2000;69:2229–2230.

Brinker F. *Herb Contraindications and Drug Interactions.* Sandy, OR: Eclectic Medical Publications; 2001.

Brockmoller J, Reum T, Bauer S, Kerb R, Hubner W-D, Roots I. Hypericin and pseudohypericin: pharmcokinetics and effects of photosensitivity in humans. *Pharmacopsychiatry.* 1997;30:94–101.

Brooks SM, Sholiton LJ, Werk EE Jr, Altenau P. The effects of ephedrine and theophylline on dexamethasone metabolism in bronchial asthma. *J Clin Pharmacol.* 1977;17:308–318.

Cadigan DA, Magaziner J, Fedder DO. Polymedicine use among community resident older women: how much of a problem? *Am J Public Health.* 1989;79:1537–1540.

Campion EW, deLabry LO, Glynn RJ. The effect of age on serum albumin in healthy males: report from the Normative Aging Study. *J Gerontol.* 1988;43:M18–M20.

Chatterjee SS, Bhattacharya SK, Wonnemann M, Singer A, Muller WE. Hyperforin as a possible antidepressant component of *Hypericum* extracts. *Life Sci.* 1998;63(6):499–510.

Chin TF, Lach JL. Drug diffusion and bioavailability: tetracycline metallic chelation. *Am J Hosp Pharm.* 1975;32:625–629.

Chrischilles EA, Segar ET, Wallace RB. Self-reported adverse drug reactions and related resource use: a study of community-dwelling persons 65 years of age and older. *Ann Intern Med.* 1992;117:634–640.

Chung KF, McCusker M, Page CP, Dent G, Guinot P, Barnes PJ. Effect of a ginkgolide mixture (BN 52063) in antagonising skin and platelet responses to platelet activation factor in man. *Lancet.* 1987; Jan. 31, 1987:248–50.

Col N, Fanale JE, Kronholm P. The role of medication noncompliance and adverse drug reactions in hospitalizations of the elderly. *Arch Intern Med.* 1990;150:841–845.

D'Arcy PF, Griffen JP. *Iatrogenic Diseases.* 3rd ed. Oxford, England: Oxford University Press; 1986.

Darnell JC, Murray MD, Martz BL, Weinberger M. Medication use by ambulatory elderly: an in-home survey. *J Am Geriatr Soc.* 1986;34:1–4.

Dauchot P, Gravenstein JS. Effects of atropine on the electrocardiogram in different age groups. *Clin Pharmacol Ther.* 1971;12:274–280.

Dresser GK, Bailey DG, Carruthers SG. Grapefruit juice-felodipine interaction in the elderly. *Clin Pharmacol Ther.* 2000;68:28–34.

Drugs that cause psychiatric symptoms. *Med Lett.* 1998;40:21–24.

Dyck DJ. Dietary fat intake, supplements and weight loss. *Can J Appl Physiol.* 2000;25(6):495–523.

Ereshefsky B, Gewertz N. Determination of SJW Differential Metabolism at CYP2D6 and CYP3A4 Using Dextromethorphan Probe Technology. *Proceedings 39th Annual Meeting.* Boca Raton, FL: New Clinical Drug Evaluation Unit; (June 1999) Poster Number 130.

Ezra A, Golomb G. Administration routes and delivery systems of bisphosphonates for the treatment of bone resorption. *Adv Drug Deliv Rev.* 2000;42:175–195.

Frishman WH. Beta-adrenergic blocker withdrawal. *Am J Cardiol.* 1987;59:26F–32F.

Fugh-Berman A. Herb-drug interactions. *Lancet.* 2000;355:134–138.

Gerety M, Cornell JE, Plichta D, Eimer M. Adverse events related to drugs and drug withdrawal in nursing home residents. *J Am Geriatr Soc.* 1993;41:1326–1332.

Grandison MK, Boudinot FD. Age-related changes in protein binding of drugs. Implications for therapy. *Clin Pharmacokinet.* 2000;38:271–290.

Graves T, Hanlon JT, Schmader KE, et al. Adverse events after discontinuing medications in elderly outpatients. *Arch Intern Med.* 1997;157:2205–2210.

Gray SL, Lai KV, Larson EB. Drug-induced cognition disorders in the elderly. Incidence, prevention and management. *Drug Safety.* 1999;21:101–122.

Gruenwald J, Brendler T, Jaenicke C (eds). *PDR for Herbal Medicines*. Montvale, NJ: Medical Economics Co., 1998.

Gulati OD, Dave BT, Gokhale SD, Shah KM. Antagonism of adrenergic neuron blockade in hypertensive subjects. *Clin Pharm Ther.* 1966;7(4): 510–514.

Gurley BJ, Gardner SF, Hubbard MA. Content versus label claims in ephedra-containing dietary supplements. *Am J Health Syst Pharm.* 2000;15;57(10): 963–969.

Gurwitz JH, Avorn J. The ambiguous relation between aging and adverse drug reactions. *Ann Intern Med.* 1991;114:956–966.

Gurwitz JH, Avorn J, Ross-Degnan D, Choodnovskiy I, Ansell J. Aging and the anticoagulant response to warfarin. *Ann Intern Med.* 1992;116:901–904.

Hanlon JT, Fillenbaum GG, Schmader KE, et al. Inappropriate medication use among community dwelling elderly residents. *Pharmacotherapy.* 2000; 20:575–8

Hanlon JT, Schmader K, et al. Adverse drug reactions. In: Delafuente JC, Stewart RB, eds. *Therapeutics in the Elderly.* 3rd ed. Cincinnati, OH: Harvey Whitney Books; 2000.

Hanlon JT, Schmader K, Lewis I. Adverse drug reactions. In: Delafuente JC, Stewart RB, eds. *Therapeutics in the Elderly.* 2nd ed. Cincinnati, OH: Harvey Whitney Books; 1995:212–227.

Hanlon JT, Schmader KE, Koronkowski MJ, et al. Adverse drug events in high risk older outpatients. *J Am Geriatr Soc.* 1997;45:945–948.

Hanlon JT, Schmader KE, Ruby C, Weinberger M. Suboptimal prescribing in older inpatients and outpatients. *J Am Geriatr Soc.* 2001;49:200–209.

Hansten PD, Horn JR. *Drug Interactions,* 7th ed. Philadelphia: Lea & Febiger; 1993.

Healthy People 2000. National health promotion and disease prevention objectives. Washington, DC: US Department of Health and Human Services; 1990. Publication No.91-50212.

Helling DK, Lemke JH, Semla TP, Wallace RB, Lipson DB, Comoni-Huntley J. Medication use characteristics in the elderly: the Iowa 65+ rural health study. *J Am Geriatr Soc.* 1987;35:4–12.

Hendricks J, Johnson TP, Sheahan SL, et al. Medication use among older persons in congregate living facilities. *J Geriatr Drug Ther.* 1991;6:47–61.

Hodding GC, Jann M, Ackerman IP. Drug withdrawal syndromes: a literature review. *West J Med.* 1980; 133:383–391.

Hoddinott BC, Gowdey LW, Coulter WK, Parker JM. *Can Med Assoc J.* 1967;97:1001–1006.

Iber FL, Murphy PA, Connor ES. Age-related changes in the gastrointestinal system. Effects on drug therapy. *Drugs Aging.* 1994;5:34–48.

Johne A, Brockmoller J, Bauer S, Maurer A, Langheinrich M, Roots I. Pharmacokinetic interaction of digoxin with an herbal extract from St John's wort (Hypericum perforatum). *Clin Pharmacol Ther.* 1999;66(4):338–345.

Kaufman P, Cseke L, Warber S, Duke J, Brielman H. *Natural Products from Plants.* Boca Raton, FL: CRC Press; 1999.

Kaye AD, Sabar R, Vig S, et al. Nutraceuticals: current concepts and the role of the anesthesiologist. Part 1. echinacea, garlic, ginger, gingko, and St. John's Wort. *Am J Anesthesiol.* 2000;27(7):405–407.

Kelliher GJ, Cohahan ST. Changes in vagal activity and response to muscarinic receptors with age. *J Gerontol.* 1980;45:842–849.

Kirk JK. Significant drug-nutrient interactions. *Am Fam Physician.* 1995;51:1175–1182.

Kremer JMH, Wilting J, Janssen LHM. Drug binding of human alpha-1-acid glycoprotein in health and disease. *Pharmacol Rev.* 1988;40:1–47.

Lamy PP. Hazards of drug use in the elderly. Common sense measures to reduce them. *Postgrad Med J.* 1984;76:50–61.

Lantz MS, Buchalther E, Giamanco V. St John's Wort and antidepressant drug interactions in the elderly. *J Geriatr Psychiatry Neurol.* 1999;12:7–10.

Lazarou J, Pomeranz BH, Corey PN. Incidence of adverse drug reactions in hospitalized patients: a meta-analysis of prospective studies. *JAMA.* 1998; 229:1200–1205.

Lieberman S. Nutriceutical review of St. John's Wort (Hypericum perforatum) for the treatment of depression. *J Women's Health.* 1998;7(2):177–182.

Liu B, Anderson G, Mittmann N, To T, Axcell T, Shear N. Use of selective-reuptake inhibitors of tricyclic antidepressants and risk of hip fractures in elderly people. *Lancet.* 1998;351:1303–1307.

MacKichan J. Influence of protein binding and use of unbound (free) drug concentrations. In: Evans WE, Schentag JJ, Jusko WJ, eds. *Applied Pharmacokinetics: Principles of Therapeutic Drug Monitoring.* 3rd ed. Vancouver, WA: Applied Therapeutics; 1992: chap 5.

Markowitz JS, DeVane CL, Boulton DW, Carson SW, Nahas Z, Risch SC. Effect of St. John's Wort (Hypericum perforatum) on cytochrome P-450 2D6 and 3A4 activity in healthy volunteers. *Life Sci.* 2000; 66:L133–L139.

May FE, Stewart RB, Cluff LE. Drug interactions and multiple drug administration. *Clin Pharmacol Ther.* 1977; 22:322–328.

Mayersohn MB. Special pharmacokinetic considerations in the elderly. In: Evans WE, Schentag JJ, Jusko WJ, eds. *Applied Pharamcokinetics: Principles of Therapeutic Drug Monitoring*. 3rd ed. Vancouver, WA: Applied Therapeutics; 1992: chap 9.

McKenna DJ, Jones K, Hughes K. Efficacy, safety, and use of ginkgo biloba in clinical and preclinical applications. *Altern Ther Health Med*. 2001 Sep-Oct; 7(5):70–86, 88–90.

Meletis CD, Jacobs T. *Interactions Between Drugs and Natural Medicines*. Sandy, OR: Eclectic Medical Publications; 1999.

Michalets EL. Update: clinically significant cytochrome P-450 drug interactions. *Pharmacotherapy*. 1998; 18:84–112.

Miller LG. Herbal medicinals—selected clinical considerations focusing on known or potential drug-herb interactions. *Arch Intern Med*. 1998; 158: 2200–2211.

Mills S, Bone K. *Principles and Practice of Phytotherapy*. Edinburgh: Churchill Livingstone; 2000.

Moore AR, O'Keefe ST. Drug-induced cognitive impairment in the elderly. *Drugs Aging*. 1999;15:15–28.

Nix DE, Schentag JJ. The quinolones: an overview and comparative appraisal of the pharmacokinetics and pharmacodynamics. *J Clin Pharmacol*. 1988;28: 169–178.

Nolan L, O'Malley K. Prescribing for the elderly. Part I. Sensitivity of the elderly to adverse drug reactions. *J Am Geriatr Soc*. 1988;36:142–149.

Nolan L, O'Malley K. Adverse drug reactions in the elderly. *Br J Hosp Med*. 1989;41:452–457.

Odar-Cederlof I, Lunde P, Sjogvist F. Abnormal pharmacokinetics of phenytoin in a patient with uremia. *Lancet*. 1970;2(7677):831–832.

Owens NJ, Silliman RA, Fretwell MD. The relationship between comprehensive functional assessment and optimal pharmacotherapy in the older patient. *DICP ANN Pharmacother*. 1989;23:847–854.

Pacifici GM, Viani A, Taddeuci-Brunelli G, Rizzo G, Carri M, Schulz HU. Effects of development, aging, and renal and hepatic insufficiency as well as hemodialysis on the plasma concentrations of albumin and α-1-acid glycoprotein: implications for binding of drugs. *Ther Drug Monit*. 1986;8: 259–263.

Packer M, Gheorghiade M, Young J, et al. Withdrawal of digoxin from patients with chronic heart failure treated with angiotensin-converting-enzyme inhibitors. *N Engl J Med*. 1993;329:1–7.

Pirotzky E, Colliez P, Guilmard C, Schaeverbeke J, Braquet P. Cyclosporine-induced nephrotoxicity: preventive effect of a PAD-acether antagonist, BN 52063. *Transplant Proc*. 1988;20(3; suppl 3): 665–669.

Planta M, Gundersen B, Petitt JC. Prevalence of the use of herbal products in a low-income population. *Fam Med*. 2000;32(4):252–257.

Polk RE, Healy DP, Sahai J, Drwal L, Racht E. The influence of chronic administration of calcium carbonate on the bioavailability of oral cirprofloxacin. *Antimicrob Agents Chemother*. 1989;33:1841–1844.

Rasmussen P. St John's Wort: a review of its use in depression. *Aust J Med Herbalism*. 1998;10(1):8–13.

Ray WA, Griffen MR, Schaffner W, Baugh DK, Melton L. Pychotropic drug use and the risk of hip fracture. *N Engl J Med*. 1987;316:363–369.

Roby CA, Anderson GD, Kantor E, Dryer DA, Burstein AH. 2000. St John's Wort: effect on CYP3A4 activity. *Clin Pharmacol Ther*. 2000;67:451–457.

Rogers EA, Gough JE, Brewer KL. Are emergency department patients at risk for herb-drug interactions? *Acad Emerg Med*. 2001;8(9):932–934.

Rowe JW, Andres R, Tobin JD, et al. The effect of age on creatinine clearance in men: a cross-sectional and longitudinal study. *J Gerontol*. 1976;31:155–163.

Schatzberg AF, Haddad P, Kaplan EM, et al. Serotonin reuptake inhibitor discontinuation syndrome: a hypothetical definition. Discontinuation Consensus panel. *J Clin Psychiatry*. 1997;58(suppl 7):5–10.

Schneider JK, Mion LC, Frengley JD. Adverse drug reactions in an elderly outpatient population. *Am J Hosp Pharm*. 1992;49:90–96.

Seppala M, Sourander L. A practical guide to prescribing in nursing homes. Avoiding pitfalls. *Drugs Aging*. 1995;6:426–435.

Simmen U, Schweitzer C, Burkard W, Schaffner W, Lundstrom K. *Hypericum perforatum* inhibits the binding of μ- and κ-opiod receptor expressed with the semliki forest virus system. *Pharm Acta Helv*. 1998;73:53–56.

Steel K, Gertman PM, Crescenzi C, Anderson J. Iatrogenic illness on a general medicine service at a university hospital. *N Engl J Med*. 1981;304:638–642.

Stewart RB, Caranasos GJ. Medication compliance in the elderly. *Med Clin North Am*. 1989;73:1551–1563.

Stewart RB, Cooper JW. Polypharmacy in the aged. Practical solutions. *Drugs Aging*. 1994;4:449–461.

Stewart RB, Moore MT, May FE, Marks RG, Hale WE. A longitudinal analysis of drug use in an ambulatory elderly population. *J Clin Epidemiol*. 1991;44: 1353–1359.

Stockley IH. *Drug Interactions*. 4th ed. London: Pharmaceutical Press; 1996.

Stough C, Clarke J, Lloyd J, Nathan PJ. Neuropsychological changes after 30-day Ginkgo biloba administration in healthy participants. *Int J Neuropsychopharmacol*. 2001 Jun;4(2):131–134.

Sugimoto K, Ohmori M, Tsuruoka S, et al. Different effects of St John's Wort on the pharmacokinetics of simvastatin and pravastatin. *Clin Pharmacol Ther.* 2001;70(6):518–524.

Taylor WF, Heimlich EM, Strick L, Busser R. Ephedrine and theophylline in asthmatic children: quantitive observations on the combination and ephedrine tachyphylaxis. *Ann Allergy.* 1965;23:437–440.

Thapa PB, Gideon P, Cost TW, Milam AB, Ray WA. Antidepressants and the risk of falls among nursing home residents. *N Engl J Med.* 1998;339: 875–882.

Thomas JA. Drug-nutrient interactions. *Nutr Rev.* 1995; 53:271–282.

Tinkelman DG, Avner SE. Ephedrine therapy in asthmatic children. *JAMA.* 1977;237(6):553–557.

Treasure J. Herbal pharmacokinetics: a practitioner update with reference to St. John's Wort (*Hypericum perforatum*) herb-drug interactions. *J Am Herb Guild.* 2000;1(1):2–11.

Ullah MI, Newman GB, Saunders KB. Influence of age on response to ipratropium and salbutamol in man. *Thorax.* 1981;36:523–529.

Veering BT, Burm AG, Souverijn JH, Serre JM, Spierdijk J. The effect of age on serum concentrations of albumin and alpha-1-acid glycoprotein. *Br J Clin Pharmacol.* 1990;29:201–206.

Vestal RE, Norris AH, Tobin JD, Cohen BH, Shock NW, Andres R. Antipyrine metabolism in man: influence of age, alcohol, caffeine and smoking. *Clin Pharmacol Ther.* 1975;18:425–432.

Vestal R, Wood A, Shand D. Reduced β-adrenoreceptor sensitivity in the elderly. *Clin Pharmacol Ther.* 1979; 26:181–186.

Vestal RE, Wood AJJ, Branch RA, Shand DG, Wilkinson GR. Effect of age and cigarette smoking on propranolol disposition. *Clin Pharmacol Ther.* 1979;26: 8–15.

Viani A, Rizzo G, Carrai M, Pacifici GM. Interindividual variability in the concentrations of albumin and alpha-1-acid glycoprotein in patients with renal or liver disease, newborns and healthy subjects: implications for binding of drugs. *Int J Clin Pharmacol Ther Toxicol.* 1992;30:128–133.

Walma E, Hoes A, Van Dooren C, et al. Withdrawal of long term diuretic medication in elderly patients: a double blind randomized trial. *BMJ.* 1997;315: 464–468.

White M, Roden R, Minobe W, et al. Age-related changes in β-adrenergic neuroeffector systems in the human heart. *Circulation.* 1994;90:1225–1238.

Wilkens JH, Wilkens H, Uffman J, Bovers J, Fabel H, Frolich JC. Effects of a PAF-antagonist (BN 52063) on bronchoconstriction and platelet activation during exercise induced asthma. *Br J Clin Pharmacol.* 1990;29:85–91.

Williamson J, Chopin JM. Adverse reactions to prescribed drugs in the elderly: a multi-centre investigation. *Age Ageing.* 1980;9:73–80.

Woodhouse K, Wynne HA. Age-related changes in hepatic function. Implications for drug therapy. *Drugs Aging.* 1992;2:243–255.

Yarnell E. Botanical hepatotoxicity: a critical review and update. *HN Rev Comp Integ Med.* 2000;7(2): 119–24.

Zhan C, Sangl J, Bierman AS, et al. Potentially inappropriate medication use in the community-dwelling elderly: findings from the 1996 medical expenditure. *JAMA.* 2001;28(22):2823–2829.

Elder Abuse and Neglect

LEARNING OBJECTIVES

1 Define elder abuse and neglect and discuss their incidence.

2 Discuss the profiles of an at-risk elder and an abuser.

3 Describe the techniques used to assess elder abuse and neglect.

4 Demonstrate sensitivity to the abused older patient.

5 Recognize the value of nonverbal communication with the abused older patient.

6 Discuss the proper documentation and reporting of elder abuse and neglect cases.

CHAPTER 14

David R. Snyder, MA, NREMT-P

CASE STUDY 1

You are dispatched to the home of an 84-year-old woman by her son. The son reports that the patient has had multiple falls over the last two weeks. History obtained from the son reveals that the patient suffers from dementia, and that she has not eaten in the last four days. Your assessment reveals a frail, malnourished-looking patient who also appears to be in a state of poor hygiene. The patient answers in one-word sentences and is oriented to her name only.

What are your initial priorities?

What are your other considerations based on your findings and the information provided?

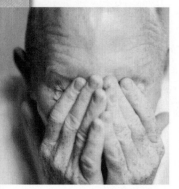

Introduction

One of the EMS provider's most important responsibilities is acting in the best interest of the patient. Nowhere is this more important than when encountering elder abuse and neglect. EMS providers must be able to recognize elder abuse and neglect. EMS providers must also provide valuable information to the hospital emergency department and others involved in elder abuse cases, such as Adult Protective Services (APS), social services, and the police. Knowing how to assess for the signs of abuse may help countless older people who are living lives of fear and deprivation.

Attitude Tip

Remember that abuse and neglect *do* occur in the older population, and that older people are just as nondeserving of it as are children and other younger patients.

When assessing and treating any older patient, always keep a critical eye for the possibility of abuse or neglect.

Background

Reports of physical, emotional, and financial elder abuse have risen significantly, increasing 150% nationwide since 1986.[1] The phenomenon of elder abuse is known as "the hidden iceberg," because estimates are that many more incidents of elder abuse take place than are reported.[2] According to the U.S. House Select Committee on Aging, elder abuse is less likely than child abuse to be reported.[3] The National Center on Elder Abuse estimated that in 1997, 2.1 million people over age 60 were abused, exploited, or neglected.[4] It has been suggested that elder abuse is suffered by between 4% and 5% of all older persons.[5]

Elder abuse is insidious. Elder abuse can occur anywhere, at any time, and spans all socioeconomic classes. It is a full-scale national prob-

lem. Like child abuse and domestic violence a decade ago, elder abuse is moving toward the front of the nation's social consciousness. Therefore, several issues involved in identifying and managing elder abuse must be confronted.

Many agencies are involved in elder abuse cases, and their roles vary depending on the circumstances of the case. **Adult Protective Services (APS)** investigates cases involving abuse and neglect and provides case management services in some instances. Local law enforcement also may be involved in the investigation of elder abuse cases. Many police departments now have an elder crimes unit that handles these cases. If the case involves a nursing home, state licensing agencies are involved in the investigation. If cases can be substantiated, county or state district attorneys will prosecute such cases.

The Long Term Care Ombudsman Program, authorized by the Older Americans Act, advocates for residents in nursing homes (and assisted-living facilities in some states) and their relatives and friends. There is an Ombudsman in every state, territory, and the District of Columbia, usually housed in the state agency handling aging services (called the State Unit on Aging in the Act). The responsibility of the Ombudsman is to be a presence in the facility, to receive and investigate quality of care and residents' rights, complaints, and concerns, and to resolve them if possible before crises occur. As with other health care professionals, if the Ombudsman detects or suspects abuse, neglect, or exploitation, a report is made to the licensing authority and law enforcement agencies.

The EMS provider's role and responsibility in elder abuse cases is not to prove that abuse or neglect has occurred, but to recognize and report suspicions. Given that many agencies may become involved in the investigation of elder abuse cases, proper documentation by the EMS provider is essential.

Attitude Tip

Acting in the patient's best interest is at the forefront of the EMS provider's responsibility. Nowhere is this more important than when encountering elder abuse and neglect.

Definitions

Elder abuse is any form of mistreatment that results in harm or loss to an older person. The following are specific types of abuse and neglect:

Physical abuse is the use of physical force that may result in bodily injury, physical pain, or impairment. Examples include shoving, pushing, hitting, shaking, hair pulling, unreasonable physical confinement, and unreasonable physical or chemical restraint.

Sexual abuse is nonconsensual sexual contact of any kind with an older person.

Psychological abuse, or emotional abuse, is the infliction of anguish, pain, or distress through verbal or nonverbal acts. Examples include verbal assaults, threats, creating fear, isolation, and withholding emotional support.

Financial/material exploitation is illegal or improper use of an older person's funds, property, or assets.

Neglect is the failure to provide needed care, services, or supervision. Two types of neglect have been identified: active neglect, which is the deliberate withholding of companionship, medicine, food, exercise, or assistance to bathroom; and passive neglect, which occurs when the older person is ignored, left alone, isolated, or forgotten (▼ Figure 14-1).[6] Passive neglect can result from inadequate knowledge, laziness, or illness on the part of the care provider.[7] Examples include the failure to provide food, clothing (including providing inappropriate or soiled clothing), shelter, safety, or medical care.

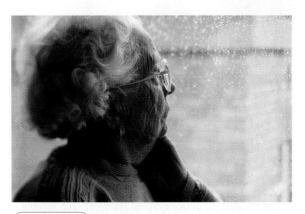

(Figure 14-1)   Passive neglect occurs when the older person is ignored, left alone, isolated, or forgotten.

Self-neglect is the behavior of an older person that threatens the older person's health or safety. Self-neglect can result from poor health, mental decline, or lack of financial resources for adequate self-care. Examples include being unable to provide for his or her own needs, such as hygiene, food, and medications. Older people living alone in the community are most at risk for self-neglect.

Abandonment is the desertion of an older person by an individual who has physical custody of the older person or by a person who has assumed responsibility for providing care.[8]

One of the problems with defining elder abuse and neglect is the lack of a national, uniform set of definitions. Also, while different types of abuse and neglect are defined separately to provide categorical understanding, more than one form of abuse can be occurring at the same time—for example, physical abuse and psychological abuse could occur concurrently.

A simple way of understanding the manifestations of any abuse or neglect is to ascribe to the principle of inadequate care. If the care of the older person appears inadequate for whatever reason, you should suspect abuse or neglect. The goal of EMS providers in abuse and neglect cases is recognition and referral. Knowing how to make appropriate referrals will begin the process of intervention. This is the first step in helping the older person to live free of abuse, fear, and intimidation.

Attitude Tip

EMS providers can be the key link in detecting elder abuse and neglect.

Theories of Abuse and Neglect

There are many theories that attempt to explain abuse and neglect. Although EMS providers are concerned with treating and managing the results of abuse and neglect, an understanding of why abuse and neglect occur is worthy of a brief discussion. Among the most prominent theories are social learning or transgenerational violence theory, stressed caregiver theory, isolation theory, dependency theory, and psychopathology of the abuser theory.

The **social learning theory**, or **transgenerational theory**, maintains that violence is learned. It states that if children are abused, they will abuse their own children. If this theory is extended to elder abuse, the theory holds that these same children will abuse their parents. The **stressed caregiver theory** contends that when the caregiver reaches a certain stress level, abuse and neglect situations will occur. **Isolation theory** maintains that the patient's diminishing social network is a major risk factor in elder abuse. The **dependency theory** maintains that frailty and medical illness set up the older person for abuse and neglect. Finally, the **psychopathology of the abuser theory** states that the abuser's problems (such as personality disorders or substance abuse) lead to abuse and neglect.[9]

Incidence

In 1996, the National Center on Elder Abuse conducted the National Elder Abuse Incidence Study. The study posed this basic question: What is the incidence of domestic elder abuse and neglect in the United States today? The findings showed that an estimated 551,011 persons age 60 and over experienced abuse, neglect, or self-neglect in domestic settings in 1996. Of this total, 21% were reported to and substantiated by APS agencies. These figures show that almost four times as many new incidents of elder abuse, neglect, or self-neglect were unreported.

Additionally, the study found that:

♦ Older women are abused at a higher rate than men, after accounting for their larger proportion in the aging population.

♦ Those age 80 and above are abused and neglected at two to three times their proportion of the older population.

♦ In almost 90% of the elder abuse and neglect incidents with a known perpetrator, the perpetrator is a family member, and two thirds of the perpetrators are adult children or spouses.

♦ Victims of self-neglect are usually depressed, confused, or extremely frail.

Abuse in the Institutional Setting

The National Elder Abuse Incidence Study did not address abuse in institutional settings. Although only about 5% of the nation's older population resides in nursing facilities, those who do often suffer multiple chronic and debilitating illnesses. Additionally, many residents of nursing facilities do not receive visits from relatives or close acquaintances. Nursing home residents who receive no visitors have a higher likelihood of abuse and neglect, because there is no outside influence to watch over the resident's care (▼ **Figure 14-2**).

Small-scale studies have been conducted to examine the prevalence of abuse in institutions. One study conducted by Pillemer and Moore surveyed 577 staff members from 31 nursing facilities to determine the extent of physical and psychological abuse perpetrated by staff.[10] In the year preceding the study, 81% of staff reported seeing at least one incident of psychological abuse, 36% witnessed physical abuse, 10% admitted to committing acts of physical abuse, and 40% admitted to committing at least one act of psychological abuse.

The Nursing Home Reform Amendments of the Omnibus Budget Reconciliation Act (OBRA) of 1987 require that nursing facilities "promote and protect the rights of each patient." The general provisions of these rights have been paraphrased in (▶ **Table 14-1**): Rights of Nursing

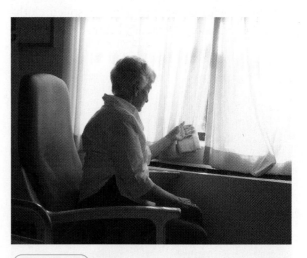

Figure 14-2   Nursing home residents who receive no visitors have a higher likelihood of abuse and neglect, because there is no outside influence to watch over the resident's care.

TABLE 14-1 Rights of Nursing Home Residents

The Nursing Home Reform Amendments of OBRA 1987 require that nursing facilities "promote and protect the rights of each resident. . ." Several important provisions of the law set the stage for the protection of these rights. The requirements of this Act have been paraphrased and are presented here to give a broad understanding to EMS providers of the rights afforded nursing home residents. For a complete citation, see *Volume 42, Code of Federal Regulations, Part 483*.

General Provisions

The general provisions of the law are as follows.

Quality of Life: The law requires nursing homes to "care for the residents in such a manner and in such an environment as will promote maintenance or enhancement of the quality of life of each resident." A new emphasis is placed on dignity, choice, and self-determination for nursing home residents.

Provision of Services and Activities: The law requires each nursing home to "provide services and activities to attain or maintain the highest practicable physical, mental, and psychological well-being of each resident in accordance with a written plan of care which . . . is initially prepared, with participation to the extent practicable of the resident or the resident's legal representative."

Participation in Facility Administration: The law makes "resident and advocacy participation" a criterion for assessing a facility's compliance with administration requirements.

Assuring Access to the Ombudsman Program: The law grants immediate access by ombudsmen to residents and reasonable access, in accordance with state law, to records. It requires facilities to inform residents how to contact an ombudsman to voice complaints or in the event of a transfer or discharge from the facility and requires state agencies to share inspection results with ombudsman.

Specific Rights

Specific nursing home residents' rights include the following.

Rights to Self-Determination: Nursing home residents have the right:

◆ to choose their personal physician;

◆ to full information, in advance, and participation in planning and making any changes in their care and treatment;

◆ to reside and receive services with reasonable accommodation by the facility of individual needs and preferences;

◆ to voice grievances about the care and treatment they do or do not receive without discrimination or reprisal, and to receive prompt response from the facility;

◆ to organize and participate in resident groups (and their families have the right to organize family groups) in the facility.

Personal and Privacy Rights: Nursing home residents have the right:

◆ to participate in social, religious, and community activities as they choose;

◆ to privacy in medical treatment, accommodations, personal visits, written and telephone conversations;

◆ to confidentiality with personal and clinical residents.

Rights Regarding Abuse and Restraints: Nursing home residents have the right:

◆ to be free from physical and mental abuse, corporal punishment, involuntary seclusion, or disciplinary use of restraints;

◆ to be free of restraints used for the convenience of the staff rather than the well-being of the residents;

◆ to have restraints used only under written physician's orders to treat a resident's medical symptoms and ensure the resident's safety and the safety of others;

◆ to be given psychopharmacologic medication only as ordered by a physician as part of a written plan of care for a specific medical symptom, with annual review for appropriateness by an independent, external expert.

Rights to Information: Nursing homes must:

◆ upon request provide residents with the latest inspection results and any plan of correction submitted by the facility;

◆ notify residents in advance of any plans to change their rooms or roommate;

◆ inform residents of their rights upon admission and provide them with a written copy of the rights, including their rights regarding personal funds and their right to file a complaint with the state survey agency;

◆ inform residents in writing, at admission and throughout their stay, of the services available under the basic rate and of any extra charges for extra services, including, for Medicaid residents, a list of services covered by Medicaid, and for those for which there is an extra charge;

(continued)

TABLE 14-1 Rights of Nursing Home Residents *(continued)*

◆ prominently display and provide oral and written information for residents about how to apply for and use Medicaid benefits and how to receive a refund for previous private payments that Medicaid will pay retroactively.

Rights to Visits: The nursing home must:

◆ permit immediate visits by a resident's personal physician and by representatives of the licensing agency and the ombudsman program;

◆ permit immediate visits by a resident's relatives, with the resident's consent;

◆ permit visits "subject to reasonable restriction" for others who visit with the resident's consent;

◆ permit an ombudsman to review resident's clinical records if a resident grants permission.

Transfer and Discharge Rights: Nursing homes "must permit each resident to remain in the facility and must not transfer or discharge the resident unless":

◆ the transfer or discharge is necessary to meet the resident's welfare and the resident's welfare cannot be met by the facility;

◆ appropriate because the resident's health has improved such that the resident no longer needs nursing home care;

◆ the health or safety of other residents is endangered;

◆ the resident has failed, after reasonable notice, to pay an allowable facility charge for an item or service provided upon the resident request;

◆ the facility ceases to operate.

Notice

Notice must be given to residents and their representatives before transfer:

◆ Timing: at least 30 days in advance, or as soon as possible if more immediate changes in health require more immediate transfer;

◆ Content: reasons for transfer, the resident's right to appeal the transfer, and the name, address, and phone number of the ombudsman program and protection and advocacy programs for the mentally ill and developmentally disabled;

◆ Returning to the facility: the right to request that a resident's bed be held, including information about how many days Medicaid will pay for the bed to be held and the facility's bed-hold policies, and the right to return to the next available bed if Medicaid bed-holding coverage lapses.

Orientation

A facility must prepare and orient to ensure safe and orderly transfer or discharge from the facility.

Protection of Personal Funds

A nursing home must:

◆ not require residents to deposit their personal funds with the facility;

◆ if it accepts written responsibility for resident's funds:

　◆ keep funds over $50 in an interest-bearing account, separate from the facility account;

　◆ keep other funds available in a separate account or petty cash fund;

　◆ keep a complete and separate accounting of each resident's funds, with a written record of all transactions, available for review by residents and their representatives;

　◆ notify Medicaid residents when their balance account comes within $200 of the Medicaid limit and the effect of this on their eligibility;

　◆ upon the resident's death, turn funds over to the resident's trustee;

　◆ purchase a surety bond to secure residents' funds in its keeping;

　◆ not charge a resident for any item or service covered by Medicaid, specifically including routine personal hygiene items and services.

Protection Against Medicaid Discrimination: Nursing homes must:

◆ establish and maintain identical policies and practices regarding transfer, discharge and the provision of services required under Medicaid for all individuals regardless of source payment;

◆ not require residents to waive their rights to Medicaid, and must provide information about how to apply for Medicaid;

◆ not require a third party to guarantee payment as a condition of admission or continued stay; not "charge, solicit, accept or receive" gifts, money, donations, or "other consideration" as a precondition for admission or for continued stay for persons eligible for Medicare.

Source: The Nursing Home Reform Amendment of OBRA 1987. *Volume 42, Code of Federal Regulations, Part 483.*

Home Residents. Unfortunately, many nursing homes fall short of the requirement.

In July 2001, the U.S. House of Representatives released a study entitled *Abuse of Residents Is a Major Problem in U.S. Nursing Homes*. This study investigated the incidence of abuse in nursing homes in the United States by evaluating state inspections of nursing homes or complaint investigations from January 1, 1999 through January 1, 2001. The study reported that 5,283 nursing homes—almost one out of every three—were cited for an abuse violation during the study period.

The study also found that more than 2,500 of the abuse violations in the last 2 years were serious enough to cause actual harm to residents or to place residents in immediate jeopardy of death or serious injury. Many of the abuse violations were discovered only after the filing of a formal complaint. The percentage of nursing homes cited for abuse violations has increased every year since 1996, and the state inspection reports and citations reviewed in the investigation describe many instances of appalling physical, sexual, and verbal abuse of residents. The report concluded that abuse of nursing home residents is a widespread and significant problem.[11]

Older people have an increased risk for abuse in nursing facilities that have a history of providing inadequate care, are understaffed, and provide poor training for their employees. Some nursing home residents who are victims of abuse may not have a way to report the abuse, may not know how to report it, may not be physically able to report it, or may fear retaliation for reporting it. Others may be the victims of abuse by visiting family members. By knowing what to look for and how to report abuse or neglect, the EMS provider can positively affect the quality of life for nursing home residents, who may otherwise remain silent sufferers.

Abuse in Assisted-Living Facilities

A new type of residence is emerging for the older person: the assisted-living facility. Assisted-living facilities combine housing, personalized support services, and health care designed to meet the needs of those who need help with activities of daily living (ADLs). Definitions of assisted-living and licensing requirements vary from state to state. Residents of assisted-living facilities are generally those who need minimum or moderate assistance with some or all of the activities of daily living (ADLs). EMS providers should become aware of such facilities in their areas. Resources for locating assisted-living facilities are state departments of aging, or local area agencies on aging.

Profiles of the Abused

Elder abuse can occur anywhere and at anytime, however, profiles of those who are most at risk can be made. Abused older people tend to be:

♦ women

♦ over age 75

♦ those with one or more chronic physical or mental impairment(s) placing them in a care-dependent position

♦ those who live with their abusers

♦ socially isolated

♦ those who exhibit problematic behavior (eg, incontinence, shouting in the middle of the night)

Profiles of the Abuser

As with the abused, profiles of abusers can be drawn. Abusers tend to:

♦ live with their victim

♦ have drug or alcohol dependency problems

♦ be over age 50

♦ be dependent on the victim for financial support

♦ have poor impulse control

♦ be ill prepared or reluctant to provide care

♦ have a history of domestic violence

♦ be adult children (39%); spouse (13%); other relatives (11%); grandchildren (8%); unrelated caregiver (5%); service provider (4%); friend/neighbor (3%); sibling (3%); and other (14%).[12]

In addition to the characteristics listed above:

♦ The majority of abusers are related to their victim.

♦ More than 50% of abusers tend to commit more than one type of abuse.[13]

Assessment for Signs of Elder Abuse and Neglect

The signs and symptoms of elder abuse and neglect can be very subtle, and in the emergency setting, can often be overlooked. Evaluate each situation involving an older person with a critical eye toward potential abuse and neglect situations.

Fulmer and O'Malley identify elder abuse and neglect as "inadequate care of the elderly."[14] They say that the reason why the inadequate care occurred is irrelevant; the end result is that the older person is not receiving the care that he or she requires to maintain optimal physical or emotional health. This simple but important concept—inadequate care of the older person—is one that EMS providers should use when encountering any older patient. Adequate care is a right that must be extended to every older person. If the environment, care, and attitudes of those surrounding the older patient are anything but adequate, suspect that something may be wrong.

How does one assess for the presence of inadequate care? Fulmer and O'Malley offer the following to define inadequate care and to detect its presence:

> Inadequate care results from the presence of unmet needs for services or assistance which threatens the physical and psychological well-being of the individual. Most older persons who are receiving inadequate care present to the medical and nursing professions with manifestations that are predictable on the basis of their functional limitations and medical problems. The most common presentations involve combinations of poor hygiene, malnutrition, unmanaged medical problems, frequent falls, and confusion. The manifestations of self abuse and neglect are primarily those of neglected medical problems, poor hygiene, malnutrition, and signs of deliberate self-injury.[14]

Assessment of Risk Factors

Older people who are at risk for abuse and neglect include:

♦ Those with chronic, progressive, disabling illnesses that impair function and create care needs that exceed or will exceed their caregivers' ability to meet them, such as:

    Dementia

    Parkinson's disease

    Severe arthritis

    Severe cardiac disease

    Severe chronic obstructive pulmonary disease (COPD)

    Severe non–insulin-dependent diabetes

    Recurrent strokes

♦ Those with progressive impairments who are without support from family or neighbors, or whose caregivers show signs of burnout.

♦ Those with a personal history of substance abuse or violent behavior or a family member with a similar history.

♦ Those who live with a family in which there is a history of child or spousal abuse.

♦ Those with family members who are financially dependent on them.

♦ Those residing in institutions that have a history of providing substandard care.

♦ Those whose caregivers are under sudden increased stress due, for example, to loss of job, health, or spouse.[15]

Most EMS providers can identify the "frequent flyers" in their community—those who often use EMS. This can be helpful in identifying abuse in older patients. Suspicion should be aroused if an older patient repeatedly presents with injuries that are inconsistent with the history stated, has experienced recurring multiple injuries, or has symptoms that cannot be explained medically. When an older person is injured, you should also note any delay in accessing the EMS system, a caregiver who will not allow the patient to provide his or her own history, and frail or cognitively impaired patients who are alone. Careful questioning and a detailed assessment will help yield clues as to the presence of elder abuse or neglect.

Proper evaluation for mistreatment has four components:[16]

1. A detailed history from the patient;
2. A corroborative history from the suspected abuser;
3. A comprehensive physical examination of the patient; and
4. Confirmatory testing and documentation.

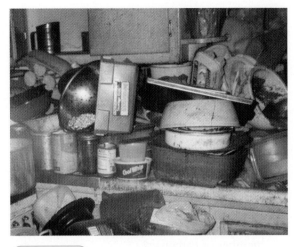

Figure 14-3   The patient's environment can provide clues to abuse or neglect.

EMS providers are able to perform all of these functions, with the exception of confirmatory testing. EMS providers also bring an advantage to the information-gathering and investigative function of elder abuse cases: they are able to gather information regarding the patient's environment that would otherwise be unknown to social service and other health care providers.

Environmental Assessment

Many of the risk factors for elder abuse—alcohol/substance abuse by the caregiver, the presence of other family violence, ineffective coping strategies of the caregiver, stress factors of the caregiver, and dependency between caregiver and victim—will be unknown to the EMS provider. Given these unknowns and the sometimes subtle nature of abuse and neglect, the assessment phase should begin with a scene size-up of the patient's environment   ▶ **Figure 14-3** . Things you should look for in the environmental assessment include:

◆ What is the physical condition of the patient's residence? Is the exterior of the home in need of repair? Is the home secure?

◆ Are hazardous conditions present? Does the home have poor wiring, rotten floors, unventilated gas heaters, broken window glass, or clutter that prevents adequate egress?

◆ Is the home too hot or too cold?

◆ Are the utilities (electricity, heat, water, toilet) working and adequate?

◆ Are there burn patterns on the floor or cabinets?

◆ Is there a fecal or urine odor in the home?

◆ Is food present in the home? Is it adequate and unspoiled?

◆ Are liquor bottles present (lying empty)?

◆ Is bedding soiled or urine soaked?

◆ If the patient has a disability, are appropriate assistive devices (such as walker or wheelchair) present?

◆ Are there restraints in the home?

◆ Does the patient have adequate access to a telephone (near the bed or other location where the patient spends time)?

◆ Are medications out of date, unmarked, or from many different doctors?

◆ Are smoke detectors present and working?

◆ If living with others, is the patient confined to one part of the home?

◆ If the patient is residing in a nursing facility, does the care appear to meet his or her needs?

Attitude Tip

Take adequate time to listen patiently to any concerns expressed by your older patients about their care (or lack of it).

Interviewing the Patient

Interviewing the older patient requires more time than interviewing younger patients (▼ **Figure 14-4**). Although patient condition and priority will determine the time that can be spent on the interview, try not to rush it. Increased age equals more history. Additionally, some aging patients tend to integrate past events with the present. That is, they may talk about previous life experiences along with events of the present. When interviewing the older patient, look for the following:

♦ Does the patient appear fearful of a family member or caregiver?

♦ Does the patient appear reluctant to respond when questioned?

♦ Does the patient appear depressed? (Symptoms of depression are discussed in Chapter 11.)

♦ Do the patient and caregiver provide conflicting accounts of the situation (history of the present illness)?

♦ Does the caregiver seem indifferent or hostile toward the patient?

♦ Does the caregiver "hover" around the patient, not allowing the EMS provider privacy with the patient?

♦ Does the caregiver seek to prevent the patient from interacting with the EMS provider?

♦ Does the caregiver seem concerned about the problem at hand, but not with the patient's overall health?

♦ Does the caregiver answer for the patient even when the patient can provide verbal history?

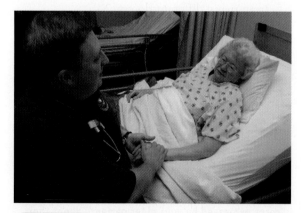

Figure 14-4 Interviewing the patient is an important part of assessment of an older patient.

♦ Does the patient look to the caregiver before answering?

♦ Does the patient sound like he or she is reciting a "script" to explain the injuries?

♦ Does the caregiver refer to the patient as accident-prone? Remember, injuries that do not fit medically or that differ from the stated history of the present illness should arouse suspicion.

The following questions may elicit a history of abuse from an older patient. If abuse or neglect is suspected, remove the patient from the potential abuser and ask the patient directly:

♦ Are you afraid of anyone at home?

♦ Has anyone ever made you do things you didn't want to do?

♦ Are you afraid of your caregiver?

♦ Have you ever been threatened or scolded by your caregiver?

♦ Has anyone ever touched you without your consent?

♦ Has anyone at home ever hurt, beaten, or struck you?

♦ Has anyone ever taken anything that was yours without asking?

♦ Have you ever signed any documents you didn't understand?

♦ Have you ever been left alone?

♦ Have you ever been restrained?

♦ Has anyone ever failed to help you take care of yourself when you needed help?

To assure your safety and that of your patient, ask these questions when you are alone with the patient. It is essential to document (in quotes) the patient's response. These are difficult questions to ask; it may be best to save these questions for the end of the interview.[17]

Dementia

Patients with **dementia** often experience delusions. However, do not be quick to dismiss abuse reports as a manifestation of the dementia. They may be true. Additionally, patients with dementia may not be able to provide details about pain or other symptoms. Abusers often rely on the fact that most people will not believe what a demented patient says. This means that EMS providers must be especially vigilant for signs of abuse in patients with dementia, who are often seen as "easy prey" and sometimes cannot report the abuse or are even unaware of it. Rely on the rest of the findings, the history of the present illness as stated, and interviews with the family or the caregiver.

Be aware that the patient's anxiety will always increase when he or she is out of a secure and familiar environment.

Interviewing Suspected Abusers

At times in suspected cases of abuse or neglect, it may be necessary to interview the patient's caregivers. Note that if a caregiver is guilty of abuse or neglect, he or she may perceive questioning as interfering or accusatory. Also note that caregiving is an extremely taxing job; a genuinely hard-working caregiver may deeply resent any intonation that he or she is neglectful or otherwise doing a bad job, so this interview must proceed in a sympathetic manner. You need to use common sense when deciding whether or not to interview a suspected abuser. Oftentimes an interview of the suspected abuser may be better left for law enforcement or APS workers. If you decide to interview the suspected abuser, remove him or her from the patient. Remember that the patient is always your first responsibility. If it is necessary to interview the suspected abuser, use the following basic principles:

♦ Avoid confrontation. Do not be accusatory, because this will put the person on the defensive and limit the amount of information that will be offered.

♦ Interview the suspected abuser alone, because this may reveal discrepancies between the patient's account and the suspected abuser's account of the situation.

♦ Focus initially on the history of the present illness, and then move to more broad questions regarding the patient's general condition. For example:

What happened to the patient today?

What is the patient's medical history?

What kind of care does the patient require?

Who provides this care?

Is there anything else I should know about the patient?

♦ If the suspected abuser is cooperative and calm during the interview, and a strong index of suspicion is present, more direct questions may be asked, such as:

Can you tell me how the patient received those bruises (or lacerations, abrasions, etc.)?

The patient appears undernourished. Can you tell me how he or she got that way?

When interviewing a suspected abuser, pay attention to the following:

♦ Does the suspected abuser offer an implausible explanation for the patient's injuries?

♦ Is the suspected abuser uncooperative or disinterested?

♦ Does the suspected abuser appear dominant and overly protective?

If the suspected abuser admits to abuse or neglect during the interview, ask him or her to specify the abusive or neglectful event(s). Record exactly (in quotes) what the abuser states. Follow this by asking the abuser if he or she would like to speak to a professional or initiate counseling. Remember that the victim is not removed permanently from his or her caregiver in all cases of documented abuse or neglect. Often, family counseling and effective coping strategies and resources will allow patient–caregiver relationships to improve. The EMS provider can positively impact these situations by showing a calm, courteous, and professional demeanor, and by knowing how and when to ask relevant questions and make appropriate referrals.

Clinical Assessment

The physical examination should be performed as with all adult patients, and in accordance with state, local, or regional protocols. Priority is given to life-threatening emergencies.

When performing a physical examination of the older patient, remember to preserve the patient's dignity. The physical examination, along with an environmental assessment and appropriate patient/caregiver interviewing, will yield important clues for the presence of elder abuse. There are, however, clinical syndromes and disease states that

CASE STUDY 2

You are dispatched to the local nursing home for a patient in respiratory distress. Before entering the patient's room, you are greeted by the nurse who states that the patient is a 68-year-old woman who has a history of a stroke, leaving the patient with aphasia and right-sided hemiparesis.

Upon entering the patient's room, you observe the patient to be slightly tachypneic and apprehensive. To examine the patient, you must move the patient's food tray, which you notice is placed on the right side of the bed, with no food consumed from the tray. You also notice a hearing aid lying on the floor next to the patient's bed. Physical examination reveals bruising to the left forearm and to the patient's neck, along with a small abrasion to the neck. The patient's nurse is unable to account for your findings.

What are the red flags in this example?

What are your responsibilities?

---

can mimic elder abuse and neglect. Some medications, for instance, cause changes in patients' clotting times and bleeding mechanisms that place some patients at risk to bruise more easily.

Context is the key in making a determination. The environmental assessment, social assessment, interaction between patient and caregiver, and the physical assessment must be weighed together.

Overall Hygiene

Look at the patient's overall hygiene and consider the following: Is the patient's clothing clean and appropriate? Is the patient dressed appropriately for the season? Are there cigarette burns on clothing? Are undergarments torn, soiled, or bloody? Does the patient have poor hygiene? Is there evidence of recent weight loss (this information may have to be obtained by asking the patient or caregiver) or malnutrition? Does the patient lack assistive devices (glasses, hearing aid, dentures, walker, wheelchair) when it is obvious that the patient requires them?

Head and Neck

When assessing a patient with a head injury ascribed to a fall, observe for other associated injuries from the fall (such as to the extremities or

trunk). A head injury ascribed to a fall with no other associated injuries may have come from an assault. Assess for the presence of facial bruises, lacerations, or abrasions; tooth fractures; ill-fitting dentures (secondary in some cases to weight loss); mandibular and maxillary fractures; poor dental hygiene; oral venereal lesions; bruising in the mouth (indicating possible forced oral copulation); and cigarette burns on the lips (this may signal either a neglect situation or a functional decline of the patient).

Assessment of the eyes may reveal trauma (recent or chronic). Findings indicative of recent trauma include subconjunctival or vitreous hemorrhage. Because a detailed ophthalmologic examination in the prehospital setting is impractical, examination of the eyes and periorbital area should be limited to pupillary assessment (pupil size and reactivity, and extraocular movements if you are trained in their assessment) and observing for signs of orbital fractures or the presence of subconjunctival bleeding.

When examining the nasal area, observe for signs of a deviated septum (a sign of repeated trauma). When examining the anterior/posterior neck, be observant for signs of circumscribed nuchal rope burns or handprints (indicative of recent strangulation attempts or bondage). If strangulation is suspected, patency of the trachea and an adequate airway must be confirmed. Bruising of the tracheal rings can result in gradual swelling that can lead to hypoxia and death. With any history of strangulation, apply oxygen by mask or nasal cannula unless contraindicated by other medical conditions. If pulse oximetry is available, it should be used when caring for victims of strangulation. Excessive shaking may lead to whiplash injuries or dislocation of cervical vertebrae, which may cause paralysis or death. In older patients with severe osteoporosis, cervical fractures or spinal cord injuries may result. If the mechanism of injury or the history of the present illness is suggestive of either, immediate cervical/spinal immobilization should occur.

Skin

Bilateral bruising on soft parts of the body (such as the inner arm or thigh) should be thought of as suspicious, as well as bruising that is clustered. The shape of skin lesions may suggest a patterned mechanism of injury, such as a belt buckle or cigarette burn. The presence of multiple bruises in various stages of healing strongly suggests abuse (▶ **Figure 14-5A and B**).

The presence of pressure ulcers and how they are cared for may be a clue of neglect. (Pressure ulcers are discussed in Chapter 12.)

Urine burns may suggest that a patient has been allowed to remain unchanged for long periods of time. Additionally, **excoriations** or chafing may also suggest poor attention to continence. **Infestations** may also be present. Assess skin turgor for signs of dehydration. Other integumentary findings relevant to elder abuse include traumatic **alopecia** (traumatic hair loss, as opposed to hair loss suggestive of normal aging); ecchymosis; burns; lacerations (▶ **Figure 14-5C**); skin disorders such as rash, impetigo, and eczema; and undiagnosed and untreated fractures. Stocking or glove injuries may suggest an immersion burn (▶ **Figure 14-6**).

Thorax and Abdomen

Blunt trauma to the thorax and abdomen may result in rib fractures and a pneumothorax or hemothorax. Serious abdominal trauma can lead to such life-threatening conditions as splenic rupture and intra-abdominal hemorrhage. Bruising

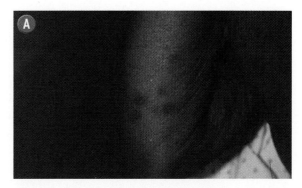
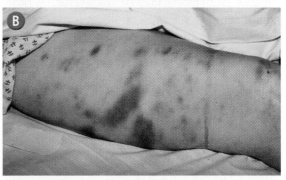
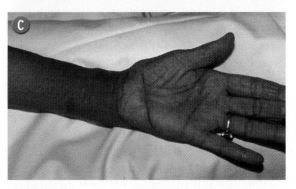

Figure 14-5   Patterned, fingertip-like contusions suggest the use of excessive force. **(A).** Bruises from being grabbed by husband from elder domestic violence. **(B).** Bruises to right lateral thigh from older brother caregiver and circular imprinting from anti-emboli stockings. **(C).** Knife wounds can also suggest abuse; this wound was inflicted by husband during elder domestic violence.

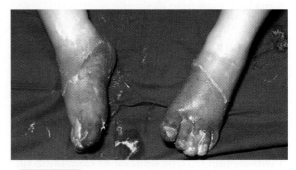

Figure 14-6   A stocking or glove injury can suggest an immersion burn.

of the abdominal flanks (<u>Grey Turner's sign</u>) and around the umbilicus (<u>Cullen's sign</u>) are suggestive of extravasation of intra-abdominal hemolyzed blood to the flank and periumbilical region, respectively. These forms of ecchymosis may not be immediately apparent.

It is important to keep in mind that EMS providers may be called for reasons unrelated to a possible finding of abuse. For example, when treating a patient for chest pain, Grey Turner's or Cullen's ecchymosis may be discovered. A thorough history of the present illness (or stated history) provides important clues when these physical signs are discovered.

Musculoskeletal System

The presence of abrasions around the wrist or ankles may indicate the use of restraints. Differentiating lower extremity abrasions, erosions, and ulcerations from burns, scratches, lacerations, statis dermatosis, and plantar ulcerations is difficult for the EMS provider. Making the emergency department staff aware of findings that may look "unusual" will suffice; it is then the responsibility of the emergency department staff to investigate further. For example, the EMS provider may note the presence of hand swelling. Whether this swelling is related to vitamin C deficiency or to trauma will need to be determined in the emergency department. The emergency department staff may be able to access additional information through the patient's medical records or private provider. It cannot be overemphasized that the scene size-up and detailed history of the present illness—weighed against physical findings—are extremely important. EMS providers lend valuable clues to emergency department staff regarding the environment of the patient and statements from those present at the scene.

Neurological System

A neurological examination in the older patient may prove difficult due to pre-existing neurological conditions. The patient's level of orientation upon presenting to EMS should be weighed against the patient's normal level of orientation. However, this may be difficult to determine unless someone well known to the patient can provide information regarding subtle cognitive changes. Focal neurological signs and symptoms may be the result of spinal cord injury or head trauma with development of concussion or subdural/epidural hematoma. Note the patient's orientation to person, place, and time and his or her recollection of the history of the present illness.

Assess the patient's ability to move all extremities, as well as grip strength in each extremity. Weigh these findings relative to the patient's overall presentation, medical history, and the reason for the call. Document findings appropriately and report any discrepancies to the emergency department staff. More appropriate mental status examinations and neurological testing can be performed at the hospital.

Genitourinary System

One must always consider sexual abuse or cancer when an older patient has vaginal or rectal bleeding. Injuries to these areas should be treated accordingly. If sexual abuse is suspected, the preservation of evidence is extremely important. Medical control should be notified and local protocols followed regarding evidence protection and patient transport.

Social Assessment

A social assessment from a patient or caregiver is usually not solicited by the EMS provider. However, when considering cases of elder abuse and neglect, a social assessment will prove valuable when taken in context with other information. Some of the most important social assessment indicators are ADLs. Patients who are unable to perform these activities usually require a caregiver. If, during your assessment, you find that a patient is unable to perform one or several of these functions, ask the following:

◆ Are these activities being provided for the patient? If so, by whom?

◆ Are there any delays in obtaining food, medication, or toileting? The patient may complain of this, or the environment may be suggestive; there may not be food in the home.

◆ In an institutional setting, is the patient able to feed himself or herself? If not, is food still sitting in the food tray? Has the patient been lying in his or her own urine or feces for long periods of time?

Emotional suffering is one of the most important clues pointing to psychological abuse, but it is also very difficult for EMS providers to assess. Examples of psychological abuse include harassment, intimidation, manipulation, belittling, and isolation. Patient responses and the observed interaction between patient and caregiver may yield clues to the presence of abuse or neglect.

Undermedication of a patient could be a sign that a caregiver is stealing or not providing the medication. Overmedication can also be a sign of abuse. Patients are sometimes sedated for the caregiver's comfort.

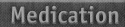

Medication Tip

Both undermedication and overmedication of a patient can be signs of elder abuse.

Lab Tests

More definitive testing, such as lab tests, for elder abuse can be conducted in the emergency department. Useful lab tests for confirming or excluding physical abuse include hematuria, myoglobinuria, elevated serum creatine phosphokinase, lactate dehydrogenase, erythrocyte sedimentation rates, microscopic hair analysis, coagulation times, bone scans, x-rays, and CT or MRI scans.

Putting It All Together

Observe the interaction between the patient and the caregiver. Does the caregiver dominate the situation or show a marked lack of concern? Does the caregiver blame the patient for his or her condition? Assess the caregiver for the presence of drug or alcohol intoxication. If the caregiver is absent, does the patient present as someone who should be left alone? Does the older person speak of the caregiver in a negative way? Assess the patient's affect and nonverbal behavior. Is the patient fearful or overly quiet?

Abuse should be suspected whenever the patient presents with multiple injuries in various stages of healing. Neglect should be suspected whenever a dependent patient (who has adequate resources and a caregiver) presents with deficiencies in hygiene, nutrition, and medical needs. If one type of abuse is present, look for other types. Frequently an older person is the victim of more than one type of abuse or neglect. Are there previous reports of similar injuries? Does the patient express fear of an intervention? After you have made your assessment and conducted patient and caregiver interviews, if your intuition tells you that all is not well between the patient and the caregiver, it probably isn't.

Evidence of abuse can be determined, in part, by the physical examination. Evidence of neglect can be determined, in part, by the failure of the caregiver to:

♦ Assist with personal hygiene, or with the provision of food, clothing, or shelter;

♦ Provide medical care for physical and mental health needs;

♦ Protect from health and safety hazards; or

♦ Prevent malnutrition.

Psychological abuse indicators (in the patient) include the following:

♦ Ambivalence

♦ Deference

♦ Passivity

♦ Fear of the caregiver or the EMS provider

♦ Fearfulness expressed in the eyes (However, in some cultures it is considered rude to look a person directly in the eye, so be careful not to confuse deference with fear.)

♦ Withdrawal

♦ Helplessness

♦ Resignation

♦ Depression

♦ Hopelessness

Intervention Decisions

EMS providers face a wide variety of situations, each of which must be evaluated on its own merits.

CASE STUDY 3

You are dispatched to the home of a 74-year-old patient. Upon arrival, you are greeted on the front lawn by the patient's son. The son states that the patient is out of control because of her dementia and has become violent. The son continues to state that he had to throw the patient to the ground to keep her under control, and would like the patient taken directly to a psychiatric facility. The son further informs you that he has the patient's full power of attorney.

You respectfully request that the son wait outside as you enter the patient's home. Once inside, you encounter the patient seated in a chair. The patient appears calm, but tearful. She is alert, oriented, and conversive, and states no complaints. The patient does inform you that her son is trying to take her finances and her home, and earlier threw her to the ground, and she fears for her safety.

Your observations reveal that the patient appears well nourished with appropriate hygiene. The home is well kept. You observe large plastic ties lying on the table. The patient states that the son threatened to tie the patient up if she did not calm herself.

What are your immediate priorities?

What concerns do you have?

However, some basic guidelines can help the EMS provider decide when it is necessary to intervene.

When immediate, life-threatening problems exist as the result of an abuse or neglect situation, EMS providers must immediately address the health crisis. Further follow up can be conducted after the patient is stabilized in the emergency department. The emergency department physician should be made aware of the circumstances of the abuse or neglect situation.

If the patient's condition is stable but he or she is in a physically unsafe environment due to lack of heat, water, or food, or the caregiver's actions, see if the older patient will accept transportation to the emergency department. If not, determine whether he or she is receptive to assistance from local APS. If the patient is receptive to assistance, notify the appropriate agency. If a caregiver seems to be the problem, notify APS or law enforcement, according to your local protocols. Remain with the patient only if it is safe to do so.

Some patients choose to remain in an abusive or neglectful situation despite offers of assistance.

If the patient is competent, often little can be done, since a competent adult's rights must be honored. Document the circumstances of these cases, and notify APS. In many states you are mandated to report suspected cases of elder abuse, and APS may be able to develop a relationship with the older person so that he or she

Controversy

Some patients choose to remain in an abusive or neglectful situation, despite an offer of assistance. If the patient is competent, often little can be done, since their rights must be honored. Document the refusal of care. If a pattern emerges of a history of refusing care, your document could help give social services evidence to open an investigation. You may not be able to help today, but documenting the patient's refusal could lead to help later.

eventually chooses to accept services. Initiate a case file so there is a record if additional EMS requests are made on behalf of the patient.

Assessing for elder abuse and neglect can be difficult and challenging. EMS is seldom called to the scene for elder abuse. Instead, abusive and neglectful situations are discovered during the patient encounter. The EMS provider is part of a multidisciplinary system in elder abuse cases. Others on the multidisciplinary team may include law enforcement, APS, physicians, nursing staff, advanced practice nurses, physician assistants, social service workers, ombudsmen, state regulatory agencies (if the abuse occurred in a nursing facility), and members of the criminal justice system. The burden of proof does not reside with the EMS provider. Awareness is key in the discovery of elder abuse and neglect. Documentation and reporting your objective findings can have significant impact on elder abuse cases. Carefully document the patient's environment and condition on your arrival. This evidence is valuable to investigators.

Many resources are available to assist the EMS provider with questions regarding specific elder abuse cases. These resources include APS, law enforcement (many police departments also have an elder crimes unit), long-term care ombudsmen, state elder abuse hotlines, state licensing agencies (for nursing home issues), area agencies on aging, and local/state departments of aging. EMS providers should become familiar with the resources their local/state agencies can provide, and have their numbers readily accessible. The National Center on Elder Abuse is an excellent resource for elder abuse information.

Documentation

Documentation is crucial when elder abuse is suspected. Detailed descriptions of the secondary findings and injuries (size, color, shape, and location) must be included. A sketch sheet is very useful. The patient care report may become evidence in a court of law. Specifically, you should document the following:

- Why EMS was called to the scene
- Chief complaint, if different from how the call was received

- Complete past medical history
- Social history/assessment findings
- Environmental assessment
- Patient's current prescribed medications, and whether these medications are being taken by the patient. This will be important later in determining whether therapeutic levels are present.
- Allergies
- Physical assessment
- Any statements made by the patient or caregiver. These statements must be written in quotes. If you ask specific questions about elder abuse, document the question that was asked as well as the response.
- Assessment of the interaction between the patient and the caregiver
- Interventions provided
- If the police were called to the location, document the responding officer's name and agency.
- Name of the physician or health care provider assuming care of the patient

Because most APS workers are not health care professionals, a well-documented assessment by the EMS provider will prepare the APS worker and aid in the diagnosis.

> **Attitude Tip**
>
> Be compassionate and sensitive to the needs of your older patients and provide them with emotional support and appropriate reassurance that you will help!

Recommendations

EMS systems should have written protocols in place that address assessment, treatment, and referral of elder abuse and neglect. The development of such protocols should be a collaborative effort involving EMS, law enforcement, APS, local/state departments of aging, the state attorney general's office, and members of the physician community. Protocols must reflect local, regional, and state laws and policies regarding reporting of elder abuse cases. Elder abuse awareness programs should be incorporated into initial EMS certification and continuing education programs. These training efforts should involve APS and social service workers to help open lines of communication and help make the identification and referral process more effective. Feedback should be given to EMS providers on cases that are reported. Good communication needs to take place among EMS, law enforcement, social service agencies, and APS workers regarding elder abuse cases.

Summary

Elder abuse and neglect are prevalent, and with the growth of the older population, the number of older people experiencing abuse and neglect is likely to increase. You, as an EMS provider, are in the unique position to detect it. Be sure to keep the signs of elder abuse and neglect in mind as you observe the patient, the caregiver, and the environment. Take precautions when interviewing potential abuse victims and abusers. Last, be sure to document any suspected abuse or neglect. The actions you take can help end an abuse or neglect situation.

Chapter Resources

Case Study Summaries

CASE STUDY 1 SUMMARY

Given that the patient has had multiple falls, your first priority is to assess for injuries. This patient also suffers from dementia and appears malnourished. It will be difficult to determine if the patient's level of orientation is a result of the progression of her dementia or malnutrition. Since you also note that the patient has poor hygiene, an index of suspicion should be raised that the patient may not be cared for properly. Remember, older patients in general have de-creased appetites. When caring for persons with dementia, meals must be provided regularly to them. Persons with dementia may lack the capacity to prepare their own meals. Given this patient's presentation, transportation to the emergency department is warranted. Inform the emergency department staff of your observations and suspicions. It may also be prudent to notify your local Adult Protective Services agency.

CASE STUDY 2 SUMMARY

Your first priority in this case is to treat the respiratory difficulty. Several red flags should appear from your observations. The patient's apprehensiveness should be the first red flag. The obvious unexplained bruising to the arm and neck, and the abrasion, should be the next flag. Do these bruises have a particular shape, such as finger marks? Other flags include the fact that although the patient has right-sided paralysis, the food tray is placed on the right side of the bed, with no food consumed. You also note a hearing aid on the floor by the patient's bed. Does this patient use assistive devices, such as a hearing aid? You will need to inquire further about this. If the patient is in any respiratory distress, transportation to the emergency department is indicated. If not, consider transportation anyway, for patient safety reasons. You will be unable to solicit a verbal history from the patient, given a history of aphasia; therefore, scene clues and the physical examination are paramount. Your concerns should be documented and relayed to the emergency department staff. Consider referring your findings to your state nursing home regulatory agency.

CASE STUDY 3 SUMMARY

This is a case that will present difficulty to the EMS provider. There is no physical injury to the patient and no strict medical condition that warrants immediate transport to the emergency department. However, many red flags are present, and should arouse a high index of suspicion that all is not well between patient and son. The first red flag is that the son stated he threw the patient to the ground, which was also confirmed by the patient. Furthermore, the patient stated that she fears for her safety. The patient also stated that her son threatened to tie her up (psychological abuse). In this case, transportation to the emergency department is warranted for safety reasons. You are removing the patient from a potentially threatening environment.

Once in the emergency department, the hospital may be able to initiate safety measures for the patient. You should also refer this case to APS.

Endnotes

1. National Center on Elder Abuse. *Elder Abuse Informational Series,* Number 1. Washington, DC: November 1997.

2. National Center on Elder Abuse. *National Elder Abuse Incidence Study.* Washington, DC: 1996.

3. House Select Committee on Aging. Washington, DC: 1990.

4. National Center on Elder Abuse. Washington, DC.

5. National Center on Elder Abuse. *Elder Abuse Informational Series,* Number 1. Washington, DC: November 1997.

6. Maryland Department of Aging. "Abuse is Wrong at Any Age" training program, 1998.

7. Fulmer TM, O'Malley TA. *Inadequate Care of the Elderly: A Health Care Perspective on Abuse and Neglect.* New York: Springer; 1987: 18.

8. National Center on Elder Abuse. *Elder Abuse Information Series;* Number 1. Washington, DC: November 1997.

9. Lachs MS, Fulmer T. Recognizing elder abuse and neglect. *Clinics in Geriatric Medicine.* 1993; 9(3):665–675.

10. Pillemer and Moore, 1989.

11. Abuse is a Major Problem in US Nursing Homes. U.S. House of Representatives. July 2001.

12. National Center on Elder Abuse. Washington, DC.

13. National Center on Elder Abuse. Washington, DC.

14. Fulmer TM, O'Malley TA. *Inadequate Care of the Elderly: A Health Care Perspective on Abuse and Neglect.* New York: Springer; 1987.

15. Fulmer TM; O'Malley TA. *Inadequate Care of the Elderly: A Health Care Perspective on Abuse and Neglect.* New York: Springer; 1987:29–30.

16. Anetzberger GJ, Lachs MS, O'Brien JG, O'Brien S, Pillemer KA, Tomita SK. Elder mistreatment: A call for help. *Patient Care,* June 15, 1993.

17. Modified from: American Medical Association. *Diagnostic and Treatment Guidelines on Elder Abuse and Neglect.* Chicago: Author, 1992:9; and Gallo JJ, Reichel W, Anderson LM. *Handbook of Geriatric Assessment.* Gaithersburg, MD: Aspen, 1995:114.

Bibliography

American Medical Association. *Diagnostic and Treatment Guidelines on Elder Abuse and Neglect.* Chicago: Author; 1992.

Baumhover LA, Beal SC. *Abuse, Neglect, and Exploitation of Older Persons.* Baltimore: Health Professions Press; 1996.

Capezuti E, Brush B, Lawson WT. Reporting elder mistreatment. *Journal of Gerontological Nursing.* July 1997:24–32.

Conlin MM. Silent suffering: a case study of elder abuse and neglect. *Journal of the American Geriatrics Society.* 1995;43(11):1303–1308.

Costa AJ. Elder abuse. *Primary Care.* 1993;20(2): 375–389.

Gallo JJ, Reichel W, Anderson LM. *Handbook of Geriatric Assessment.* Gaithersburg, MD: Aspen; 1995.

Janing J. Reflections on aging: communicating with elderly patients. *Journal of Emergency Medical Services.* June 1991:34–44.

Jones JS, Walker G, Krohmer JR. To report or not to report: emergency services response to elder abuse. *Prehospital and Disaster Medicine.* 1995;10(2): 96–100.

Lachs MS, Pillemer K. Abuse and neglect of elderly persons. *New England Journal of Medicine.* 1995; 332(7): 437–443.

Marshall CE, Benton D, Brazier JM. Elder abuse: using clinical tools to identify clues of mistreatment. *Geriatrics.* 2000;55(2):42–53.

Missouri Department of Social Services, Division of Aging. *Indicators of Abuse, Neglect, and Exploitation of the Elderly.* Summer 1981.

National Center for Victims of Crime. Excerpts from *Focus on the Future: A Systems Approach to Prosecution and Victim Assistance, A Training and Resource Manual*. Grant Number 92-MU-MU-K003. U.S. Department of Justice, Office for Victims of Crime.

Paris BE, Meier DE, Goldstein T, Weiss M, Fein, ED. Elder abuse and neglect: how to recognize warning signs and intervene. *Geriatrics*. 1995;50(4):47–51.

Police Executive Research Forum. *Improving the Police Response to Domestic Elder Abuse*. Washington, DC: Author; 1993.

Pritchard J, ed. *Elder Abuse Work: Best Practices in Britain and Canada*. Philadelphia: Jessica Kingsley Publishers; 1999.

US Code of Federal Regulations. *The Nursing Home Reform Amendments of OBRA*. 1987.

Improving Quality of Life

LEARNING OBJECTIVES

1 Discuss the responsibilities of EMS to improve the quality of life of older patients.

2 Discuss the importance of the social aspect of an older patient's life in determining his or her quality of life.

3 Describe how home safety affects quality of life.

4 Discuss the importance of compassion when working with older patients.

5 Discuss community strategies for change.

CHAPTER 15

David L. Seabrook, MPA, EMT-P

Sue Fryer Ward, MSW, LCSW, BCD

CASE STUDY 1

You are dispatched to the home of an 84-year-old woman who fell in the kitchen and injured her shoulder and upper arm. There is deformity and increased pain with any movement. This fall happened while she was preparing breakfast, and there are two cats who seem quite interested in the milk and eggs that have spilled on the floor. Your patient is dressed only in a short nightgown and slippers and the room is cool.

She has significant pain in her shoulder and obviously needs to be treated and transported, but she is reluctant and gives multiple reasons why this would be inconvenient. She asks that you call her son at work and have him come to help her. The vital signs are within normal limits and the patient is alert and oriented. ALS providers are on scene and preparing to move the patient from the floor.

> **What are some reasons why this person may be reluctant to consent to transport?**
>
> **What can you do to alleviate the patient's concerns?**
>
> **What are some considerations in management, treatment, and transport of this patient?**

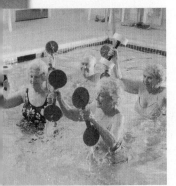

Introduction

You should remember that an older patient is first and foremost a person. This is an obvious statement, but as an EMS provider caring for older patients, you will do well to remember that your patients are whole persons, and more than a health care problem. As with most adults, older people lead lives that focus more on social, economic, or spiritual matters than on the state of their health (▼ **Figure 15-1**). EMS providers can greatly assist their patients by paying attention to matters that are not usually viewed as health care issues, but that are nevertheless important to patients.

> ### Attitude Tip
>
> By improving your attitudes and the attitudes of other EMS and health care providers toward the older population, you will positively affect the quality of life enjoyed by the older patients in your community.

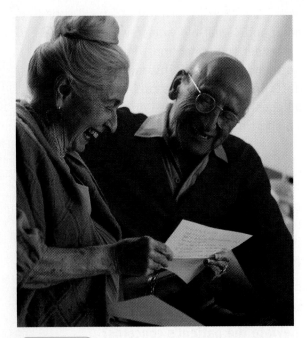

Figure 15-1   Most older people lead lives that focus more on social, economic, or spiritual matters than on the state of their health.

Elements of Quality of Life

The World Health Organization (WHO) defines health as "not merely the absence of disease or infirmity, but a state of complete physical, mental, and social well-being." Another concept used by researchers is "health-related quality of life." This concept narrows down the WHO definition and focuses on how the patient feels about his or her own health and level of functioning, and as such, is highly individualized. EMS providers can view **quality of life** as having four interrelated factors: physical and emotional health, social connections, economic security, and safety. Thus, an agenda focusing on improving quality of life is one that aims to add life to years, rather than just years of life alone. This is particularly important to the older population we serve.

Quality of life for older people includes living with as much choice, independence, and dignity as possible. EMS providers can assist with improving or maintaining that quality by consistently showing respect for the patient, letting the patient know what emergency care is being provided and why, talking with the patient rather than over or around them, addressing them using Mr. or Ms. and their last name, or "sir" or "ma'am," and not taking the patient for granted. If the patient seems unconscious, direct communication is still essential, because he or she may be able to perceive that something is happening. For example, "Mr. Smith, I'm going to take your blood pressure now." Or, in working with a colleague, you can say, "Joe is going to take your blood pressure now, Ma'am."

> ### Communication Tip
>
> If the patient seems unconscious, direct communication is still essential, because he or she may be able to perceive that something is happening.

Even when speed is necessary, talking people through the procedure adds no extra time and provides reassurance to the person being examined or transported. Refer to Chapter 3 for more comprehensive information about communicating with older patients.

Health

The overall health of older people includes physical, mental, social, and spiritual well-being. Ask what health problems they have, and particularly which ones are most bothersome to them or interfere with their functioning and happiness. By soliciting the patient's interpretation of which health problems most affect their quality of life, the EMS provider and other health care providers can prioritize their treatments to be consistent with the patient's goals of care. The EMS provider can ask the following questions to determine whether the patient feels if he or she is being given adequate medical care: "Do you have a doctor?" Or, "Do you feel you have the right amount of medical attention currently?" Negative answers to these questions may provide an opportunity for the EMS provider to improve health-related quality of life by making appropriate referrals.

Asking these questions respectfully will also communicate an interest in the patient and help establish a relationship. In addition, you should begin assembling the personal items, such as glasses, dentures, and walking aids, that should go with the person if transportation is indicated.

In communicating with the patient, the EMS provider may develop a good sense of an older person's mental health and self-confidence (▼ Figure 15-2). If the individual is aware of his or her surroundings, recognizes you as an EMS provider, and cooperates in the history and the care, you may presume that the person is mentally healthy and self-confident. If the person has slow responses, intense sadness, or seems belligerent with no apparent reason, one may be concerned that quality of life is problematic.

Nutrition and Hydration

Adequate nutrition is imperative for older individuals, because undernutrition and dehydration can cause both physical illnesses and mental aberrations. Poor nutritional intake among the older population may be fairly common, regardless of income. In a quick assessment of the person's living situation, especially if he or she lives alone, glance into the refrigerator and freezer, and into cupboards to see if food is available. If you suspect that the person is not eating well or is not drinking enough fluids, ask what they had for breakfast/lunch/dinner, depending on the time of day. Of course, poverty may be a factor in poor eating habits, as well as difficulty getting to the store, preparing meals, or poor dental care.

Social Connections

Isolation and loneliness have an adverse impact on quality of life for many older people. Connections with social groups are important factors for you to look for (▼ Figure 15-3). If transport is indicated, the family/friend/neighbor network can be of major assistance to the person and to the EMS provider. If there is no one with the person when you arrive, ask a series of questions, starting with

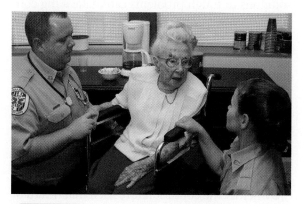

Figure 15-2   In communicating with the patient, the EMS provider may develop a good sense of an older person's mental health and self-confidence.

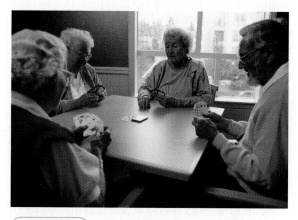

Figure 15-3   Connections with social groups are important factors for you to look for.

the immediate and then looking at a broader social system. Your purpose is to find people who can be relied on by the individual and who should be called for help, as well as to determine if the person is socially isolated. Ask questions such as:

♦ Does someone live here at the house with you? (If yes) Who is it?

♦ Do you have family nearby?

♦ Is there someone you would like me to call?

♦ Does someone come in to help you?

♦ Do you have friends you can call on if you need help?

The person's responses to your questions about community will also tell you a great deal about the relationships. Warm responses indicate warm relationships. Angry responses like "I have a daughter who never comes to see me" may indicate difficulties with family or personality difficulties with the individual.

If the person will be transported to a hospital, it is important to know if someone can be there with the person and, if necessary, provide transportation home if admission is not planned. Get names and phone numbers, either for you to call or to give to the hospital for followup. If the answers provided suggest social isolation, referral to appropriate social services is indicated. Referral resources are discussed later in this chapter.

Other questions that may help determine if the patient is socially isolated are, "How do you spend your time? Do you go to church, synagogue, or other religious meetings?" If the person says he or she used to but cannot go anymore, ask if anyone from the religious group visits and how often. "What do you do for fun? What hobbies do you have? Do you do any volunteer work? Do you belong to any clubs?" Based on the answers to these questions, various other referrals could be suggested to the patient to enhance their quality of life. For instance, an isolated person who says they enjoy playing cards might derive a significant benefit from joining a local senior center.

Economic Security

Economic security is also an element in quality of life. Older people in poverty are predominantly older women, women living alone, and minority women. You can get a sense of how the person is faring economically by quick observation. Does the person's house appear to be in good—or adequate—repair? Is the fence sagging? Is the house badly in need of painting? Do the lights work? Does the phone work? Do the appliances appear dangerous (frayed cords, broken oven or refrigerator door)? Is the house warm (or cool in the summer)? Is there adequate food in the house? Is the smoke detector working?

Questioning the person about these matters requires delicacy. You may encounter defensiveness or resistance about any information that seems related to finances. Neutral questions such as, "Do you like living here? If you had your choice, where would you like to live?" may be more successful. Many people are not aware that economic assistance and other resources are available to help people maintain independence in their homes. The Area Agencies on Aging, discussed later in this chapter, can help older persons find solutions to economic problems.

Quality of the Patient's Environment

When EMS providers respond to a patient's home, they sometimes find more problems than they were specifically called for. The EMS provider may recognize problems in the patient's environment that could contribute to health-related problems. Many EMS providers feel they have inadequate training to deal with such issues. However, EMS providers may be the only members of the community with insight into the patient's living conditions. EMS providers who help patients find solutions to tough problems can make a big contribution toward improving the quality of life for the patient. This section reviews assessment of the patient's environment, and suggests resources that may be available to help EMS providers assist their patients.

It should first be acknowledged that some home environments occur as the result of choice. Different people have different standards with respect to housekeeping and personal hygiene. The key issues that the EMS provider must consider are whether the conditions are such that health or safety is jeopardized. With regard to safety, the EMS provider must recognize that different people have different tolerance of risk. The EMS provider should avoid a strict "better safe than sorry" approach, and should avoid being overly judgmental. EMS providers may assume that the wishes of most people will be to maintain independence in their own homes as long as possible. EMS providers are encouraged to confirm this assumption through dialogue with the patient and the patient's family. The assessment of the patient's environment is done to support the patient's quality-of-life choices.

Environmental assessment may be the only clear indicator of an abuse or neglect situation (▼ **Figure 15-4**). Less obvious but also problematic are the situations that represent self-neglect. Problems of abuse and self-neglect are covered in Chapter 14. EMS providers should also note situations that represent potential health and safety problems. For example, EMS providers may notice an absence of food in the home, moldy remnants of old meals, and stacks of unwashed dishes. There may be improper waste disposal, the presence of vermin, or copious amounts of pet urine and feces. There may be inadequate toilet facilities, or mismanagement of incontinence. Such conditions may be a result of inadequate education, sloppy habits, or a psychiatric-behavioral disorder. The problem may also be due to a functional decline that prevents the patient from doing the things they would normally do.

In cases where the problem results from a psychiatric disorder, such as compulsive/obsessive "hoarding" syndrome, a referral to the mental health system is indicated. When there is doubt

> **Attitude Tip**
>
> In addition to participating in injury prevention, home safety evaluation, and medical information access programs in your community, you should support programs that promote EMS drop-in visits (between calls) to older patients living alone, at risk for health declines, or who are frequent consumers of EMS in your area.

whether the patient is mentally or legally competent, a referral to an appropriate agency should be made as well.

If the basis of the problem is functional disability, it may be that assisting the patient to access home care, chore services, or home-delivered meals will provide the stability needed to maintain the preferred living situation. A great variety of state-sponsored and local volunteer services are available to assist older persons who want to stay in their own homes but need a little help to do so. Appendix A: Organizations and Services for Older People lists some of these services.

A growing number of EMS systems are adopting innovative programs to connect older persons with other health care and social service agencies that help older people maintain independence and dignity. (▶ **Table 15-1**) describes three programs.

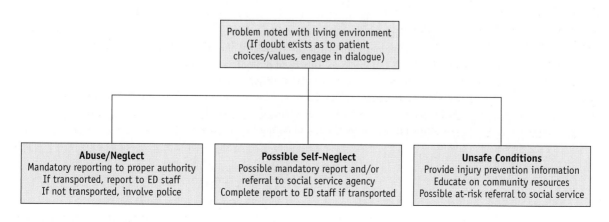

Figure 15-4   GEMS Living Environment Assessment.

TABLE 15-1   Innovative Integration Between Fire/EMS and Social Service Agencies

Examples of Innovative Programs to Assist Elder Persons

Agency and Name of Program	Program Description	Contact for Further Information
"Older Persons Are Important" Program Vancouver Fire Department (VFD) (Washington)	Specialized training program about geriatric emergencies as well as practical exercises that attempt to influence attitudes toward older persons. An enhanced relationship with Washington Department of Social & Health Service's Home & Community Services. This agency serves as a "one-stop" referral source. An at-risk referral form may be completed on-scene with a copy accompanying the patient to the ED. Fire Department personnel participate in monthly interorganizational meetings to brainstorm solutions to problem cases. Firefighters can provide on-scene injury prevention and public education, assisted by the "Firefighters Safety Guide for Senior Citizens."	Vancouver Fire Dept. Capt. Dave Seabrook 7110 N.E. 63rd St. Vancouver, WA 98661 360-892-4323 dave.seabrook@ vancouver.ci.wa.us www.vanfire.org
"Carpe Diem" (Seize the Day) Acadian Ambulance (Louisiana)	This six-hour program focuses the attention of participants on the emotional and physical needs of the older patient. In an effort to provide the highest quality of care possible, EMS providers are taught to understand the importance of their interaction with these patients and the significance of things that are often overlooked. Emotionally powerful case studies, role-playing exercises, and direct experience are used to give participants a better appreciation of the challenges that many older persons confront. EMS providers and paramedics alike are also strongly reminded of the need to make every effort to maintain the dignity, pride, and respect that these patients deserve.	Acadian Ambulance & Air Med Services Dee Dee Sewell, Employee Relations Representative P.O. Box 98000 Lafayette, LA 70509 337-291-1507 dsewell@acadian.com www.acadian.com
REACH program—Reaching Elders with Additional needs through Community Help Harwich Fire Department/Cape and Islands EMS System (Massachusetts)	This program informs EMS providers about the changes in our health care system and in the social fabric that place seniors at greater risk. Fire/EMS providers are increasingly responding to "public assistance" requests that are not medical emergencies but are nevertheless needed services. The REACH program attempts to build a network from involved agencies. The direct involvement of the Fire/EMS providers is a key component of the network because they are so trusted by the community. On-scene Fire/EMS responders can complete an at-risk referral form or may request a response from volunteers with the Harwich Council on Aging to assist with tough cases. This then prompts an assessment from the Visiting Nurse Association. Other important members of the network include Elder Services of Cape Cod, the Alzheimer's Association of Cape Cod and the Islands, and Hospice Palliative Care of Cape Cod, and Cape Cod Health Care.	Harwich Fire Dept. Capt. William Flynn 175 Sisson Road Harwich, MA 02646 508-430-7546 wflynn.fd@verizon.net

Where unsafe conditions exist because of behavioral choice, it may be that education by the EMS provider will promote change. Appendix C: Home Safety Checklist can be used to assist you in evaluating an older person's home. The EMS provider can help the patient to see the probable consequences of risky choices, and suggest that a modification of the living environment is needed to help maintain independence. When injury prevention education is delivered at the time and place of a recent injury, it is said to be a "teachable moment."

Attitude Tip

As an advocate for your older patients, in addition to providing care for any immediate problem or need, remember that providing resource referral for the patient or their family is a valuable support service with which you can assist.

CASE STUDY 2

A direct call to your station by a concerned citizen prompts a visit to the home of an 84-year-old man. The concerned neighbor meets you outside a small home in a poor neighborhood. He tells you that he has noticed a decline in his neighbor's ability to take care of himself. Of primary importance to the neighbor is the presence of a dead dog inside the home for several days.

You knock on the door and a disheveled older man greets you politely. You are also greeted by an extremely offensive odor. You explain that there is concern for his well-being and ask for permission to enter. With permission, you enter to do a basic home safety check.

Inside the home you note multiple piles of old newspapers and magazines. Multiple dirty dishes with half-eaten and moldy food are stacked on top of horizontal surfaces. The sofas and chairs have yellowish stains indicating possible incontinence. There are several piles of dog feces on the kitchen floor. In the bathroom, you discover a large stack of soiled adult diapers in the bathtub, and the toilet and sink are equally soiled. In the kitchen you find very little food and more evidence of unhealthy conditions.

Not really knowing where to start, you ask him about his dog and he explains that he has in fact moved the dog's body to the back yard. You tell the client that it appears he could use some help around the house and he agrees, saying that since his wife died things have gone downhill. You perform a basic medical assessment. Past and recent medical history is denied, but you discover some expired prescription bottles for the patient. The vital signs are within normal limits. The patient is oriented to person, place, and events, but you suspect depression or other mental health problems.

What other information should you try to get from the patient?

Should you recommend transport to the hospital for this patient?

If the patient is transported, what are your responsibilities?

If the patient declines transport, what then would you do?

Advocacy Issues/ Appropriate Patient Interaction

In addition to remembering that patients are persons first, EMS providers should recognize that older persons may have different values and as a result may make different health-related choices than EMS providers might choose for themselves. When delivering care to an older person, EMS providers must pay careful attention to ethical principles such as the right to autonomy. When the situation allows, EMS providers can and should make efforts to determine what the patient's wishes are. In this way, EMS providers help to minimize any potentially negative effects of the EMS experience on the patient's quality of life.

When formulating treatment plans, try to involve the patient. Once initial contact has been made, the lead EMS provider should advise the patient of how the assessment will progress and then find out whether this matches the patient's expectations. Similarly, the general treatment plan should be discussed with the patient at the earliest time possible. For example, an ALS provider could advise the patient that an IV should be started and let the patient know why. This would be better than only providing warning immediately prior to the needle stick.

> ### Communication Tip
>
> Once initial contact has been made, the lead EMS provider should advise the patient of how the assessment will progress and then find out whether this matches the patient's expectations.

Allow the patient to have some control about how treatment occurs. For example, when starting an IV, it may be possible to ask the person in which arm he or she would prefer to have the IV. If the patient indicates a need to use the bathroom prior to transport, give careful consideration to whether this is possible. Even with an IV line or ECG cables trailing, this may be the last chance for quite some time to take care of this physiological need. EMS providers should remember that some older persons have a decreased bladder capacity. EMS providers who help the older person to avoid unnecessary embarrassment are greatly improving the patient's self-esteem and quality of life.

When exposing patients during assessment, remember that older persons are not only prone to hypothermia, but also have at least as strong a sense of modesty as a younger person. Try to be as discreet as possible. Allow the patient to don a favorite robe or slippers unless this would be problematic. Prior to transport, be sure to ask whether items such as hearing aids, dentures, assistive devices, or a purse or wallet are needed. Ask whether lights should be turned off and if pets' needs are taken care of, especially if the patient lives alone. Check to see that portable heating devices and cooking appliances have been turned off. Lastly, ask the patient if he or she is comfortable and offer extra padding for bony areas or places where pressure ulcers are present.

> ### Communication Tip
>
> **The Little Things Make a Big Difference**
> - Communicate openly and respectfully.
> - Provide information about your assessment and proposed plan of action.
> - Respect the patient's autonomy, and honor competent choices.
> - Allow some control over when, how, or if minor procedures occur.
> - Give prior explanation for assessments and treatment.
> - Allow for elimination prior to transport.
> - Remember to ask about hearing aids, dentures, and other personal needs.
> - Provide for comfort and warmth with extra blankets or padding.

Resources

A basic and universal resource for older people is the State or **Area Agency on Aging (AAA)**. Under the Older Americans Act, all state and local agencies provide information services that can lead to

CASE STUDY 3

You are dispatched at about 2:00 a.m. to the home of a 92-year-old man who needs help getting back into bed after he slipped to the carpeted floor while on his way back from the bathroom. He had struggled for about four hours to get himself up, but finally resorted to activating his medical alert device. Instructions on where to find the hidden key to the locked door were relayed from the medical alarm company.

Although the patient lives alone, he has daily home care aide service. A review of his medications reveals that he is taking diazepam as a sleep aid. A quick check of the environment reveals a well-kept home, no obvious fall hazards, and adequate food. You do notice that the single smoke detector's cover is hanging down and it is missing a battery. On the kitchen counter is a journal used by the home care and home health workers. They apparently use this to communicate with each other about the patient. Your review of the last few days' notes shows no decline in the patient's health. It is noted that he has a history of mild dementia and diabetes.

The patient denies injury and you find none on exam. You ask for consent to check his vital signs and blood sugar. These are within normal limits. Once helped to his feet, the patient ambulates acceptably with his walker and gets himself back to bed. He denies need for further medical assistance. He asks that you turn out the lights and lock the door on your way out.

As the lead EMS provider on this call, do you feel comfortable leaving this patient at home?

If you have concerns, what are they, and how will you address them?

public and private resources close to where the person is. Telephone numbers usually are found under the government or organizational listing for the state or local jurisdiction, under Aging Services, Aging: Area Agency, or Office on, or Bureau of, or there may be a listing for Senior Information. The national Eldercare Locator is a toll-free number (1-800-677-1116) that can lead you to your state unit on aging or local AAA as well as other services.

When looking for resources, the AAA is a good place to start. They have senior information programs that track all resources in the community. The programs are variously called Information and Referral (I&R) or Information and Assistance (I&A). AAAs also sponsor nutrition programs, senior centers (locations where seniors can gather for meals, physical and social activities, and educational and volunteer opportunities), and transportation services.

The Long-Term Care Ombudsman at each local AAA reviews complaints in nursing homes and other long-term care facilities and tries to resolve them before crises occur, calling on the licensing agency or law enforcement if abuse is suspected. Some area agencies serve as public guardians of last resort if assigned by the Court; some have employment services; some do geriatric care management. Some AAAs provide services directly and some contract out the services, but the information program staff have knowledge about local available resources, public or private.

Senior centers welcome talks by community resources such as EMS. Other groups welcoming your presentations would be resident councils in apartments, senior citizen clubs, and service organizations. The AAA can be of assistance in connecting you to such groups.

Attitude Tip

To increase your awareness, understanding, and appreciation of the mobility problems and other sensory deficits faced by the older people, participate in geriatric empathy-training programs and workshops.

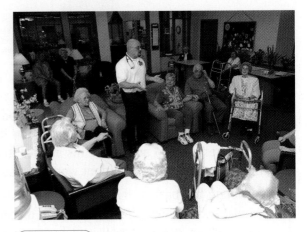

Figure 15-5 Talking with older people in the community can help prevent emergencies and provides a social connection.

Summary

EMS providers have an important role to play in improving the quality of life for older people. In prevention, you are invaluable in educating homeowners about home safety, and EMS providers can offer to do home safety checks. You can also talk with the older community about your role in saving lives, and what EMS providers can and cannot do. People generally are more comfortable if they know the process to be followed, so by educating the public, you can make your job more efficient in the long term **▲ Figure 15-5**.

Chapter Resources

Case Study Summaries

There are many reasons why this person may be reluctant to leave her home and go to the hospital. There may be denial as to the serious potential of her injury. EMS providers should avoid overly optimistic assessments and give honest information. At the same time, they should attempt to alleviate the patient's fears of hospitalization, surgery, or of nursing homes. A common fear of older people is going to a nursing home. Many nursing homes are just used for rehabilitation, and then the patient can return home. Addressing this fear directly can greatly reassure a patient.

Other reasons that the patient may be reluctant could include a concern for leaving a mess on the floor, concern for the welfare of her cats, or concern that she needs to make contact with family members. The EMS provider can help provide solutions to these concerns. Creative problem solving in this case could include the EMS providers doing the following: (1) cleaning up the spilled mess; (2) making sure that the cats have food, water, and access to their litter box; and (3) contacting the patient's son to advise him of the situation and where the patient will be transported.

Another concern the patient probably has is the probable increase in pain that will come from being moved during management and transport. The EMS providers can do much to reassure the patient that everything possible will be done to minimize discomfort. They can describe how splinting and the sling and swathe will help control the shoulder pain. ALS providers should consider providing IV analgesia prior to splinting or moving the patient.

This case represents extreme conditions that EMS providers occasionally encounter. Despite olfactory overload or basic disgust, the EMS providers must proceed in a systematic way to evaluate the situation, engage the client or patient in frank discussion, and create a plan of action. As health care providers, we must first determine whether a medical emergency exists and decide if, when, or how the patient will be medically evaluated. Remember that consent to perform a medical evaluation should be obtained before the evaluation. In this case, our patient was cooperative. This is not always the case, and the EMS providers must be tactful in establishing trust and rapport on first contact. EMS providers can ask whether the patient has any family members in the local area and if so, his frequency of contact with them. The patient should be asked about ADLs and IADLs (discussed in Chapter 2). This information will help social workers determine what level of assistance the patient will need. Ask for the name of the patient's doctor. It would also be good to know if the patient seems generally open to the idea of getting help or not.

In this case, the EMS provider might feel that at the least, the patient's incontinence requires medical evaluation. For this and the possible mental health issues, transport to the emergency department (ED) could be justified. If so, the EMS provider must make sure that ED staff is aware of the home environment and that something must be done to remedy the situation. A separate and direct report from the EMS agency to the appropriate social service agency may also be indicated. Depending on the client's willingness to accept help, a social service agency such as Adult Protective Services can arrange for cleaning the home as well as assistance for daily home care chores such as cleaning, bathing, dressing, or toileting.

If the patient is not transported to an ED, then the EMS provider must decide whether the patient represents an imminent danger to himself or others. In some cases a police officer may help make this determination, and in most cases would be required if the patient was to be involuntarily removed from the home. In some areas, an immediate response from a mental health professional may be available and helpful. If the EMS provider believes that the patient is not in imminent danger but requires expedient assistance, then a referral should be made based on the assessment that unsafe conditions exist and the patient is engaged in self-neglect.

Local and state factors will determine the appropriate agency for the referral. The social service agency may only take calls Monday through Friday during regular hours. The EMS provider might need to phone several agencies before finding the right person to help the client. It is recommended that a written referral accompany a telephone referral. The persistence of the EMS provider will hopefully be rewarded by a resolution of the situation. Be sure to ask for feedback from the social worker so that you can learn how your patient was helped. In this case, it would also be good to contact the concerned neighbor and let him know about the plan of action. In general, EMS providers can encourage neighbors and families to help.

In this case, the providers decided that the client was not in imminent danger but they communicated their findings in detail to Adult Protective Services. Within three days, a company was hired to clean out the home and the dog was taken for cremation. Meals on Wheels service was started, and a home care agency was hired to help with daily chores. The patient was evaluated for depression, dementia, and incontinence issues.

In cases like this, EMS providers may be the first ones to notice a problem in an older person's home environment. The observations of the EMS providers should lead to action. The actions and communications of individual EMS providers can make a huge difference in getting people the help they need.

CASE STUDY 3 SUMMARY

If a person denies injury and wishes to get back to bed and sleep, it may be that transport to an ED is not indicated. EMS providers should make an effort to determine whether there has been a decline in health or function that would indicate a need for evaluation. In this case, as evidenced by the home health journal, it seems that the patient has not had a sudden decline in function. In the absence of such information from formal care providers, it may be advisable for EMS providers in this situation to seek confirmation of the patient's usual health from the patient or by contacting family members or a neighbor. Consent to contact others should be obtained from the patient first.

In this case, the EMS provider might wonder whether the sleep aid tranquilizer contributed to the patient's fall. It is known that in the older population, the use of some medicines is associated with a greater risk of falling. Although there was no apparent injury with this fall, it may be that future falls would involve injury. The EMS providers were also concerned about leaving the resident without a working smoke detector, and they supplied a battery, tested the unit, and made sure the resident knew what to do if the alarm sounded.

EMS providers can and should concern themselves with injury prevention. In this case, EMS providers communicated with the patient's home health workers by leaving a note on or near the journal. They related the specifics of their observations and the services rendered. They also communicated their concern that the medicine may be placing the patient at risk for future falls.

Bibliography

Fleisher FI, White LJ, McMullen MJ, Chambers R. The geriatric obstacle course: A training session designed to help prehospital personnel recognize geriatric stereotypes and misconceptions. *The Journal of Emergency Medicine.* 1996;14(4):439–444.

Gerson LW, Schelbe DT, Wilson JE. Using paramedics to identify at-risk elderly. *Annals of Emergency Medicine.* 1992;21(6):688–691.

Hogan, TM. *Geriatric Emergencies: An EMT Teaching Manual.* 2nd ed. Turlock, CA: Medic Alert Foundation; 1996.

Hsiao AK, Hedges JR. Role of the emergency medical service system in regionwide health monitoring and referral. *Annals of Emergency Medicine.* 1993; 22(11):1696–1702.

International Association of Firefighters. Emergency Medical Services: Adding Value to a Fire-based EMS System, Monograph 7. Washington, DC: Author; 1997.

Janicki MP, Keefe RM. *Integration Experiences Casebook: Program Ideas in Aging and Developmental Disabilities.* Community Integration Project, New York State Office of Mental Retardation and Developmental Disabilities; 1992.

Jones JS, Walker G, Krohmer JR. To report or not to report: Emergency services response to elder abuse. *Prehospital and Disaster Medicine.* 1995;10(2): 96–100.

Kane RL. Home and community care of the elderly: Framing the issues. In JA Barondess, DE Rogers, KN Lohr, eds.: *Care of the Elderly Patient: Policy Issues and Research Opportunities.* Forum of the Council on Health Care Technology, Institute of Medicine. Washington, DC: National Academy Press; 1989.

Kassner E, Martin J. *Decisions, Decisions: Service Allocation in Home and Community-Based Long-Term Care Programs. A Four State Analysis.* Washington, DC: Public Policy Institute, American Association of Retired Persons; 1996.

Kaye LW, Applegate JS. *Men as Caregivers to the Elderly: Understanding and Aiding Unrecognized Family Support.* Lexington, MA: Lexington; 1990.

Kellogg Foundation. *Timely Opportunities: What Works in Community Care for the Elderly.* Battle Creek, MI: W.K. Kellogg; 1995.

Litwin H, ed. *The social networks of older people: A cross national analysis.* Westport, CT: Praeger; 1996.

McConnel CE, Wilson RW. The demand for prehospital emergency services in an aging society. *Social Science Medicine.* 1996;46(8):1027–1031.

Netting FE, Williams FG. Establishing interfaces between community and hospital-based service systems for the elderly. *Health and Social Work.* May 1989:134–139.

Newman SJ. *The Effects of Supports on Sustaining Older Disabled Persons in the Community.* Washington, DC: Public Policy Institute, American Association of Retired Persons; 1995.

O'Looney J. Beyond privatization and service integration: Organizational models for service delivery. *Social Service Review.* December 1993:501–534.

Pelham A, Clark W. *Managing Home Care for the Elderly: Lessons from Community-based Agencies.* New York: Springer; 1986.

Sanders AB. The training of emergency medical technicians in geriatric emergency medicine. *The Journal of Emergency Medicine.* 1996;14(4):499–500.

Stuck AE, Aronow HU, Steiner A. A trial of in-home comprehensive geriatric assessment for elderly people living in the community. *The New England Journal of Medicine.* 1995;333(18):1184–1189.

Wofford JL, Schwartz E, Byrum JE. The role of emergency services in health care for the elderly: A review. *The Journal of Emergency Medicine.* 1993; 11:317–326.

Procedures and Home Health Devices

Vicki Bacidore, RN, MS

Roxy Barnes, RN

Chris Coughlin, MEd, CEP

James Upchurch, MD

Contents

PROCEDURE 1
Urinary Catheters

Introduction

Catheterization of the bladder involves introducing a rubber or plastic tube through the urethra and into the bladder. Bladder catheterization is an invasive procedure that carries some associated risks. Special training and authorization from medical direction is required to perform bladder catheterization. There are several different types of urinary catheters.

Single-Use Straight Catheter

This catheter is used for only a short time to drain the bladder, and then it is removed. Some patients or caregivers are taught to insert the single-use straight catheter on their own.

Indwelling Foley Catheter

This catheter (▶ **Figure P1-1**) has a small inflatable balloon that encircles the catheter at the tip. When the balloon is inflated with sterile saline, it rests against the bladder outlet to anchor the catheter in place. The indwelling Foley catheter may also have as many as three separate lumens within the body of the catheter.

Condom Catheter (Texas Catheter)

The condom catheter is used for male patients who are incontinent or comatose. These patients still have complete and spontaneous bladder emptying.

Suprapubic Catheter

This catheter (▶ **Figure P1-2**) is surgically inserted into the bladder through the lower abdomen above the symphysis pubis. It is generally used for short periods with patients who have had gynecological or bladder surgery. It may be

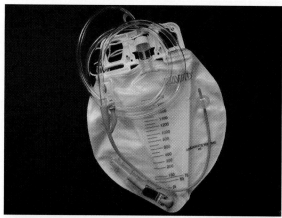

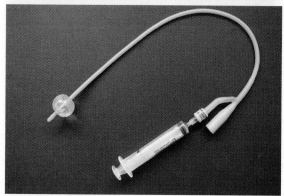

Figure P1-1 **(A)** Foley catheter and bag. **(B)** Foley catheter with the balloon inflated with sterile saline.

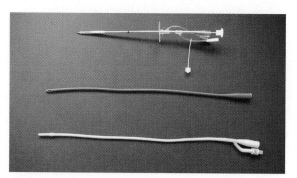

Figure P1-2 A suprapubic catheter shown at top, with Foley catheters beneath.

Urinary Catheters

319

used for patients who require a long-term alternative to catheterization due to incapacity to hold a Foley catheter in place. The suprapubic catheter is more comfortable than other catheters, as the patient may void naturally when the catheter is clamped.

Rationale

The urinary catheter provides a continuous flow of urine for patients unable to control the bladder, for patients with an obstruction, or for patients who are unable to ambulate. It usually remains in place until the patient can void voluntarily.

Preparation

Most patients will be apprehensive and frightened of bladder catheterization. The EMS provider should fully explain the procedure, reassure the patient, and make every effort to ensure privacy.

Equipment

Catheterization equipment includes personal protective equipment as well as a urinary catheter set containing:

- ◆ Sterile gloves
- ◆ Antiseptic solution
- ◆ Sterile cleansing sponges
- ◆ Sterile drapes or towels
- ◆ Syringe containing 5 mL of sterile water
- ◆ Connecting tubing and collection bag
- ◆ Water-soluble sterile lubricant
- ◆ Urinary catheter with 5-mL Foley balloon (usually 16F for males, 14F for females)

Procedure: Male Catheterization

1. Place the patient in supine position and remove the patient's pants and undergarments.
2. Open the catheterization set using sterile technique.
3. Wash hands and don sterile gloves.
4. Place one sterile drape under the patient's penis and another above the penis to cover the abdomen.
5. Open a package of antiseptic solution and saturate sterile sponges or cotton balls.
6. Attach the syringe to the catheter and test the balloon to make sure it inflates.
7. Open a package of water-soluble lubricant and lubricate the first several inches of the catheter.
8. Grasp the patient's penis with one hand and retract the foreskin (if present).
9. With the other hand, cleanse the glans with a sterile sponge (maintaining hand sterility) and then discard the sponge. Repeat the procedure.
10. Raise the shaft of the penis upright to straighten the penile urethra and pass the tip of the catheter through the hole in the tip of the penis.
11. Continue passing the catheter with gentle, steady pressure, advancing the catheter 7 to 9 inches or until urine flows out the distal end of the catheter. Once urine appears, advance the catheter another 2 inches. If mild resistance is felt at the external sphincter, slightly increase traction on the penis and continue with steady, gentle pressure on the catheter. (If significant resistance is met, withdraw the catheter and consult with medical control.)
12. Attach the syringe to the catheter and inflate the balloon with 3 to 5 mL of sterile water.
13. Gently pull back on the catheter until the balloon rests against the prostatic urethra. (Resistance will be encountered.) Reposition the retracted foreskin of an uncircumcised patient. Attach the drainage bag to the catheter.
14. Run the catheter tubing along the patient's leg and tape the connecting tubing to the patient's thigh. Do not place any tension on the catheter.
15. Attach the collection bag to the bed or stretcher at a level below that of the patient to facilitate drainage by gravity.

Procedure: Female Catheterization

1. Place the patient in supine position and remove the patient's pants and undergarments. Female patients should be positioned with knees bent, hips flexed, and feet resting about 24 inches apart.

2. Open the catheterization set using sterile technique.

3. Wash hands and don sterile gloves.

4. Place one sterile drape just under the patient's buttocks; position the drape with a central opening over the perineum, exposing the labia.

5. With one hand, separate the patient's labia to expose the opening of the urethra.

6. Cleanse the surrounding area with a sterile sponge or cotton ball (maintaining hand sterility) in downward strokes from anterior to posterior and then discard sponge. Repeat the procedure.

7. Introduce the tip of the well-lubricated catheter into the urethra using aseptic technique. Continue to advance the catheter 2 to 3 inches with gentle, steady pressure until urine flows out of the distal end of the catheter. Once urine appears, advance the catheter another 2 inches.

8. Attach a syringe to the catheter and inflate the balloon with 3 to 5 mL of sterile water.

9. Gently pull on the catheter until resistance is encountered.

10. Attach the collection tubing and bag to the catheter and secure the collection tubing to the patient's thigh as described above. Position the collection bag to facilitate drainage.

Possible Complications

Urinary Tract Infection

Urinary tract infection (UTI) is common and occurs in both sexes. The organisms most frequently associated with UTI are gram-negative organisms normally found in the gastrointestinal (GI) tract, including *Escherichia coli*, *Klebsiella*, *Proteus*, *Enterobacter*, and *Pseudomonas*. These fre-

quently are introduced from the hands of health personnel at the time of bladder catheterization. If allowed to progress, UTI may lead to septic complications (urosepsis), which can be especially dangerous in the older patient. Steps to help prevent UTI include:

- Never raise the bag above the level of the patient's bladder.

- The bag should be emptied every 8 hours via the drainage valve using an alcohol wipe to clean the drainage tube before emptying.

- Hands should be washed and gloves worn before and after handling the catheter, bag, or tubing.

- Urine should not be allowed to collect in the tubing.

- Know and recognize the signs and symptoms of a UTI: cloudy urine, hematuria, fever, chills, anorexia, malaise, and pain/burning sensation.

Traumatic Removal of Indwelling Foley Catheter

When the catheter is pulled out with the balloon still inflated, the urethra can be traumatized. Cover the penis or vagina with a loose dressing and transport, replacing fluids if necessary. If the catheter is not totally dislodged, check with medical control to determine if the balloon should be deflated. After deflation, the catheter should not be pulled out.

Other Emergencies

Bladder distention from blockages can occur from the tubing becoming kinked or compressed externally, or disfigured internally from blood or sediment. The patient should be transported. Another emergency is the inability of the patient to self-catheterize. If this occurs, there is no field treatment other than to transport the patient.

Transport Considerations

When transporting a patient with a catheter in place, make sure that the tubing is secured to the leg of the patient, protect the patient's modesty, and do not pull on the tubing during transport.

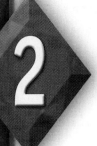

PROCEDURE
Ureterostomy

Introduction

A urinary diversion refers to the rerouting of the urinary tract when it is necessary to remove or bypass the bladder. The bladder may be removed due to cancer. A bypass procedure may be indicated in neurogenic bladder. The **ileal conduit** and the **ureterostomy** are the two most common types of urinary diversion.

The most common type of urinary diversion in adults is the ileal conduit. An ileal conduit is not a new bladder, but a tube or conduit constructed of small bowel that allows urine to drain to the outside of the body. Urine drains continuously through the stoma and requires an external pouch.

A ureterostomy may be seen in adult patients when the ileal conduit cannot be constructed. The ureter is brought to the abdominal wall to form a stoma. The ureterostomy has a higher rate of stenosis (narrowing), infection, and pouching difficulties.

Contraindications

Obesity makes it more difficult to construct a good stoma. Obesity is also associated with more tension on the mesentery, leading to stomal **necrosis**. Bowel that has received radiation treatments should not be used for the conduit and may indicate the use of a higher segment of ileum or jejunum for the conduit.

Possible Complications

- The stoma may be a source of bleeding. If the bleeding is visible, apply pressure and transport.
- The stoma is not sensitive to touch, but the skin around the stoma can become sensitive if irritated by urine or the adhesive of the urostomy pouch.
- Normally there should not be emergencies related to this device. The patient or family may have questions or concerns.

Colostomy/Ileostomy

Introduction

Certain illnesses or injuries prevent the normal passage of intestinal contents through the large and small bowel. A **colostomy** is a diversion involving the colon, in which a segment of diseased or injured colon is bypassed or removed and an end (or loop) of colon is brought through a small opening in the abdominal wall, forming a stoma. The removal of the entire colon and rectum results in the ileum being brought through the abdominal wall, forming an **ileostomy** stoma. The bowel usually discharges liquid or solid feces into the bag (pouch) once or twice a day; the bag is then changed. Colostomy irrigation, ostomy care, and pouch changes are usually performed for home care patients by the patients themselves, family members, and home health practitioners. These procedures require special training, and usually are not considered an acute intervention for EMS practice.

Possible Complications and Emergency Care

Possible complications include:

♦ Bowel perforation

♦ Significant fluid/electrolyte imbalances from colostomy irrigation or diarrhea

♦ Stomal problems (eg, bleeding, necrosis, retraction, stenosis, prolapse)

♦ Infection

♦ Obstruction

If the stoma is bleeding, apply pressure and transport. The stoma is not sensitive to touch, but the skin around the stoma can become sensitive if irritated by the appliance. The patient should be evaluated by obtaining a focused history and performing a physical examination to determine the need for immediate transport to a hospital.

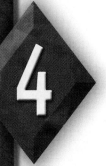

PROCEDURE

Tracheostomy

Introduction

A <u>tracheostomy</u> is a temporary or permanent surgical opening (stoma) through the third or fourth tracheal ring. Tracheostomies are performed when an endotracheal tube is contraindicated, cannot be passed, or when sustained ventilatory support is required. Patients who require a tracheostomy fall into one of two categories. Patients in the first group have an obstruction at or above the level of the larynx, such as foreign body obstruction, carcinoma of the larynx, severe infection, or trauma to the tongue or mandible. Patients in the second group have no actual obstruction, but are unable to clear their own secretions and are in danger of hypoxia if secretions accumulate and are not removed from the chest. These patients include those with paralysis of the chest muscles and diaphragm, patients who are unconscious or semiconscious with head injuries, and patients with fractured ribs or other chest injuries causing severe pain that inhibits them from coughing.

Tracheostomy tubes may be constructed of polyvinyl chloride (PVC) or silastic (silicone rubber) and may be single or double construction. The single tube has a built-in tracheal cuff and an obturator or stylet used for insertion. A double tube has a similar attached cuff but also has an inner cannula. The inner cannula is designed to be easily removed, cleaned, or replaced to maintain good air exchange. The cuff is inflated to prevent aspiration of upper airway secretions. Some tracheostomy tubes have a small opening in the cannula that enables the patient to whisper or talk by moving air through the larynx. Once the tube is inserted in the neck, it is secured with sutures or soft cloth ties.

Rationale

The tracheostomy tube is inserted to allow passage of air and the removal of tracheobronchial secretions.

Possible Complications and Emergency Care

Most complications occur within the first 24 hours of the procedure. Three common complications are obstruction, dislodgment, and infection. Less common complications are hemorrhage, subcutaneous emphysema, and mediastinal emphysema. Prehospital management consists of an appropriate assessment and maintaining an open airway. If the patient with a tracheostomy experiences acute respiratory distress, consider the following possible causes.

Obstruction

The tube may be obstructed from excessive secretions, accumulated dry secretions, pressure on the tube from foreign bodies, or airway edema. When mucus obstructs a double tube, the inner cannula can be removed and rinsed with sterile water or saline. The inner cannula can also be left in place and cleaned of mucus with suction. If the airway remains obstructed, it may be necessary to remove the tracheostomy tube and replace it with an endotracheal tube. This is a risky procedure and should not be performed without specific training and medical direction.

Infection

The stoma itself may become infected, leading to redness, swelling, pus, and fever. Improper suctioning techniques may cause pulmonary infections and sepsis. By using aseptic technique and good wound care, the risk of infection is reduced.

Tracheal Stenosis

Stenosis occurs when the trachea narrows at the site of the cuff, and may develop weeks or years after the tube has been inserted. Due to the reduced diameter of the trachea, the patient may develop dyspnea, stridor, decreased exercise tolerance, and recurring respiratory infections.

Tracheal Necrosis

Necrosis is associated with excessive cuff pressure, and may occur as early as 3 to 5 days after insertion of the tube. In some patients, the necrosis may extend through the posterior wall of the trachea, causing an opening to develop between the trachea and esophagus. Necrosis may also cause erosion through the anterior wall of the trachea and into an artery, although this is rare. If this occurs, the tube may pulsate and/or show bright red blood.

Opening Between the Trachea and Esophagus

This opening or fistula allows air to escape into the stomach, which can cause oral and gastric secretions to be aspirated into the lungs. The patient may experience dyspnea, stridor, or evidence of aspiration pneumonia. If suction is not adequate to keep the tube clear, consider inserting a slightly smaller endotracheal (ET) tube through the tracheostomy tube until the tip is just above the carina. If external bleeding is noted, use an absorbent dressing and apply slight pressure.

Subcutaneous/Mediastinal Emphysema

This is rare and usually appears immediately after initial insertion or reinsertion. It can occur when the tube is displaced and air leaks into the surrounding tissues. The patient may experience mild to severe respiratory distress. The area beneath the skin may appear puffy and a crackling sensation (crepitus) may be palpated. Provide respiratory support and monitor the patient carefully. Refrain from using positive-pressure ventilation as this may increase the extent of the air leak.

PROCEDURE
Respirators/Ventilators

Introduction

Historically, mechanical ventilators were only available in the intensive care units (ICUs) of hospitals. Portable units are now widely available for interfacility patient transport and home use. Mechanical ventilators are classified according to preset parameters that control the mechanism of the inspiratory phase (volume cycled, pressure cycled, and time cycled).

- *Volume ventilators* deliver a predetermined volume of gas with each cycle, after which inspiration is terminated. These types of ventilators deliver a constant tidal volume regardless of changes in airway resistance or compliance of the lungs and thorax. The volume stays the same unless high airway pressures are reached, in which case safety release valves stop the flow.

- *Pressure ventilators* are pressure-cycled devices that terminate inspiration when a preset pressure is reached. At this point, the gas flow ceases and the patient passively exhales. These types of ventilators are most often used for patients whose ventilatory resistance is not likely to change.

- *Negative-pressure ventilators* have settings for the respiratory rate and pressure of the negative force exerted. They use negative pressure to raise the rib cage and lower the diaphragm to create negative pressure within the lungs so that air flows into the lungs. These types of ventilators are used for patients with healthy lungs who have a muscular inability to inhale (spinal cord injury, neuromuscular disease).

- *Continuous positive airway pressure (CPAP) ventilatory support systems* are for patients who require continuous positive airway pressure. CPAP assists breathing by raising pressure in the nose and pharynx, forcing air into the lungs during inspiration. After inspiration, pressure returns to a lower level. It can be delivered through mask CPAP or nasal CPAP.

- *Bilevel positive airway pressure (BiPAP) ventilatory support systems* deliver two different levels of positive airway pressure. The system cycles spontaneously between a preset level of inspiratory positive airway pressure (IPAP) and expiratory positive airway pressure (EPAP). BiPAP is intended only to augment the patient's breathing. Patients with chronic obstructive pulmonary disease (COPD) or sleep apnea may benefit from BiPAP.

Rationale

Mechanical ventilators are used for home or transport patients who are unable to maintain spontaneous respiration for any length of time. Management goals are to improve airway patency, ventilation, and oxygenation.

Emergency Care

When caring for a patient with a ventilator, evaluate the patient's work of breathing, tidal volume, peak flow, oxygen saturation, and quality of breath sounds. Signs and symptoms of hypoxia should be recognized and treated:

- Restlessness
- Headache
- Confusion and mental status changes
- Hyperventilation
- Tachycardia
- Hypertension
- Dyspnea
- Cyanosis

The family may be familiar with the machine, but the onset of problems may initiate a call to EMS. Having a back-up ventilator is essential. You may encounter a wide variety of ventilators, but always remember to treat the patient and not the machine. Disconnect the ventilator from the tracheostomy tube and attach a bag-valve-mask (BVM) device. The initial oxygen delivery ventilatory rate should be similar to the patient's ventilator settings or as advised by medical control. Assess the patient's response via vital signs, skin color, and pulse oximetry, and adjust ventilatory rate and oxygen delivery accordingly.

Tip

Ventilator Alarms

Ventilators are equipped with alarms to signal problems with ventilator function, including alarms for loss of power, frequency alarms (indicating changes in respiratory rate), volume alarms (indicating low-exhaled volume or low/high minute-ventilation), and high-pressure alarms. If alarms are sounding, check for the following causes:

- Kinks in ET tubes
- Disconnected ventilator tubing or poor connections
- Water in ventilator tubing
- Excessive secretions
- Pneumothorax
- Patient anxiety

After consulting with medical control, acute interventions may include providing temporary ventilation assistance with a BVM device, repositioning the ET tube, correcting poor ventilator tube connections, emptying water from tube or water traps, suctioning the airway, thoracic decompression, and possible sedation.

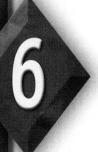

6 PROCEDURE
Patient-Controlled Analgesic Pumps

Introduction

Patient-controlled analgesia (PCA) provides safe, effective, and consistent pain relief to manage postoperative and chronic pain. The patient is allowed to have control over medication administration, with predetermined safety limits. A PCA pump is an electrically controlled infusion pump that will administer a preset amount of pain medication by continuous infusion or by self-administration of a preset bolus dose. A timing device sets the interval between patient-administered doses. The timer can be set to a specific interval that prevents additional doses from being administered until the time interval expires, regardless of how many times the button is pushed. Most pumps have a locked safety system to prevent tampering. At no time should anyone but the patient push the medication button. This prevents overmedication and is why it is called "patient-controlled analgesia."

The patient and caregivers can be valuable information resources concerning the PCA pump and medication. There should be written doctor's orders in the home or on the medication cartridge stating the type of analgesic, loading dosage, concentration of analgesic mixture, and "lock-out interval" (minimum time allowed between doses). Overdose is uncommon, but should be considered in the patient who presents with an altered mental status that is not his/her baseline status.

The pump can administer medication via intravenous (IV) lines, subcutaneous needle, or epidural catheter.

Rationale

Patient-controlled analgesia provides safe, effective, and consistent pain relief and allows the patient to control delivery of pain medication in a safe, consistent, effective, and reliable manner.

Equipment

Equipment that may be found in the patient's home includes the following:

- PCA infusion pump
- PCA administration set (pump tubing)
- IV tubing and fluid as applicable
- PCA infuser key
- PCA flow sheet
- Ordered narcotic analgesic vial, syringe, or cassette (mixed by pharmacy)
- Patient information booklet
- IV start kit (unless venous access is already available)

Possible Complications

Infiltration of Intravenous Administration Site

This can occur when IV fluids enter the subcutaneous space around the venipuncture site. Look for swelling and pallor (blanching) around the site, or note if the patient complains of a painful, burning sensation. Discontinue the infusion by shutting off the pump, and raise the extremity to promote venous drainage. Contact medical control.

Phlebitis

Phlebitis is inflammation of the vein, and may be caused by the type of catheter, chemical irritation by medications, or the anatomical position of the catheter. The patient may complain of pain and tenderness at the vein site. The skin over the vein may be warm and red. Discontinue the infusion and apply warm, moist compresses over the site to provide relief.

Introduction

Enteral feedings are administered through a tube placed in the stomach or small intestine via the esophagus or directly through the abdominal wall. Common conditions that warrant enteral nutritional support include:

- Dysphagia
- Stroke
- Cancer
- Gastrointestinal disease
- Coma
- Cardiac or respiratory failure
- Depression

A gastric tube, or feeding tube, is a small polyurethane or silicone tube that is inserted through the nose to the stomach (nasogastric) or through the mouth to the stomach (orogastric) to provide liquid nutrition. Long-term effectiveness of these tubes is limited due to patient discomfort and irritation. This type of tube is used if the patient requires tube feeding for less than 6 weeks.

A gastrostomy, or G-tube, is used when prolonged or permanent (longer than 6 weeks) enteral feedings are needed. While the patient is under general or local anesthesia, a physician makes a small opening in the abdominal wall and inserts a special gastrostomy catheter through the wall and into the stomach. The tube usually extends 12 to 15 inches from the skin and is sutured into place. For more active patients, a "button" device can be placed. This provides a skin-level gastrostomy and eliminates the cumbersome external catheter. The button allows the attachment of a safety cap after removing the feeding tube.

A jejunostomy, or J-tube, is an intestinal tube that passes through the stomach into the portion of the small intestine called the jejunum. This type of tube is used if the patient is at risk for aspiration or has severe esophageal reflux, obstruction, stricture (abnormal narrowing of duct), fistulae (abnormal passages in the GI tract), or ileus of the upper GI tract.

Rationale

Enteral feedings can be used to provide liquid nutrition for patients who have a healthy GI system, but are unable to swallow due to injury, paralysis, or unresponsiveness.

Indications

- **Malnutrition risk or presence**
- **Inadequate intestinal digestion and absorption**
- **Absence of bowel obstruction**

Possible Complications

Possible complications include:

- Pulmonary aspiration of formula
- Chronic leakage around the stoma site
- Dehydration
- Nausea
- Diarrhea
- Bacterial contamination
- Electrolyte imbalance
- Tube displacement

If the tube has been displaced and bleeding is present, apply direct pressure with a sterile dressing. If any complications present a danger, transport of the patient is required.

PROCEDURE
Vascular Access Devices

Introduction

Many patients with cancer and other chronic illnesses require prolonged and frequent access to venous circulation. In the past, it was necessary for the patient to remain hospitalized or suffer repeated needle sticks to obtain blood or receive antibiotics at home. Medications, parenteral nutrition, and blood transfusions can be administered through a variety of vascular access devices (VADs).

These tubes are inserted into the central circulation where they remain for weeks or months, allowing reliable access to circulation. This allows more patients to be managed at home, and as a result, EMS providers encounter increasing numbers of patients with VADs. The use of VADs in the prehospital setting was strongly discouraged, but in critical situations, VADs may provide immediate and life-saving venous access.

Rationale

For the patient who requires immediate vascular access and offers no peripheral route, a VAD can provide a safe, rapid solution. However, only those who have received specialized training and whose protocols allow it should attempt VAD access.

Although many types of VADs are currently in use, they may be classified into three general categories:

♦ Central venous catheters (CVC)

♦ Implanted ports

♦ Peripheral inserted central catheters (PICC)

Each category includes several types of catheters with a variety of uses and functions. Although the specifics are complex, a working knowledge of the general types and functions of VADs is valuable for the EMS provider.

Features

Catheters implanted for long-term use have many common features. Most are constructed of radiopaque silicone or, less often, polyurethane. Silicone is strong, flexible, and less likely to cause clot formation than other materials. The location of the catheter will vary based on patient characteristics, patient preference, type and duration of therapy, and self- and home-care capabilities.

The venous catheter is inserted with the tip in the superior vena cava just above the right atrium, thus the descriptive name of central venous catheter. The insertion site is usually one of the major veins of the chest or upper neck, or, in the case of peripheral access, one of the large veins of the arm or leg.

VADs are used for both bolus injections and continuous IV infusions. Examples include IV solutions, medications, total parenteral nutrition (TPN), blood, and blood products. Blood samples for laboratory studies are obtainable through most VADs. The catheter may have one, two, or three lumens.

Central Venous Catheters

Central venous catheters (CVCs) may also be referred to by the manufacturer's name (eg, Broviac, Hickman, Groshong, Corcath). A CVC may be a single-lumen or a multiple-lumen catheter (▶ **Figure P8-1**). The multiple-lumen catheter is used for patients requiring complex therapy. Lumen sizes vary from 21- to 14-gauge. A small cap (referred to as an intermittent injection cap, buffalo cap, or heparin lock) covers each lumen and is filled with a heparin or saline solution to keep blood clots from blocking the catheter.

These catheters are inserted through the skin, and then tunneled through the subcutaneous tissue to the site in which the catheter enters the vein (▶ **Figure P8-2**). A cuff located in the subcutaneous portion of the catheter helps the catheter to imbed itself in tissue. Fibrous tissue then

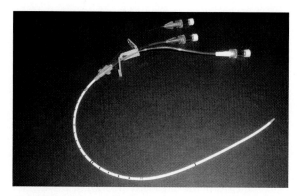

Figure P8-1   A CVC may be a single-lumen or a multiple-lumen catheter. Here, a three-lumen catheter is shown.

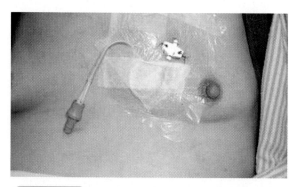

Figure P8-2   Central venous catheters (CVCs) are inserted through the skin and then tunneled through the subcutaneous tissue to the site in which the catheter enters the vein; a Groshong catheter is shown here.

grows around the cuff, stabilizing the catheter and creating a barrier against infection.

Implanted Ports

Unlike a CVC, there is no external infusion site with an implanted, or subcutaneous, port. This port is like a tiny drum; it has a solid bottom and sides and is covered on top by a flexible material called the septum. This port is located at the distal end of the catheter and is implanted approximately 0.5 inch under the skin. The port is palpated through the skin, and a needle is inserted into the self-sealing septum.

Although not required, a dressing is often placed over the access site to add further protection. In routine circumstances, a special "Huber" needle is used to extend the life of the septum ▶ Figure P8-3 .

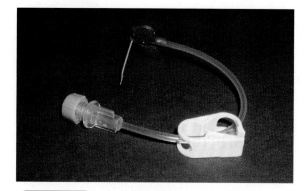

Figure P8-3   A Huber needle.

Peripheral Inserted Central Catheter

Peripheral inserted central catheters (PICCs) are small (23- to 16-gauge) single- or double-lumen catheters ▼ Figure P8-4 . Because of the smaller size, they are often used for neonates, very young children, or patients who require only short-term therapy.

PICC lines are less expensive than CVCs and have fewer major complications such as hemothorax, pneumothorax, and air emboli. They are also called nontunneled catheters, because they enter the skin near the point at which they enter the vein. PICC lines are often inserted at the antecubital space into the basilic or cephalic vein. Once inserted, the catheter may be sutured in place for stability.

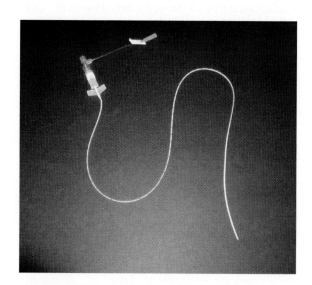

Figure P8-4   A peripheral inserted central catheter (PICC).

Medication Tip

Several medications can be administered through an endotracheal tube when IV access is not available.

Preparation

1. Rapid venous access is important in many medical and traumatic emergencies.

2. Standard methods of venous access, such as peripheral and external jugular IVs, and the intraosseous route (typically reserved for pediatric patients), should always be attempted before using a VAD.

3. It is also important for the EMS provider to remember that several medications can be administered through an endotracheal tube when IV access is not available.

4. The patient, family members, and other caregivers can often provide valuable information about the patient's medical condition and the use of the VAD, despite their limited knowledge of emergency situations.

Procedure

For the patient who requires immediate vascular access and offers no peripheral route, a VAD can provide a safe, rapid solution. However, only those who have received specialized training and protocols should attempt this.

1. Because of the extremely high risk of infection and sepsis, careful aseptic technique, including sterile gloves, must be used at all times.

2. The EMS provider should identify the location of the catheter or palpate the site of the implanted port.

3. The catheter can be clamped by folding it over, and smooth hemostats (no teeth) can be used to prevent infusion of air.

4. When clamping, use care to prevent tearing the catheter. If an infusion is in progress or a pump is attached, the rescuer should ask for help from those familiar with the pump; the pump should be turned off, clamped, or the line coming from it disconnected.

5. If the VAD has multiple lumens, the pump may be left on and a "free" lumen can be used.

6. The EMS provider should remove the small injection cap covering the hub of the lumen and attach the syringe or IV tubing directly to the catheter.

7. The cap can also be left in place, and after cleaning the cap with alcohol or povidone-iodine, a needle (20 g or smaller) can be inserted through.

8. The EMS provider should then remove the clamp or unpinch the catheter.

9. Using a syringe, aspirate 3 to 5 mL of blood slowly, to avoid collapsing the catheter. This confirms placement and clears the line of heparin.

10. If called for in local protocols, blood samples can be obtained using a syringe or vacutainer.

11. A vacutainer should not be used for PICC lines.

12. Be sure to pinch or clamp the lumen when attaching and removing syringes to avoid taking air into the catheter.

13. Using at least 10 mL of normal saline, the catheter should be flushed of blood.

14. Then connect the IV tubing and carefully tape it, using a loop of tubing to prevent inadvertent disconnection.

15. The infusion site should be monitored and the patient reassessed.

16. An implanted port may be used in much the same way as a central line or PICC.

17. The port is usually implanted in the rib area or antecubital space.

18. Using a sterile gloved hand, the paramedic should apply pressure around the edges of the port to slightly "stretch" the skin over the injection site.

19. If a Huber needle is not available, as small a needle as possible (preferably a 21 g or smaller) should be used to avoid port damage and leakage at the injection site.

20. The needle and syringe or IV tubing should be flushed first.

Skill Drill P8-1 — Huber Needle Insertion into a Subcutaneous Port

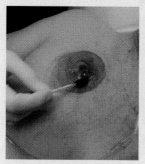 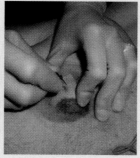 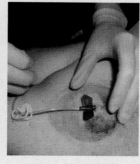 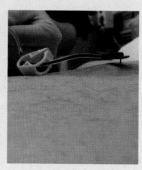

1. Prep the site.

2. Apply pressure around the edges of the port to stretch the skin over the injection site.

3. Insert the needle.

4. Aspirate for blood.

21. The needle must be inserted until it touches the back of the port; this may require a great deal of pressure to puncture the skin, scar tissue, and septum (▲ Skill Drill P8-1).

22. Then aspirate blood; if it does not return freely, the device should not be used.

23. The port should again be flushed and infusion of medications or fluids begun.

Possible Complications and Emergency Care

Patients with VADs may call EMS for a variety of reasons. Because many patients with VADs have chronic illnesses, they may seek help for complications of cancer, AIDS, or sickle cell disease. Patients with VADs may be injured or have problems with unassociated illnesses.

Several difficulties related directly to the presence of a VAD may occur. The more common possibilities include:

♦ Infection of the exit site, tunnel, or port

♦ Systemic infection that develops from bacteria ascending through the catheter and entering the patient's circulation

♦ Catheter clot

♦ Venous thrombosis

♦ Catheter displacement

♦ Catheter leak

♦ Air embolus

Management of local infections may begin in the prehospital setting with simple dressing changes and caution to avoid further spread of infection. Systemic sepsis or septic shock will require standard management of airway, breathing, and circulation (ABCs). The VAD itself may be used because IV access for fluid resuscitation of the critical patient may be difficult or impossible, and aseptic technique is essential (eg, sterile gloves, alcohol, povidone-iodine). It is important for the EMS provider to remember that the VAD itself may be the site of infection. If any clinical signs suggest this, the VAD should not be used for access.

Communication Tip

The patient, family members, and other caregivers can often provide valuable information about the patient's medical condition and the use of the VAD.

VADs are usually flushed with a heparin or saline solution to prevent clotting. Despite proper care, clots may form in the catheter, disrupting the flow of solutions and medications. Sluggish flow or inability to infuse solutions requires rapid intervention. Never attempt to force or dislodge the clot. The catheter may require declotting with thrombolytics or may have to be replaced.

Thrombosis can develop in the vessel in which the catheter is inserted. The patient may complain of local tenderness or swelling in the arm, neck, or shoulder near the device. In addition, the patient or family may notice that the flow of solution or medication through the catheter is sluggish. Prehospital management of a thrombosis is similar to that of a deep vein thrombosis: the area should not be massaged; instead, the area or extremity must be immobilized, low-flow oxygen administered, and the patient transported to definitive care.

It is rare for the catheter or port to migrate or become displaced because VADs are secured, usually with sutures. However, physical exercise or accidental "tugging" on the external apparatus can displace the catheter. The patient may complain of bleeding, burning upon infusion, or swelling from infiltrated fluid. Upon palpation of an implanted port, the patient may have pain, swelling, and bruising in the area. In extreme cases, the tip of the catheter can migrate and puncture or become lodged in a major vessel wall or the myocardium, leading to more severe symp-toms. Patients who complain of shortness of breath, chest pain, dizziness, tachycardia, or hypotension should be treated by standard emergency protocols, with an awareness that the symptoms can result either from complications related to a special device or from an unrelated and potentially life-threatening event.

Occasionally a catheter develops a leak or tear, perhaps related to improper use. When this occurs, fluids or medications infiltrate into the surrounding tissues. The surrounding area appears swollen and tender, and the patient may complain of burning. The infusion should be stopped immediately; certain medications may cause significant irritation and even necrosis of tissues when infiltration occurs. An appropriate dressing can be applied to the area to help prevent infection and necessary measures should be used to stop bleeding.

Either improper occlusion of the catheter port or a tear in the catheter can lead to an air embolus. Because exact prehospital diagnosis is impossible, management is by standard protocol based on a complete patient assessment. The patient should be transported in a left lateral position with the legs slightly elevated and head lowered, to prevent an air embolus from migrating to the brain and causing a stroke. Oxygen, cardiac monitor, venous access, and rapid transport are indicated in these patients.

Introduction

The kidneys remove toxic materials from the body and maintain fluid, electrolyte, and acid-base balance. Dialysis uses the principles of osmosis, diffusion, and ultra-filtration to eliminate toxic materials from the body for patients with acute or chronic renal failure. Despite advances in therapies and transplants, nearly every patient with end-stage renal disease requires some form of dialysis. The two techniques are peritoneal dialysis and hemodialysis.

Peritoneal dialysis requires an implanted catheter, constructed of nylon or silicone rubber, which is fed into the abdominal cavity. Sterile dialyzing fluid (dialysate) bathes the peritoneal membranes that cover the abdominal organs and supporting capillary beds. Blood toxins travel from the abdominal capillaries into the dialysate fluid, which is then drained back through the catheter. This process lasts approximately 1 hour and is often repeated many times daily or throughout the night while the patient sleeps.

Hemodialysis involves shunting the patient's blood through a dialysis machine to facilitate removal of waste and toxins (▶ **Figure P9-1**). Once the blood has been "detoxified," it is returned to the patient's circulation. There are three common methods of vascular access for hemodialysis:

- *Arteriovenous (AV) fistula*—AV fistulas are created by establishing a surgical connection between an artery and an adjacent vein (anastomosed). The high pressures associated with arterial flow creates a "bulge" or swelling of the vein known as a pseudoaneurysm (▶ **Figure P9-2A**). Outflow of blood is accomplished by inserting a large-bore needle into this "bulge."

- *Arteriovenous (AV) graft*—AV grafts are the most frequently used access points for chronic renal dialysis. Synthetic materials such as Gore-Tex or biological materials such as human umbilical veins are surgically im-

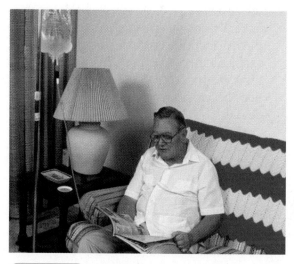

Figure P9-1 Hemodialysis involves shunting the patient's blood through a dialysis machine to facilitate removal of waste and toxins.

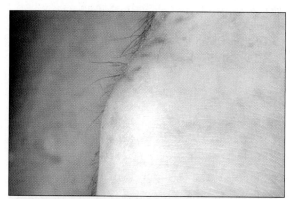

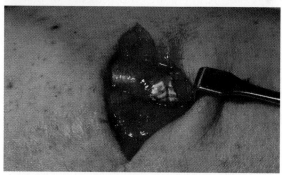

Figure P9-2 With an AV fistula, a bulge is created by arterial pressure **(A)**. An arteriovenous graft creates a raised area that looks like a large vessel **(B)**.

Dialysis

335

planted in the limb to create a U-shaped tunnel. This graft is connected to the vein and artery, then secured just under the surface of the skin, which creates a raised area that looks like a large vessel (◄ **Figure P9-2B**).

♦ *External arteriovenous (AV) shunt*—External AV shunts are seldom used today because of the advent of vascular access devices such as femoral and subclavian catheters. Similar to the AV graft, the external AV shunt joins the vein and artery together. The tubing extends from each vessel tip outside the body and may be connected with a heparinized "T" device.

Rationale

To maintain patency of access for dialysis and to detect complications of a hemodialysis access site related to infection, thrombosis, occlusion, bleeding, or cannula separation.

Assessment

Assessment should focus on the following:

♦ Status of the fistula, graft, or cannula site and dressing
♦ Location of shunt, fistula, or graft
♦ Vital signs
  ♦ *Blood pressure assessments in the shunted extremity should be avoided because this procedure will obstruct blood flow.*
♦ Pulses distal to shunt, fistula, or graft
♦ Color, temperature, and presence of pain or numbness in the extremity in which the access is located

Possible Complications

♦ Infection, thrombosis, occlusion, bleeding, or separation of the cannula
♦ Too much water removal (hypovolemia, hypotension)
♦ Too little water removal (pulmonary edema, congestive heart failure)
♦ Electrolyte imbalances

Complications Specific to Peritoneal Dialysis

♦ Peritonitis (infection of the peritoneal cavity)
♦ Dialysate may fail to drain from the peritoneal cavity due to catheter occlusion or the catheter tip lodging against the abdominal wall. Turning the patient from side to side or gently pressing on the abdomen may alleviate the fluid accumulation. It may be necessary for a physician to irrigate or replace the catheter.
♦ Mild pain or discomfort with the procedure [severe pain is not normal; consider the possibility of GI bleeding, myocardial infarction (MI), or aortic dissection]
♦ Respiratory distress due to increase in pressure on diaphragm as dialysate is infused. Respiratory distress can be further compounded in the patient who is overhydrated (consider other causes of respiratory distress).

> ### Tip
>
> Peritonitis is most often associated with organisms that have been introduced through the catheter itself, and can cause severe sepsis and shock in a relatively short period of time. The patient experiences generalized abdominal tenderness and exhibits guarding upon exam.
>
> Management of the septic patient includes the ABCs, intravenous fluid administration (normal saline is the crystalloid of choice; lactated Ringer's should be avoided because of the higher concentration of potassium), cardiac monitoring, and rapid transport.

Prehospital Use of Dialysis Vascular Access Devices

Preparation

1. The decision to use a dialysis access device in the prehospital setting must be made based on training and local protocols.
2. Family or home caregivers may be able to provide useful information regarding the type and placement of the device.

Indications

♦ **To be utilized in the critical patient only after failure to obtain peripheral intravenous access (including the external jugular vein) and when the intraosseous or endotracheal route is not an option.**

♦ **In the critical patient when routine access is not available, AV grafts, fistulas, and shunts can provide rapid and safe vascular access.**

Contraindications

The rescuer should note that a peritoneal dialysis catheter cannot be used for vascular access.

Equipment

Povidone-iodine prep (alcohol should never be used as it will damage synthetic materials)

14- or 16-gauge needle (standard steel or Teflon IV catheters may be used)

5-mL syringe for discard

Syringe or vacutainer for blood samples

0.9% normal saline IV solution

IV tubing (primed)

Tape

Constricting band (optional)

3. The area should be gently palpated to locate the fistula or graft. A "thrill" or vibration should be felt over the fistula.

4. Any area that is red, tender, swollen, or draining, or shows other evidence of infection, should not be used.

Procedure

1. Usually the vein is sufficiently distended, but a constricting band can be placed proximal to the insertion site if needed.

2. Prep the site with povidone-iodine.

3. Stabilize the site before inserting the IV needle.

4. Insert the needle in the direction of venous flow (toward the head) at a slight angle (15 to 20 degrees), to prevent penetrating the posterior lumen of the vessel (► **Skill Drill P9-1**).

5. The needle should be directed and the Teflon catheter advanced in the same manner as with standard IVs (watch for a "flashback" in the hub).

6. Next, 3 to 5 mL of blood should be aspirated and then discarded to confirm correct placement as well as clear the shunt of heparin (grafts and fistulas are not heparinized).

7. Obtain the necessary blood samples per local protocol.

8. Remove the constricting band.

9. Attach the IV tubing and begin the infusion of normal saline or medications.

10. Use caution when administering fluids to avoid inadvertently overhydrating the patient.

11. Tape the IV tubing carefully and reassess the infusion site as well as the patient.

Skill Drill P9-1 Accessing a Dialysis Shunt

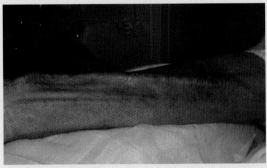

1. In accessing a dialysis shunt, locate the site.

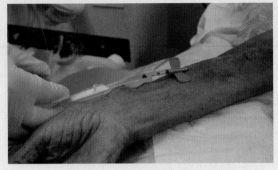

3. Aspirate 3 to 5 mL of blood to confirm correct placement and clear the shunt.

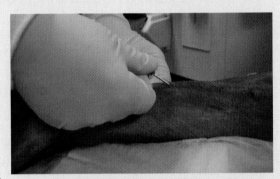

2. Insert the needle in the direction of venous flow (toward the head) at a slight angle (15 to 20 degrees), to prevent penetrating the posterior lumen of the vessel.

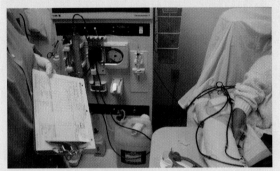

4. Continue to reassess the infusion site and the patient.

Introduction

A ventricular shunt is an implanted drainage system used to remove excess cerebrospinal fluid (CSF) in the brain. In patients with hydrocephalus, excess fluid in the brain can lead to increased intracranial pressure (ICP). A ventricular shunt consists of a primary catheter, a reservoir, a one-way valve, and the terminal (drainage) catheter. The primary catheter is surgically implanted into the lateral ventricle of the brain. The reservoir collects the fluid and the one-way valve prevents cerebral spinal fluid from flowing back into the brain. Once implanted, the reservoir can be easily palpated through the skin, usually over the mastoid or parietal bone just behind the ear. The terminal (drainage) end of the catheter empties into the jugular vein or in the peritoneal cavity.

Rationale

Increased ICP is a true medical emergency and requires rapid recognition and intervention to prevent brain stem herniation.

Possible Complications

- Plugging of the catheter with clotted blood or other thickened fluid
- Displacement of the primary or terminal end
- Dislodgment or damage to one or more components
- Infection

Emergency Care

1. Recognize signs of increased intracranial pressure.
2. Manage the airway with high-flow oxygen.
3. Intubate and hyperventilate as needed per local protocols.
4. Obtain venous access, but limit flow rate.
5. A plugged shunt may be pumped (per local protocol and medical direction).
   A. Locate the reservoir with palpation.
   B. Using one or two fingers, gently compress and release the reservoir several times.
   C. Pumping the reservoir may provide temporary relief.
   D. Do not delay airway management or rapid transport.

Tip

Early signs of increasing ICP:

- **Headaches**
- **Visual disturbances**
- **Irritability**
- **Vomiting**
- **Nausea**

Late signs of increasing ICP (Cushing's Triad):

- **Rising systolic blood pressure**
- **Abnormal respirations**
- **Bradycardia**

PROCEDURE
Automatic Implantable Cardioverter Defibrillators

Introduction

More than 300,000 people die each year from sudden cardiac death. Of those resuscitated, over 50% will experience a second arrest within 2 years. The automatic implantable cardioverter defibrillator (AICD) was developed for high-risk patients with recurrent ventricular tachycardia or ventricular fibrillation. More than 14,000 have been implanted.

The AICD consists of a pulse generator, sensing electrodes, and two large patches. The unit is capable of sensing and terminating ventricular tachycardia, ventricular fibrillation, and bradyarrhythmias. The device, which is smaller than a deck of cards, is inserted under the skin in the upper chest area, and then wires are tunnelled and inserted into the atria and ventricles. Once implanted, the generator can be palpated under the surface of the skin. The device is programmed to sense tachycardia and the width of QRS complexes. It will discharge when the ventricular rate exceeds set parameters (usually 170 beats/min) for 10 to 30 seconds. The shock is usually set at 25 to 30 joules, and given four times within a 2-minute period. The AICD is then programmed to reset, recharge, and deliver a series of four more shocks after 35 seconds of a normal rhythm has been sensed. Most modern devices are capable not only of defibrillation and cardioversion, but also of pacing.

Rationale

AICDs are used in patients who experience lethal arrhythmias despite medical management to control ventricular tachycardia or ventricular fibrillation.

Possible Complications

♦ Most of the complications with the AICD occur in the inpatient setting. Most are related to a collection of blood at the site of AICD insertion (hematoma) or dislodgment of the wires.

♦ The AICD may fail to fire if it has lost stored energy or battery power; if the sensing electrodes are damaged, disconnected, or displaced; or if the maximum rate is not set correctly despite evidenced ventricular tachycardia or ventricular fibrillation.

♦ The AICD may fire when no discharge is indicated, causing the patient fear and discomfort. The patient may experience a "jolt" because the discharge usually does not cause unconsciousness. It can also discharge because of certain upper extremity movements or for no apparent reason. The greatest danger is that the discharge might cause an "R-on-T phenomenon" and actually cause ventricular tachycardia or ventricular fibrillation. This happens if the leads sense a supraventricular rhythm that is faster than the prescribed parameter. If complications occur, the patient will have to be monitored to determine causes of inappropriate discharges or failures.

Emergency Care

1. The AICD will not interfere with basic life support.
2. Follow the same arrhythmia protocols as for the patient without an AICD.

3. The presence of an AICD is not a contraindication for standard external defibrillation.

4. If the patient has received one or more internal countershocks, initial external shocks should be delivered at the maximum output (follow your local protocols).

5. Paddles or patches should not be placed directly over the generator as this may cause permanent damage to the device.

6. If the first and second external countershocks are unsuccessful, consider using anterior-posterior placement of the defibrillator paddles or patches.

Controversy

While the AICD may discharge while treating a patient, studies show that this is not a hazard as only approximately 2 joules of energy reach the body's surface, causing only a minor shock with no significant danger or physical harm.

Communication Tip

Provide emotional support to the patient and caregiver on any AICD-related call.

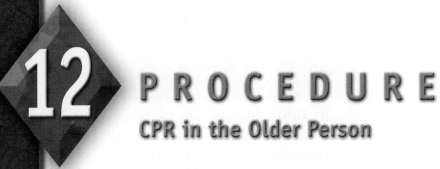

PROCEDURE
CPR in the Older Person

Introduction

The primary cause of cardiac arrest or "sudden death" in the older population is usually a lethal cardiac arrhythmia, such as ventricular fibrillation or pulseless ventricular tachycardia. As a result, successful resuscitation requires early defibrillation. Defibrillation is far more likely to be effective if adequate cardiopulmonary resuscitation (CPR) is initiated rapidly. Early initiation of effective CPR is the most important treatment for cardiac arrest in an older person until an automated external defibrillator (AED) or advanced life support personnel are available.

Rationale

CPR is administered to patients who are in cardiac arrest in an effort to restore breathing.

Preparation

1. Place the patient supine on a firm surface. This may dictate moving the patient, or placing a backboard under the patient.
2. Request additional resources, such as an AED, transportation, and advanced cardiac life support (ACLS) backup, as soon as possible.

Tip

The risk of injury to someone who receives CPR unnecessarily is far less than the risk of death to a cardiac arrest victim who does not receive CPR rapidly.

Indications

Unresponsive, apneic, and pulseless

Contraindications

- Signs of circulation
- Spontaneous breathing
- Movement
- Coughing
- Palpable carotid pulse

Equipment

- Body substance isolation equipment
- Gloves
- Eye protection
- Barrier device with one-way-valve or BVM device with supplemental oxygen
- Appropriate size mask
- Airway adjuncts
- AED

Controversy

There is no set standard defining what is considered a "futile" attempt at resuscitation outside of the obvious signs of irreversible biological death (such as rigor mortis and dependent lividity). Therefore, resuscitation should be initiated even in situations where resuscitation seems unlikely.

Procedure

1. *Initial Assessment:* Establish responsiveness of the patient. If the patient is unresponsive, activate EMS.

2. *Airway:* Open the airway using the head tilt-chin lift maneuver if no spinal injury is suspected. If trauma is suspected, use the jaw-thrust maneuver. Remove any obvious obstructions, such as dentures, food, or vomit.

3. *Breathing:* With the airway already open, look, listen, and feel for breathing. If spontaneous breathing is absent, or inadequate (such as agonal respirations), begin rescue breathing with two slow breaths. Provide a ventilatory volume that is sufficient to cause the chest to gently rise and fall. Provide rescue breathing at a rate of one breath every five seconds, or 10 to 12 breaths/min. Patients who are found to be breathing spontaneously should be placed in the recovery position unless spinal injury is suspected. Be sure to monitor the patient for any change in condition.

4. *Circulation:* Check for signs of circulation. If there is no pulse, begin chest compressions. Provide compressions at a rate of approximately 100 per minute using a 15 compressions to 2 ventilations ratio. Remember, 15:2 is the correct ratio for both one- and two-person adult CPR for patients who are not intubated. The depth of compression should be that which is adequate to produce a palpable carotid pulse (about $1\frac{1}{2}$ to 2 inches). Do not use the "chest compression only" CPR technique. This technique is only appropriate when a rescuer is unwilling or unable to perform rescue breathing, such as dispatcher-assisted CPR with an untrained caller.

5. *Reassessment:* Perform four complete cycles of 15:2 compressions and ventilations, then reassess the patient for signs of breathing and circulation.

6. *Second EMS provider:* When a second EMS provider becomes available, he or she should assist in two-rescuer CPR by taking over chest compressions.

7. *AED:* Use of an AED should be initiated without delay as soon as it is available. It is appropriate to continue CPR until the AED is attached and ready to analyze the patient's rhythm. Do not delay use of the AED to finish a cycle of CPR.

> **Tip**
>
> Do not allow the fear of harming the patient prevent you from performing effective CPR. Even the best CPR will provide only a fraction of normal cardiac output. The CPR you provide must be proficient if the patient is to have any chance of survival.

> **Tip**
>
> Do not delay CPR to determine the status of the patient's do not resuscitate (DNR) order. Every state that allows EMS providers to recognize a DNR order requires that it be verified in some way. Become familiar with your local and state protocols.

Possible Complications

- Gastric distention
- Vomiting
- Rib fracture
- Fractured sternum
- Punctured lung
- Lung contusion
- Laceration of the liver
- Ruptured spleen

> **Tip**
>
> Complications from CPR can be greatly reduced in the older patient by providing slow breaths (about two seconds each) and proper hand position while performing chest compressions.

PROCEDURE

Death Notification

Introduction

As the older population grows, so will the number of out-of-hospital deaths involving DNR orders. Prehospital professionals are being called upon more frequently to make the notification of death to family members. Unlike many paramedic skills, it is not possible to develop a step-by-step skill sheet to follow when making a death notification. Each situation must be evaluated independently for the best approach. In all cases, the EMS provider's approach should be based on the following factors:

1. Provider safety
2. Compassion
3. Unmistakable terms

Safety

It is not always possible to predict how people will respond to the news that a loved one has died. Many people tend to internalize their grief, or connect with other family members for support. Some people may act out in a more physical manner, presenting a potential risk to the EMS provider. Someone who acts out physically following a death notification may or may not actually intend harm to the person making the notification. When making the notification, position yourself near an exit, but not directly between the survivor and the exit.

Compassion

Death notification should not be made in a group setting. Determine who is who among the survivors. Identify the most immediate family member or members, and locate a private place to make the notification. Often, the closest family member will prefer to tell the others in his or her own way.

Do not just "wing it." Consider what you will say in advance, but do not deliver the news in a rehearsed or detached manner. Do not stand over the survivor; place yourself at eye level when possible. Using soft eye contact and a gentle touch (holding their hand or touching their shoulder) while delivering the news will help express your genuine concern for their well-being. If the family member is alone, take the time to contact a friend, family member, neighbor, or clergy member to provide support. Many EMS systems have internal social service resources that can respond directly to the scene and offer additional support.

> **Tip**
>
> In some cases, family members may request time with the patient to say goodbye. This is a very important part of the grief process, and should be allowed when possible.

Unmistakable Terms

Introduce yourself by name and title, for example, "My name is Nathan. I'm a paramedic with the fire department." Use very clear, understandable terms such as "died" or "dead." In some cases, the survivor may not comprehend your meaning at first. Make certain they understand what you are telling them. Do not use platitudes. Platitudes are trite remarks delivered with the intention of sounding profound, but that in reality mean nothing. Examples of platitudes include "He is in a better place now" or "She will always be with you." There is nothing wrong with the survivors expressing such beliefs, but it is not appropriate for EMS providers to do so. In fact, some survivors may take offense at such remarks.

Let the survivors know that there was nothing more that could have been done. Offer the full resources of your agency, such as spending additional time on the scene, offering to make phone calls to family members, providing transportation, or requesting social service intervention. Let the survivor know what to expect next, such as the arrival of local authorities, the medical examiner, or coroner.

Tip

Once resuscitation attempts have been discontinued, your immediate concern becomes the well-being of the survivors. The survivors should be able to expect your support as they come to grips with the loss of a loved one. Occasionally, survivors may develop a medical condition that requires your medical attention. Do not forget about this important part of your role as an EMS provider. Your handling of the situation will undoubtedly be remembered by the survivors for some time to come.

Controversy

Each EMS system has its own protocol for when field termination of resuscitation is appropriate. It is important to have a clear understanding of what is expected from your EMS system and medical director. Check your local protocol.

Tip

Physical manifestations of grief include thrashing, kicking, running, or throwing things. Be prepared for anything when making a death notification. Deliver the news in a safe environment for you and the survivor.

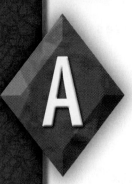

APPENDIX

Organizations and Services for Older People

For a complete listing of resources, including addresses, telephone numbers, and websites for older people, go to www.GEMSsite.com.

General Aging Resources

Administration on Aging
Washington, DC

Aging Network Services
Bethesda, MD

Alzheimer's Association
Chicago, IL

American Association of Homes and
  Services for the Aged
Washington, DC

American Association of Retired Persons
Washington, DC

American Federation for Aging Research
New York, NY

American Geriatrics Society
New York, NY

American Senior Fitness Association
New Smyrna Beach, FL

American Seniors Housing Association
Washington, DC

American Society on Aging
San Francisco, CA

ARCH National Respite Network
Chapel Hill, NC

Assisted Living Federation of America
Fairfax, VA

Children of Aging Parents
Levittown, PA

Family Caregivers Alliance
San Francisco, CA

Gerontological Society of America
Washington, DC

Hospice Foundation of America
Washington, DC

Indian Health Services
Rockville, MD

National Adult Day Services Association
McLean, VA

National Aphasia Association
Millersville, MD

National Asian Pacific Center on Aging
Seattle, WA

National Association of Area Agencies
  on Aging
Washington, DC

National Association for Home Care
Washington, DC

National Association of State Units on Aging
Washington, DC

National Center on Elder Abuse
Washington, DC

National Citizens' Coalition for
  Nursing Home Reform
Washington, DC

National Council on Aging
Washington, DC

National Hospice Foundation
Alexandria, VA

National Institute on Aging
Bethesda, MD

National Stroke Association
Englewood, CO

US Bureau of the Census
Suitland, MD

APPENDIX B
Medication Guide

In order for medications to work properly, they must be taken correctly. Many things can affect how medications work:

♦ Diet—some foods affect the effectiveness of medicine.
♦ Lifestyle—standing up, lying down, and even the time a medicine is taken may be important.
♦ Other medications—drug-to-drug interactions are a concern. Some interactions may cause serious medical conditions.

Because older people take many medications, they are more likely to experience medication interactions. Also, the medications they take may affect their medical treatment at the hospital. For these reasons, it is important for you to collect a thorough medication history from all older patients. However, patients may not have this information readily available, making it difficult or impossible for you to obtain.

When interacting with older people, you have an opportunity that many health care providers do not—you observe the person first hand. If the patient is not transported to the emergency department, you may be the only person who interacts with him or her. You can affect how well older patients keep track of their medications by photocopying the reverse side of this page and distributing it to older patients when time permits. Explain to your older patients the importance of keeping track of their medications, and ask them to use the form. This measure takes only a minute, but may save a life.

My Drug and Supplement Diary

In order for medications to work properly, they must be taken correctly. Many things affect how medications work:

Diet—some foods affect how well a medicine works

Lifestyle—standing up, lying down, and the time of day when a medication is taken are important

Other medications—drug-to-drug interactions are a concern. Some interactions may cause serious medical conditions.

Make sure that your doctor knows exactly what drug you are taking, including non-prescription drugs and any dietary supplements such as vitamins, minerals, and herbals. Use this form to write down what medications you are taking, the dosage, and when you take it. Be sure to keep this record up-to-date, and to keep a copy with you at all times, as well as a copy at home.

By providing your doctor with this completed record during each of your appointments, you are ensuring that they are able to properly prescribe medications for you.

_____

Your Name

_____

Address

_____

Phone Number

_____

Doctor's Name

_____

Doctor's Phone Number

Name _____
Dose _____ When Taken _____

Name _____
Dose _____ When Taken _____

Name _____
Dose _____ When Taken _____

Name _____
Dose _____ When Taken _____

Name _____
Dose _____ When Taken _____

Name _____
Dose _____ When Taken _____

Name _____
Dose _____ When Taken _____

Name _____
Dose _____ When Taken _____

Name _____
Dose _____ When Taken _____

Name _____
Dose _____ When Taken _____

Resource produced by:

The AGS Foundation for Health in Aging
The Empire State Building
350 Fifth Avenue, Suite 801
New York, NY 10118
212-775-6810
email staff@healthinaging.org   www.healthinaging.org

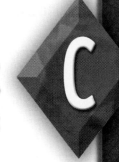
Use this checklist from the U.S. Consumer Product Safety Commission (CPSC) to spot possible safety problems that may be present in your home. Check YES or NO to answer each question. Then go back over the list and take action to correct those items that may need attention. Keep this checklist as a reminder of safe practices, and use it periodically to re-check your home.

This checklist is organized by areas in the home. However, there are some potential hazards that need to be checked in more than just one area of your home. These are highlighted at the beginning of the checklist and short reminders are included in other sections of the checklist.

ALL AREAS OF THE HOME

In all areas of your home, check all electrical and telephone cords; rugs, runners and mats; telephone areas; smoke detectors; electrical outlets and switches; light bulbs; space heaters; woodburning stoves; and your emergency exit plan.

CHECK ALL CORDS

1. **QUESTION:** Are lamp, extension, and telephone cords placed out of the flow of traffic?

   YES ___ NO ___

RECOMMENDATION: Cords stretched across walkways may cause someone to trip.

   ♦ Arrange furniture so that outlets are available for lamps and appliances without the use of extension cords.

   ♦ If you must use an extension cord, place it on the floor against a wall where people cannot trip over it.

   ♦ Move the phone so that telephone cords will not lie where people walk.

2. **QUESTION:** Are cords out from beneath furniture and rugs or carpeting?

   YES ___ NO ___

RECOMMENDATION: Furniture resting on cords can damage them, creating fire and shock hazards. Electric cords which run under carpeting may cause a fire.

   ♦ Remove cords from under furniture or carpeting.

   ♦ Replace damaged or frayed cords.

3. **QUESTION:** Are cords attached to the walls, baseboards, etc., with nails or staples?

   YES ___ NO ___

RECOMMENDATION: Nails or staples can damage cords, presenting fire and shock hazards.

   ♦ Remove nails, staples, etc.

   ♦ Check wiring for damage.

   ♦ Use tape to attach cords to walls or floors.

4. **QUESTION:** Are electrical cords in good condition, not frayed or cracked?

   YES ___ NO ___

RECOMMENDATION: Damaged cords may cause a shock or fire.

   ♦ Replace frayed or cracked cords.

5. **QUESTION:** Do extension cords carry more than their proper load, as indicated by the ratings labeled on the cord and the appliance?

   YES ___ NO ___

RECOMMENDATION: Overloaded extension cords may cause fires. Standard 18 gauge extension cords can carry 1250 watts.

   ♦ If the rating on the cord is exceeded because of the power requirements of one or more appliances being used on the cord, change the cord to a higher rated one or unplug some appliances.

   ♦ If an extension cord is needed, use one having a sufficient amp or wattage rating.

CHECK ALL RUGS, RUNNERS, AND MATS

1. **QUESTION:** Are all small rugs and runners slip-resistant?

   YES ___ NO ___

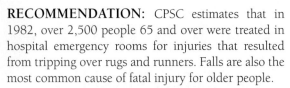

RECOMMENDATION: CPSC estimates that in 1982, over 2,500 people 65 and over were treated in hospital emergency rooms for injuries that resulted from tripping over rugs and runners. Falls are also the most common cause of fatal injury for older people.

♦ Remove rugs and runners that tend to slide.

♦ Apply double-faced adhesive carpet tape or rubber matting to the backs of rugs and runners.

♦ Purchase rugs with slip-resistant backing.

♦ Check rugs and mats periodically to see if backing needs to be replaced.

♦ Place rubber matting under rugs. (Rubber matting that can be cut to size is available.)

♦ Purchase new rugs with slip-resistant backing.

NOTE: Over time, adhesive on tape can wear away. Rugs with slip-resistant backing also become less effective as they are washed. Periodically, check rugs and mats to see if new tape or backing is needed.

2. **QUESTION:** Are emergency numbers posted on or near the telephone?

YES ___ NO ___

RECOMMENDATION: In case of emergency, telephone numbers for the police, fire department, and local poison control center, along with a neighbor's number, should be readily available.

♦ Write the numbers in large print and tape them to the phone, or place them near the phone where they can be seen easily.

3. **QUESTION:** Do you have access to a telephone if you fall (or experience some other emergency which prevents you from standing and reaching a wall phone)?

YES ___ NO ___

RECOMMENDATION:

♦ Have at least one telephone located where it would be accessible in the event of an accident which leaves you unable to stand.

CHECK SMOKE DETECTORS

1. **QUESTION:** Are smoke detectors properly located?

YES ___ NO___

RECOMMENDATION: At least one smoke detector should be placed on every floor of your home.

♦ Read the instructions that come with the smoke detector for advice on the best place to install it.

♦ Make sure detectors are placed near bedrooms, either on the ceiling or 6 to 12 inches below the ceiling on the wall.

♦ Locate smoke detectors away from air vents.

2. **QUESTION:** Do you have properly working smoke detectors?

YES ___ NO ___

RECOMMENDATION: Many home fire injuries and deaths are caused by smoke and toxic gases, rather than the fire itself. Smoke detectors provide an early warning and can wake you in the event of a fire.

♦ Purchase a smoke detector if you do not have one.

♦ Check and replace batteries and bulbs according to the manufacturer's instructions.

♦ Vacuum the grillwork of your smoke detector.

♦ Replace any smoke detectors that cannot be repaired.

NOTE: Some fire departments or local governments will provide assistance in acquiring or installing smoke detectors.

CHECK ELECTRICAL OUTLETS AND SWITCHES

1. **QUESTION:** Are any outlets and switches unusually warm or hot to the touch?

YES ___ NO ___

RECOMMENDATION: Unusually warm or hot outlets or switches may indicate that an unsafe wiring condition exists.

♦ Unplug cords from outlets and do not use the switches.

♦ Have an electrician check the wiring as soon as possible.

2. **QUESTION:** Do all outlets and switches have cover plates, so that no wiring is exposed?

YES ___ NO ___

RECOMMENDATION: Exposed wiring presents a shock hazard.

♦ Add a cover plate.

3. **QUESTION:** Are light bulbs the appropriate size and type for the lamp or fixture?

YES ___ NO ___

RECOMMENDATION: A bulb of too high wattage or the wrong type may lead to fire through overheating. Ceiling fixtures, recessed lights, and "hooded" lamps will trap heat.

♦ Replace with a bulb of the correct type and wattage. (If you do not know the correct wattage, use a bulb no larger than 60 watts.)

CHECK SPACE HEATERS

1. **QUESTION:** Are heaters which come with a 3-prong plug being used in a 3-hole outlet or with a properly attached adapter?

   YES ___ NO ___

RECOMMENDATION: The grounding feature provided by a 3-hole receptacle or an adapter for a 2-hole receptacle is a safety feature designed to lessen the risk of shock.

♦ Never defeat the grounding feature.

♦ If you do not have a 3-hole outlet, use an adapter to connect the heater's 3-prong plug. Make sure the adapter ground wire or tab is attached to the outlet.

2. **QUESTION:** Are small stoves and heaters placed where they cannot be knocked over, and away from furnishings and flammable materials, such as curtains or rugs?

   YES ___ NO ___

RECOMMENDATION: Heaters can cause fires or serious burns if they cause you to trip or if they are knocked over.

♦ Relocate heaters away from passageways and flammable materials such as curtains, rugs, and furniture.

3. **QUESTION:** If your home has space heating equipment, such as a kerosene heater, a gas heater, or an LP [liquid propane] gas heater, do you understand the installation and operating instructions thoroughly?

   YES ___ NO ___

RECOMMENDATION: Unvented heaters should be used with room doors open or windows slightly open to provide ventilation. The correct fuel, as recommended by the manufacturer, should always be used. Vented heaters should have proper venting, and the venting system should be checked frequently. Improper venting is the most frequent cause of carbon monoxide poisoning, and older consumers are at special risk.

♦ Review the installation and operating instructions.

♦ Call your local fire department if you have additional questions.

CHECK WOODBURNING HEATING EQUIPMENT

1. **QUESTION:** Is woodburning equipment installed properly?

   YES ___ NO ___

RECOMMENDATION: Woodburning stoves should be installed by a qualified person according to local building codes.

♦ Local building code officials or fire marshals can provide requirements and recommendations for installation.

NOTE: Some insurance companies will not cover fire losses if wood stoves are not installed according to local codes.

CHECK THE EMERGENCY EXIT PLAN

1. **QUESTION:** Do you have an emergency exit plan and an alternate emergency exit plan in case of a fire?

   YES ___ NO ___

RECOMMENDATION: Once a fire starts, it spreads rapidly. Since you may not have much time to get out and there may be a lot of confusion, it is important that everyone knows what to do.

♦ Develop an emergency exit plan.

♦ Choose a meeting place outside your home so you can be sure that everyone is capable of escape quickly and safely.

♦ Practice the plan from time to time to make sure everyone is capable of escape quickly and safely.

Remember periodically to re-check your home.

KITCHEN

In the kitchen, check the range area, all electrical cords, lighting, the stool, all throw rugs and mats, and the telephone area.

CHECK THE RANGE AREA

1. **QUESTION:** Are towels, curtains, and other things that might catch fire located away from the range?

   YES ___ NO ___

RECOMMENDATION: Placing or storing non-cooking equipment like potholders, dish towels, or plastic utensils on or near the range can result in fires or burns.

◆ Store flammable and combustible items away from range and oven.

◆ Remove any towels hanging on oven handles. If towels hang close to a burner, change the location of the towel rack.

◆ If necessary, shorten or remove curtains which could brush against heat sources.

2. **QUESTION:** Do you wear clothing with short or close-fitting sleeves while you are cooking?

YES ___ NO ___

RECOMMENDATION: CPSC estimates that 70% of all people who die from clothing fires are over 65 years of age. Long sleeves are more likely to catch fire than are short sleeves. Long sleeves are also more apt to catch on pot handles, overturning pots and pans and causing scalds.

◆ Roll back long, loose sleeves or fasten them with pins or elastic bands while you are cooking.

3. **QUESTION:** Are kitchen ventilation systems or range exhausts functioning properly and are they in use while you are cooking?

YES ___ NO ___

RECOMMENDATION: Indoor air pollutants may accumulate to unhealthful levels in a kitchen where gas or kerosene-fire appliances are in use.

◆ Use ventilation systems or open windows to clear air of vapors and smoke.

4. **QUESTION:** Are all extension cords and appliance cords located away from the sink or range areas?

YES ___ NO ___

RECOMMENDATION: Electrical appliances and power cords can cause shock or electrocution if they come in contact with water. Cords can also be damaged by excess heat.

◆ Move cords and appliances away from sink areas and hot surfaces.

◆ Move appliances closer to wall outlets or to different outlets so you won't need extension cords.

◆ If extension cords must be used, install wiring guides so that cords will not hang near sink, range, or working areas.

◆ Consider adding new outlets for convenience and safety; ask your electrician to install outlets equipped with ground fault circuit interrupters (GFCIs) to protect against electric shock. A GFCI is a shock-protection device that will detect electrical fault and shut off electricity before serious injury or death occurs.

For more information on cords, refer to the beginning of the checklist.

5. **QUESTION:** Does good, even lighting exist over the stove, sink, and countertop work areas, especially where food is sliced or cut?

YES ___ NO ___

RECOMMENDATION: Low lighting and glare can contribute to burns or cuts. Improve lighting by:

◆ Opening curtains and blinds (unless this causes too much glare).

◆ Using the maximum wattage bulb allowed by the fixture. (If you do not know the correct wattage for the fixture, use a bulb no larger than 60 watts.)

◆ Reducing glare by using frosted bulbs, indirect lighting, shades or globes on light fixtures, or partially closing the blinds or curtains.

◆ Installing additional light fixtures, eg, under cabinet/over countertop lighting. (Make sure that the bulbs you use are the right type and wattage for the light fixture.)

6. **QUESTION:** Do you have a step stool which is stable and in good repair?

YES ___ NO ___

RECOMMENDATION: Standing on chairs, boxes, or other makeshift items to reach high shelves can result in falls. CPSC estimates that in 1982, 1,500 people over 65 were treated in hospital emergency rooms when they fell from chairs on which they were standing.

◆ If you don't have a step stool, consider buying one. Choose one with a handrail that you can hold onto while standing on the top step.

◆ Before climbing on any step stool, make sure it is fully opened and stable.

◆ Tighten screws and braces on the step stool.

◆ Discard step stools with broken parts.

Remember: Check all of the product areas mentioned at the beginning of the checklist.

LIVING ROOM/FAMILY ROOM

In the living room/family room, check all rugs and runners, electrical and telephone cords, lighting, the fireplace and chimney, the telephone area, and all passageways.

1. **QUESTION:** Are chimneys clear from accumulations of leaves and other debris that can clog them?

   YES ___ NO ___

RECOMMENDATION: A clogged chimney can cause a poorly burning fire to result in poisonous fumes and smoke coming back into the house.

   ◆ Do not use the chimney until the blockage has been removed.

   ◆ Have the chimney checked and cleaned by a registered or licensed professional.

2. **QUESTION:** Has the chimney been cleaned within the past year?

   YES ___ NO ___

RECOMMENDATION: Burning wood can cause a buildup of a tarry substance (creosote) inside the chimney. This material can ignite and result in a serious chimney fire.

   ◆ Have the chimney checked and cleaned by a registered or licensed professional.

CHECK THE TELEPHONE AREA

For information on the telephone area, refer to the beginning of the checklist.

CHECK PASSAGEWAYS

1. **QUESTION:** Are hallways, passageways between rooms, and other heavy traffic areas well lit?

   YES ___ NO ___

RECOMMENDATION: Shadowed or dark areas can hide tripping hazards.

   ◆ Use the maximum wattage bulb allowed by the fixture. (If you do not know the correct wattage, use a bulb no larger than 60 watts.)

   ◆ Install night lights.

   ◆ Reduce glare by using frosted bulbs, indirect lighting, shades or globes on light fixtures, or partially closing blinds or curtains.

   ◆ Consider using additional lamps or light fixtures. Make sure that the bulbs you use are the right type and wattage for the light fixture.

2. **QUESTION:** Are exits and passageways kept clear?

   YES ___ NO ___

RECOMMENDATION: Furniture, boxes, or other items could be an obstruction or tripping hazard, especially in the event of an emergency or fire.

   ◆ Rearrange furniture to open passageways and walkways.

   ◆ Remove boxes and clutter.

Remember: Check all of the product areas mentioned at the beginning of the checklist.

BATHROOM

In the bathroom, check bathtub and shower areas, water temperature, rugs and mats, lighting, small electrical appliances, and storage areas for medications.

CHECK BATHTUB AND SHOWER AREAS

1. **QUESTION:** Are bathtubs and showers equipped with non-skid mats, abrasive strips, or surfaces that are not slippery?

   YES ___ NO ___

RECOMMENDATION: Wet soapy tile or porcelain surfaces are especially slippery and may contribute to falls.

   ◆ Apply textured strips or appliques on the floors of tubs and showers.

   ◆ Use non-skid mats in the tub and shower, and on the bathroom floor.

2. **QUESTION:** Do bathtubs and showers have at least one (preferably two) grab bars?

   YES ___ NO ___

RECOMMENDATION: Grab bars can help you get into and out of your tub or shower, and can help prevent falls.

   ◆ Check existing bars for strength and stability, and repair if necessary.

   ◆ Attach grab bars, through the tile, to structural supports in the wall, or install bars specifically designed to attach to the sides of the bathtub. If you are not sure how it is done, get someone who is qualified to assist you.

3. **QUESTION:** Is the temperature 120°F or lower?

   YES ___ NO ___

RECOMMENDATION: Water temperature above 120°F can cause tap water scalds.

   ◆ Lower the setting on your hot water heater to "Low" or 120°F. If you are unfamiliar with the controls of your water heater, ask a qualified person to adjust it for you. If your hot water system is controlled by the landlord, ask the landlord to consider lowering the setting.

NOTE: If the water heater does not have a temperature setting, you can use a thermometer to check the temperature of the water at the tap.

♦ Always check water temperature by hand before entering bath or shower.

♦ Taking baths, rather than showers, reduces the risk of a scald from suddenly changing water temperatures.

CHECK LIGHTING

1. **QUESTION:** Is a light switch located near the entrance to the bathroom?

   YES ___ NO ___

RECOMMENDATION: A light switch near the door will prevent you from walking through a dark area.

♦ Install a night light. Inexpensive lights that plug into outlets are available.

♦ Consider replacing the existing switch with a "glow switch" that can be seen in the dark.

CHECK SMALL ELECTRICAL APPLIANCES

1. **QUESTION:** Are small electrical appliances such as hair dryers, shavers, curling irons, etc., unplugged when not in use?

   YES ___ NO ___

RECOMMENDATION: Even an appliance that is not turned on, such as a hairdryer, can be potentially hazardous if it is left plugged in. If it falls into water in a sink or bathtub while plugged in, it could cause a lethal shock.

♦ Unplug all small appliances when not in use.

♦ Never reach into water to retrieve an appliance that has fallen in without being sure the appliance is unplugged.

♦ Install a ground fault circuit interrupter (GFCI) in your bathroom outlet to protect against electric shock.

CHECK MEDICATIONS

1. **QUESTION:** Are all medicines stored in the containers that they came in and are they clearly marked?

   YES ___ NO ___

RECOMMENDATION: Medications that are not clearly and accurately labeled can be easily mixed up. Taking the wrong medicine or missing a dosage of medicine you need can be dangerous.

♦ Be sure that all containers are clearly marked with the contents, doctor's instructions, expiration date, and patient's name.

♦ Dispose of outdated medicines properly.

♦ Request non–child-resistant closures from your pharmacist only when you cannot use child-resistant closures.

NOTE: Many poisonings occur when children visiting grandparents go through the medicine cabinet or grandmother's purse. In homes where grandchildren or other youngsters are frequent visitors, medicines should be purchased in containers with child-resistant caps, and the caps properly closed after each use. Store medicines beyond the reach of children.

Remember: Check all of the product areas mentioned at the beginning of the checklist.

BEDROOMS

In the bedroom, check all rugs and runners, electrical and telephone cords, and areas around beds.

CHECK AREAS AROUND BEDS

1. **QUESTION:** Are lamps or light switches within reach of each bed?

   YES ___ NO ___

RECOMMENDATION: Lamps or switches located close to each bed will enable people getting up at night to see where they are going.

♦ Rearrange furniture closer to switches or move lamps closer to beds.

♦ Install night lights.

2. **QUESTION:** Are ash trays, smoking materials, or other fire sources (heaters, hot plates, teapots, etc.) located away from beds or bedding?

   YES ___ NO ___

RECOMMENDATION: Burns are a leading cause of accidental death among seniors. Smoking in bed is a major contributor to this problem. Among mattress and bedding fire related deaths in a recent year, 42% were to persons 65 or older.

♦ Remove sources of heat or flame from areas around beds.

♦ Don't smoke in bed.

3. **QUESTION:** Is anything covering your electric blanket when in use?

YES ___ NO ___

RECOMMENDATION: "Tucking in" electric blankets, or placing additional coverings on top of them can cause excessive heat buildup which can start a fire.

♦ Avoid "tucking in" the sides or ends of your electric blanket.

♦ Use electric blankets according to the manufacturer's instructions.

♦ Don't allow anything on top of the blanket while it is in use. (This includes other blankets or comforters, even pets sleeping on top of the blanket.)

♦ Don't set electric blankets so high that they could burn someone who falls asleep while they are on.

4. **QUESTION:** Do you ever go to sleep with a heating pad that is turned on?

YES ___ NO ___

RECOMMENDATION: Never go to sleep with a heating pad if it is turned on because it can cause serious burns even at relatively low settings.

5. **QUESTION:** Is there a telephone close to your bed?

YES ___ NO ___

RECOMMENDATION: In case of an emergency, it is important to be able to reach the telephone without getting out of bed.

Remember: Check all of the product areas mentioned at the beginning of the checklist.

BASEMENT/GARAGE/ WORKSHOP/STORAGE AREAS

In the basement, garage, workshop, and storage areas, check lighting, fuse boxes or circuit breakers, appliances and power tools, electrical cords, and flammable liquids.

CHECK LIGHTING

1. **QUESTION:** Are work areas, especially areas where power tools are used, well lit?

YES ___ NO ___

RECOMMENDATION: Power tools were involved in over 5,200 injuries treated in hospital emergency rooms to people 65 and over in 1982. Three fourths of these were finger injuries. Good lighting can reduce the chance that you will accidentally cut your finger.

♦ Either install additional light, or avoid working with power tools in the area.

2. **QUESTION:** Can you turn on the lights without first having to walk through a dark area?

YES ___ NO ___

RECOMMENDATION: Basement, garages, and storage areas can contain many tripping hazards and sharp or pointed tools that can make a fall even more hazardous.

♦ Keep an operating flashlight handy.

♦ Have an electrician install switches at each entrance to a dark area.

CHECK THE FUSE BOX OR CIRCUIT BREAKERS

1. **QUESTION:** If fuses are used, are they the correct size for the circuit?

YES ___ NO ___

RECOMMENDATION: Replacing a correct size fuse with a larger size fuse can present a serious fire hazard. If the fuse in the box is rated higher than that intended for the circuit, excessive current will be allowed to flow and possibly overload the outlet and house wiring to the point that a fire can begin.

♦ Be certain that correct-size fuses are used. (If you do not know the correct sizes, consider having an electrician identify and label the sizes to be used.)

NOTE: If all, or nearly all, fuses used are 30-amp fuses, there is a chance that some of the fuses are rated too high for the circuit.

CHECK APPLIANCES AND POWER TOOLS

1. **QUESTION:** Are power tools equipped with a 3-prong plug or marked to show that they are double insulated?

YES ___ NO ___

RECOMMENDATION: These safety features reduce the risk of an electric shock.

♦ Use a properly connected 3-prong adapter for connecting a 3-prong plug to a 2-hole receptacle.

♦ Consider replacing old tools that have neither a 3-prong plug nor are double insulated.

2. **QUESTION:** Are power tool guards in place?

YES ___ NO ___

RECOMMENDATION: Power tools used with guards removed pose a serious risk of injury from sharp edges or moving parts.

♦ Replace guards that have been removed from power tools.

3. **QUESTION:** Has the grounding feature on any 3-prong plug been defeated by removal of the grounding pin or by improperly using an adapter?

YES ___ NO ___

RECOMMENDATION: Improperly grounded appliances can lead to electric shock.

♦ Check with your service person or an electrician if you are in doubt.

CHECK FLAMMABLE AND VOLATILE LIQUIDS

1. **QUESTION:** Are containers of volatile liquids tightly capped?

YES ___ NO ___

RECOMMENDATION: If not tightly closed, vapors may escape that may be toxic when inhaled.

♦ Check containers periodically to make sure they are tightly closed.

NOTE: CPSC has reports of several cases in which gasoline, stored as much as 10 feet from a gas water heater, exploded. Many people are unaware that gas fumes can travel that far.

2. **QUESTION:** Are gasoline, paints, solvents, or other products that give off vapors or fumes stored away from ignition sources?

YES ___ NO ___

RECOMMENDATION: Gasoline, kerosene, and other flammable liquids should be stored out of living areas in properly labeled, non-glass safety containers.

♦ Remove these products from the areas near heat or flame such as heaters, furnaces, water heaters, ranges, and other gas appliances.

STAIRS

For all stairways, check lighting, handrails, and the condition of the steps and coverings.

CHECK LIGHTING

1. **QUESTION:** Are stairs well lighted?

YES ___ NO ___

RECOMMENDATION: Stairs should be lighted so that each step, particularly the step edges, can be clearly seen while going up and down stairs. The lighting should not produce glare or shadows along the stairway.

♦ Use the maximum wattage bulb allowed by the light fixture. (If you do not know the correct wattage, use a bulb no larger than 60 watts.)

♦ Reduce glare by using frosted bulbs, indirect lighting, shades or globes on light fixtures, or partially closing blinds and curtains.

♦ Have a qualified person add additional light fixtures. Make sure that the bulbs you use are the right type and wattage for the light fixture.

2. **QUESTION:** Are light switches located at both the top and bottom of the stairs?

RECOMMENDATION: Even if you are very familiar with the stairs, lighting is an important factor in preventing falls. You should be able to turn on the lights before you use the stairway from either end.

♦ If no other light is available, keep an operating flashlight in a convenient location at the top and bottom of the stairs.

♦ Install night lights at nearby outlets.

♦ Consider installing switches at the top and bottom of the stairs.

3. **QUESTION:** Do the steps allow secure footing?

YES ___ NO ___

RECOMMENDATION: Worn treads or worn or loose carpeting can lead to insecure footing, resulting in slips or falls.

♦ Try to avoid wearing only socks or smooth-soled shoes or slippers when using stairs.

♦ Make certain the carpet is firmly attached to the steps all along the stairs.

♦ Consider refinishing or replacing worn treads, or replacing worn carpeting.

♦ Paint outside steps with paint that has a rough texture, or use abrasive strips.

4. **QUESTION:** Are steps even and of the same size and height?

YES ___ NO ___

RECOMMENDATION: Even a small difference in step surfaces or riser heights can lead to falls.

♦ Mark any steps which are especially narrow or have risers that are higher or lower than the others. Be especially careful of these steps when using the stairs.

5. **QUESTION:** Are the coverings on the steps in good condition?

YES ___ NO ___

RECOMMENDATION: Worn or torn coverings or nails sticking out from coverings could snag your foot or cause you to trip.

♦ Repair coverings.

♦ Remove coverings.

♦ Replace coverings.

6. **QUESTION:** Can you clearly see the edges of the steps?

YES ___ NO ___

RECOMMENDATION: Falls may occur if the edges of the steps are blurred or hard to see.

♦ Paint edges of outdoor steps white to see them better at night.

♦ Add extra lighting.

♦ If you plan to carpet your stairs, avoid deep pile carpeting or patterned or dark colored carpeting that can make it difficult to see the edges of the steps clearly.

7. **QUESTION:** Is anything stored on the stairway, even temporarily?

YES ___ NO ___

RECOMMENDATION: People can trip over objects left on stairs, particularly in the event of an emergency or fire.

♦ Remove all objects from the stairway.

REMEMBER PERIODICALLY TO RE-CHECK YOUR HOME.

Source: U.S. Consumer Product-Safety Commission. Safety for older consumers home safety checklist; CPSC Document 701. Washington, DC: Available at: http://www.cpsc.gov/cpscpub/pubs/701.html.

Glossary

A

abandonment As it relates to elder abuse, a situation in which an older person is left at the emergency department by a family member or caretaker.

acetabulum The depression on the lateral pelvis where its three component bones join, in which the femoral head fits snugly; hip socket.

active adult community A community that offers age-restricted housing specifically for seniors who enjoy participating in physical and social activities. Also called active adult living and active retirement community.

active metabolites Byproducts of a drug, after it has been partially or fully degraded, that have drug effects on the body.

active neglect The refusal or failure to fulfill a caretaking obligation; a conscious or intentional attempt to inflict physical or emotional stress. Examples include abandonment and denial of food- or health-related services.

activities of daily living (ADLs) Basic everyday activities needed to sustain life, such as feeding oneself, walking, dressing, getting up from a chair, and toileting.

acute myocardial infarction (AMI) Heart attack; death of heart muscle following obstruction of blood flow to it. Acute in this context means "new" or "happening right now."

acute pain Pain with a rapid onset; the body's means of indicating the presence of a new injury.

acute pulmonary edema Fluid accumulation in the lungs.

acute respiratory distress syndrome (ARDS) A condition of severe lung injury after an acute event such as smoke inhalation, near drowning, aspiration, or severe bloodstream infection (sepsis).

addiction An overwhelming desire or need to continue using a substance at whatever cost with a tendency to increase the amount or dose.

Adult Protective Services (APS) An organization that investigates cases involving abuse and neglect and provides case management services in some instances.

advance directive Written documentation that specifies medical treatment for a competent patient should the patient become unable to make decisions.

adverse drug withdrawal event (ADWE) A set of clinical signs or symptoms caused by discontinuing a drug.

ageism Stereotyping of, and discrimination against, people who are old.

alopecia Hair loss, especially from the head, suggestive of normal aging (as opposed to traumatic alopecia, indicative of abuse).

Alzheimer's care facility Specialized facilities for those with signs of Alzheimer's disease or dementia.

andropause A lessening of testosterone and sexual activity in males later in life; also known as male menopause.

anemia A deficiency in red blood cells or hemoglobin in the blood, resulting in a decrease in oxygen delivery to the tissues.

aneurysm A swelling or enlargement of part of a blood vessel, resulting from weakening of the vessel wall.

angina pectoris Chest pain or discomfort due to inadequate blood and oxygen supply to the heart tissue.

anhedonia The sense that nothing is enjoyable anymore.

anorexia Lack of appetite.

anticholinergic Medications with properties that, among other effects, block the parasympathetic nerves. Common drugs of this type include diphenhydramine (Benadryl), at-ropine, and certain tricyclic antidepressants.

aphasia A language impairment that causes the inability to understand or produce speech; aphasia is caused by injury to the brain, most commonly, stroke.

apraxia An impairment in carrying out purposeful movements, and which can also manifest as a speech impairment, with inability to produce speech with the correct rhythm and timing, as well as highly inconsistent errors.

Area Agency on Aging (AAA) A basic and universal resource that provides information services for older people; AAAs have senior information programs that track all resources in the community, and sponsor nutrition programs, senior centers and transportation services.

arrhythmia An abnormal or irregular heart rhythm resulting from an electrical disturbance in conduction. Atrial fibrillation, bradyarrhythmia, ventricular fibrillation, and ventricular tachycardia are arrhythmias.

arterial ulceration The presence of an ulcer, or disintegrated tissue, caused by a decrease in oxygen supply to that tissue; usually located in the toe or anterior tibial area.

ascites Fluid in the abdomen.

aspiration pneumonia Pneumonia resulting from inhaling an object or secretions into the lungs.

assisted living A residential facility that provides residents with assistance with activities of daily living. Also known as residential care, board and care, and boarding house.

asthma Acute constriction of the air passages in the lungs.

atelectasis Partial lung collapse.

atherosclerosis A disorder in which cholesterol and calcium build up inside the walls of the blood vessels, forming plaque, which eventually leads to partial or complete blockage of blood flow. An atherosclerotic plaque can also become a site where blood clots can form, break off, and embolize elsewhere in the circulation.

atrial fibrillation Disorganized contraction of the atria, often described as chaotic twitching, that results in ineffective pumping of blood into the ventricles.

atrophy Wasting or shrinkage of an organ.

audiologist A health care professional who evaluates and tests people with hearing difficulties and rehabilitates those whose impaired hearing cannot be improved medically or surgically.

autonomy The right of an individual to make choices freely, in accordance with the individual's own goals and values.

B

baroreceptors Sensory mechanisms in the aortic arch and carotid sinus that sense blood pressure changes and trigger a response to adjust the pressure.

Battle's sign Bruising behind the ear over the mastoid process that may indicate skull fracture.

bereavement An extremely stressful time after a loss during which grief is experienced, and includes the adaptation to that loss. Bereavement increases the risk of sleep disorders, suicide attempts, substance abuse (including alcohol, tobacco, and illicit drugs), and overall mortality.

beta blocker A heart medication that blocks the activity of a beta receptor in the heart and smooth muscle; used to control hypertension, anxiety, and various heart conditions, and to reduce the risk of a second heart attack.

biliary colic Sharp or crampy right upper quadrant pain that may radiate to the back and right shoulder; a classic symptom of gallbladder disease.

bilious Characterized by or relating to bile.

bowel perforation An opening or hole in the tissue of the bowel, which can be a complication of peptic ulcer disease, which occurs more commonly in older patients.

brain herniation The protrusion of the brain through the foramen magnum, or the opening at the base of the skull. Critical brain tissue is compressed as this occurs, which is often fatal.

bruit A whooshing sound heard upon auscultation with each heartbeat.

burst fracture A fracture of a vertebra in which pieces of it move out in horizontal directions and may result in spinal cord damage; typically results from a high-energy mechanism, such as a motor vehicle crash or fall from substantial height.

C

candida A fungal organism that usually grows in moist areas such as the groin and other skin folds.

cardiac output Amount of blood pumped out of the heart in 1 minute.

cellulitis A diffuse, acute inflammation within the skin caused by a bacterial infection.

central cord syndrome A condition that causes diminished neurological function in the upper extremities associated with an exaggerated sensation of pain in the arms from light touch, while having normal neurological function in the lower extremities.

chemoreceptor A sensory organ that responds to chemical stimuli.

cholecystitis Infection of the gallbladder.

chronic bronchitis Irritation of the major lung passageways, from either infectious disease or irritants such as smoke.

chronic obstructive pulmonary disease (COPD) A slow process of dilation and disruption of the airways and alveoli, caused by chronic bronchitis, emphysema, or asthma.

chronic pain Pain experienced repeatedly and includes behavioral as well as physical factors.

chronic respiratory failure A recurring condition in which respiratory function is inadequate and can neither maintain enough oxygen to meet the body's demand, nor sufficiently remove carbon dioxide; often a complication of COPD.

cirrhosis A chronic disease of the liver resulting in degenerative changes and death of functioning liver cells.

collagen The substance that makes the skin and other connective tissues strong; both it and elastin decrease with age.

colostomy A diversion involving the colon in which a segment of diseased or injured colon is bypassed or removed and an end or loop of colon is brought through a small opening in the abdominal wall and sutured, forming a stoma.

communication The transmitting of information from a sender to receiver and verification that the receiver received and understood the information.

compression fracture A stable injury in which one bone presses against another and results in a fracture; often only the anterior third of the vertebrae is collapsed, often results from minimal trauma, and is the most common type of spine fracture seen in the older patient population.

contact dermatitis Skin rash caused by contact with an irritating substance.

crackles High-pitched, popping breath sounds that occur during inspiration.

critical incident stress debriefing (CISD) A process that confronts the responses to critical incidents and defuses them, directing the emergency services personnel toward physical and emotional equilibrium.

Cullen's sign Bruising around the umbilicus; seen when there is blood in the free abdominal space (peritoneum).

cyanosis   Skin color that appears bluish or gray in color, caused by decreased levels of oxygen in the blood.

D

deep venous thrombosis (DVT)   A blood clot in the leg or pelvis; may result from prolonged immobility.

delirium tremens   A severe, potentially life-threatening withdrawal syndrome that can occur 24 hours to 1 week after an individual stops drinking.

dementia   Slow onset of progressive disorientation, shortened attention span, memory impairment, and loss of cognitive function.

dependency theory   A theory that attempts to explain the cause of elder abuse; maintains that frailty and medical illness set up the older person for abuse and neglect.

depression   Persistent mood of sadness, despair, discouragement; depression may be a symptom of many different mental and physical disorders, or it may be a disorder on its own.

dermis   The inner, living layer of the skin.

diabetic ketoacidosis (DKA)   A hyperglycemic, acidotic state in which cells resort to burning fat for energy when scarcity of insulin makes glucose use impossible.

diabetic neuropathy   Nerve damage resulting from diabetes, causing pain and sometimes including inflammatory lesions.

diuretics   Medications that cause the body to excrete an increased volume of water; also called water pills.

diverticulitis   Infection of a diverticulum.

diverticulosis   The presence of diverticula (pouch-like protrusions) on the bowel.

do not resuscitate (DNR) order   Written documentation giving permission to medical personnel not to attempt resuscitation in the event of cardiac arrest.

dorsiflex   To flex the foot upward.

duodenum   The first section of the small intestine; begins after the stomach.

durable power of attorney   A type of advance directive that names a future decision maker and anticipates a future situation in which decisions about CPR and other forms of life-sustaining treatment must be made, but the patient is unable at that time to make them. Also called a health care proxy or a health care agent.

dysarthria   A disorder of speech production, resulting from weakness, slowness, or incoordination of the speech mechanism due to damage to the nervous system; speech errors are highly consistent from one occasion to the next.

dyspepsia   A gnawing, burning pain in the upper abdomen.

dyspnea   Difficulty breathing; shortness of breath.

E

ecchymosis   Bruising or discoloration associated with bleeding within or under the skin.

elastin   The substance that makes the skin pliable; both it and collagen decrease with age.

elder abuse   An all-inclusive term representing all types of mistreatment toward older adults; can be an act of commission (abuse) or omission (neglect), intentional or unintentional, and of one or more types: physical, psychological (or emotional), sexual, or financial, resulting in unnecessary suffering, injury, pain, loss or violation of human rights, and decreased quality of life.

emphysema   A disease in which alveoli are destroyed with resulting loss of lung elasticity.

enabling behavior   Someone who promotes a continued self-destructive behavior of an individual. Example: Spouse continues to makes excuses for continued alcohol ingestion, stating "He needs his beer daily to keep him happy."

encephalitis   Infection or inflammation of the brain.

encephalopathy   Any degenerative disease of the brain.

endoscopic examination   An inspection of the inside of a hollow organ or body cavity, performed with an endoscope in the hospital environment.

enteral   Pertaining to products used for people with feeding tubes.

epidemiology   Patterns of occurrence.

epidermis   The outer, protective layer of the skin.

epigastric pain   Pain in the upper middle region of the abdomen, which can indicate a heart attack.

erythema   An abnormal redness of the skin caused by congestion of the capillaries; may be a symptom of cellulitis.

eschar   A covering of black dead tissue. This can form over a pressure ulcer, making it difficult to determine how deep the ulcer is.

esophageal reflux   Regurgitation of food or acid from the stomach into the esophagus.

esophageal varices   Enlarged venous channels in the esophagus that have the potential to rupture and cause uncontrolled, life-threatening bleeding.

ethnogeriatrics   Health care for older people from diverse ethnic populations.

etiology   Origins of a disease or condition.

excoriation   Abrasion of the epidermis or of the coating of any organ by trauma, chemicals, burns, or other causes.

F

fecal impaction   Hardened feces lodged or collected in the rectum or sigmoid; results in fecal incontinence and is usually treatable.

financial/material exploitation   Illegal or improper use of an older person's funds, property, or assets. Examples include cashing checks without permission, forging signatures, misusing money or possessions, forcing or deceiving into signing legal documents, improper use of guardianship, and power of attorney.

G

gait A person's manner of walking.

GEMS diamond A concept developed to assist the prehospital professional when encountering the older patient. The GEMS diamond has four components: G—geriatric patients; E—environmental assessment; M—medical assessment; S—social assessment.

geriatrics The branch of medicine concerned with the health of older people.

gerontology The study of aging.

greater trochanter A bony prominence on the proximal lateral side of the thigh, just below the hip joint.

Grey Turner's sign Bruising of the abdominal flanks.

Guillain-Barré syndrome A syndrome that typically occurs after a patient has had a viral respiratory illness that begins with weakness in the lower extremities that progresses toward the patient's head and may lead to respiratory insufficiency or aspiration of stomach contents from the loss of the ability to cough.

H

hard site An area of soft tissue lying over a bony prominence; a high-risk spot for development of pressure ulcers.

heat cramps Muscle cramps that commonly occur during intense physical activity in a hot, humid environment.

heat exhaustion A form of heat injury in which the body loses significant amounts of fluid and electrolytes because of heavy sweating; also called heat prostration or heat collapse.

heatstroke A life-threatening condition of severe hyperthermia caused by exposure to excessive natural or artificial heat, marked by warm, dry skin; severely altered mental status; and often irreversible coma; 80% of resulting deaths are in people over the age of 50.

hematemesis Vomiting red blood.

hemodynamic Relating to circulation of the blood.

hemoptysis Coughing up of blood.

hepatic metabolism The liver's use of enzymes to break drugs down into more water-soluble compounds.

herpes zoster A painful skin condition caused by reactivation of a virus.

home care In-home services offered to patients with acute illness, long-term health conditions, permanent disability, or terminal illness. Services may include assistance with activities of daily living, administration of medication therapy, and IV therapy. Also known as home health care, personal care, or in-home care.

hospice care In-home or hospice care facility services provided to patients with a terminal illness. Services include supportive medical, social, and spiritual services to patients, and support for the patient's family.

hypercarbia Increased carbon dioxide in the bloodstream.

hyperglycemia An abnormally high level of blood glucose.

hypertension High blood pressure.

hyperthyroidism Low levels of thyroid hormones, usually caused by overuse of medications in patients with hypothyroidism.

hypertrophy Enlargement of a muscle due to excessive strain put on that muscle.

hypnotic A substance that induces sleep

hypoglycemia An abnormally low level of blood glucose.

hypothalamus Organ at the base of the brain that controls many body functions through hormone systems.

hypothyroidism Low levels of thyroid hormones, caused by changes in the thyroid gland.

hypoxia A condition in which the body's cells and tissues do not have enough oxygen.

I

idiopathic Of unknown cause.

ileal conduit A tube constructed of small bowel that allows for urine to drain to the outside of the body.

ileostomy The removal of the entire colon and rectum, with the ileum being brought through the abdominal wall, forming a stoma.

immunity Provisions that are meant to protect EMS providers from the risk of being sued under certain circumstances; usually protects against both being sued and disciplinary action by a licensing or certification agency.

infestation The harboring of animal parasites. Common infestations in the setting of abuse and neglect are "bed bugs" (*Cimex lectularius*). The result of these infections is hemorrhages in the skin, or wheals.

inflammatory bowel disease Chronic inflammation of the gastrointestinal tract; ulcerative colitis and Crohn's disease are two types of inflammatory bowel disease.

informed consent doctrine Allows a patient to decide against unwanted medical interventions.

instrumental activities of daily living (IADLs) Basic everyday activities that require a higher level of function, such as going shopping, making a meal, cleaning up, or using a telephone, which may become more difficult with age.

ischemia A lack of oxygen that deprives tissues of necessary nutrients, resulting from partial or complete blockage of blood flow.

isolation theory A theory that attempts to explain the cause of elder abuse; maintains that the patient's diminishing social network is a major risk factor in elder abuse.

K

kyphosis   A condition in which the back becomes hunched over due to an abnormal increased curvature of the spine.

kyphotic   Characterized by exaggerated curvature of the spine.

L

listening   The act of receiving information. It includes observation of more than just the words; it is also the volume, pitch, inflection, tone, and nonverbal aspects.

living will   A type of advance directive that documents decisions about particular end-of-life treatments in particular situations should the patient become incompetent. Depending on the law in each state, it can cover CPR and other forms of life-sustaining treatment in the event of terminal condition, permanent unconsciousness, and fatal illness prior to the terminal phase. Also called an instructional directive.

lung infarction   Death of an area of lung tissue because of loss of circulation to the area.

M

macular degeneration   Deterioration of the central portion of the retina.

medication misuse   Unintentional or willful use of a medication in a way that differs from the prescribed dose or intent.

medication/substance abuse   Deliberate use of a drug for non-medicinal reasons.

melanin   The pigment that provides color to the hair and skin.

melena   Dark tarry stools that indicate bleeding somewhere within the gastrointestinal tract.

meningitis   An inflammation of the meningeal coverings of the brain; usually caused by a virus or a bacterium.

menopause   The process later in a woman's life during which menstruation ceases.

mesentery   The membrane(s) that connect organs to the abdominal wall.

metastasis   The transfer of disease from one part of the body to another.

morbidity   Poor health because of a chronic illness.

myasthenia gravis   A condition where patients complain of rapid muscle fatigue and loss of strength following the use of a muscle or group of muscles; occurs from the formation of immune system antibodies to the patient's own neurotransmitter (acetylcholine) receptors that allow muscles to receive the signal to contract.

myocardial infarction (MI)   Death of heart muscle caused by hypoxia, as a result of obstruction of blood flow to the heart.

N

necrosis   Cell death.

neglect   Refusal or failure on the part of the caregiver to provide life necessities, such as food, water, clothing, shelter, personal hygiene, medicine, comfort, and personal safety.

nephrons   The basic filtering units in the kidneys.

neurons   Cells that make up nerve tissue and receive and transmit impulses.

nonadherence   Failure to comply with a medication regimen, whether by not taking medications or taking them only occasionally.

non-blanching erythema   Tissue redness that does not blanch (turn white) when pressed with a finger.

nonketotic diabetic acidosis   Metabolic acidosis in a person with type II diabetes caused by hyperglycemia and dehydration, not by the formation of ketones; patients with type II diabetes have insulin in their systems, and therefore are not prone to the formation of ketones.

nonketotic hyperglycemic-hyperosmolar coma (NKHHC)   A syndrome characterized by hyperglycemia, extreme dehydration, and hyperosmolar plasma, leading to impaired consciousness.

non-steroidal anti-inflammatory drugs (NSAIDs)   Medications designed to decrease inflammation, stiffness, and pain in the joints and muscles, but whose regular use may cause bleeding from irritation of the lining of the stomach or from ulcers in the stomach or duodenum. Over-the-counter examples include aspirin, ibuprofen, and naproxen.

nonverbal communication   Hand gestures, body position, or facial expressions used to send a message. Nonverbal communication can be either intentional or unintentional.

nursing home   A facility where residents receive 24-hour nursing care. Also known as skilled nursing facility, convalescent home, or long-term care facility.

nystagmus   A lateral twitching of the eyes as the patient tracks your finger across his visual field from side to side.

O

old-age dependency ratio   The number of older people for every 100 adults between the ages of 18 and 64.

orthopnea   Difficulty breathing in the reclined position.

orthostatic hypotension   A decrease of 20 mm Hg in systolic blood pressure when moving from a sitting to a standing position; also called postural hypotension.

osteoarthritis (OA)   A progressive joint disease seen in older people resulting in the destruction of cartilage, the formation of bone spurs in joints, and joint stiffness; thought to result from "wear and tear" and, in some instances, by repetitive trauma to the joints.

osteoblast   A cell that contributes to the body's continual process of remodeling bone by depositing newly formed bone.

osteoclast   A cell that that contributes to the body's continual process of remodeling bone by absorbing bone.

osteomyelitis   Inflammation of the bone caused by infection; a frequent complication of pressure ulcers that can affect ulcer healing if the infection is not appropriately treated.

osteoporosis   A condition characterized by a decrease in bone mass, leading to a reduction in bone strength and a greater susceptibility to fracture even after minimal trauma.

P

palliative care   Care of patients whose disease is not responsive to curative treatment. Such care can include providing relief from pain and other distressing symptoms; neither hastening nor prolonging death; offering a support system to help the family cope; and integrating psychological and spiritual aspects of patient care.

palmar erythema   Red palms.

palpitation   A subjective feeling of the heart "not beating right." This can manifest as skipped beats, rapid heart rate, or pounding in the chest.

pancreatitis   Irritation or inflammation of the pancreas usually caused by infection, chronic alcohol use.

papules   Small red spots.

paraplegia   Paralysis of the lower half of the body, usually due to disease or injury of the spinal cord.

parkinsonism   Brain dysfunction that causes a loss of normal flexibility and fluidity of posture and movement and the development of a hand tremor due to a decrease in dopamine levels within the brain caused by either a primary disease process, such as Parkinson's disease, or as the result of trauma, medication use, or toxins.

Parkinson's disease   A disease that is caused by degeneration of the dopamine-producing neurons within the brain, which leads to the development of Parkinsonism.

passive neglect   An unintentional refusal or failure to fulfill a caretaking obligation, which results in physical or emotional distress to the older person. Examples include abandonment and the non-provision of food and health services that are the result of the caretaker's lack of knowledge, laziness, infirmity, or addiction to drugs or alcohol.

pedal edema   Swelling of the feet and ankles caused by collection of fluid in the tissues; a possible sign of congestive heart failure (CHF).

penumbra   Tissue surrounding the central area of a tissue involved in a stroke.

peptic ulcer disease (PUD)   Ulcerations or erosions occurring in the gastric mucosa causing irritation or bleeding. Common causes may include increased acidity, certain medications.

percussion   A physical examination technique in which the examiner places one hand on the patient's chest and strikes a finger of that hand with a finger of the other hand.

periorbital ecchymosis   Bruising around the eye socket.

peritoneal signs   Indications of peritoneal irritation, such as a rigid abdomen and scarce bowel sounds.

peripheral edema   Swelling in the abdomen or lower extremities; can be a sign of right-sided heart failure.

peripheral vascular disease   Damage to peripheral blood vessels causing decreased blood flow to the areas these vessels supply; can occur from a number of causes, most importantly from cigarette smoking.

pharmacodynamics   The pharmacologic or therapeutic effect of a medication or combination of medications.

pharmacokinetics   Absorption, distribution, metabolism, and elimination of a drug.

physical abuse   Force resulting in bodily injury, that is, from hitting, slapping, burning, unwarranted administration of drugs and physical restraints, force feeding, or physical punishment.

plantar flex   To bend the foot downward.

pleural effusion   Accumulation of fluid in the chest around the lungs.

pleural friction rub   A loud, harsh, short chest sound that usually occurs in late inspiration, caused by friction between the two pleural surfaces and often associated with pleuritic pain.

pleuritic chest pain   Chest pain related to breathing; usually indicative of lung, chest wall, or other non-cardiac problems.

pneumonia   An infectious disease of the lung that damages lung tissue.

polypharmacy   Simultaneous use of many medications.

portal hypertension   Increased resistance to venous blood flow through the portal vein and liver, displacing fluid in the abdomen, causing liver enlargement and increased size of venous channels in the esophagus.

posttraumatic stress disorder (PTSD)   A delayed stress reaction to a prior incident. This delayed reaction is the result of one or more unresolved issues concerning the incident that might have been alleviated with the use of critical incident stress management.

presbycusis   Hearing loss as a result of aging.

pressure ulcer   A sore, initially of the skin, due to prolonged pressure, usually in a person who is lying down, and possibly at any site but most commonly over bony prominences. The combination of pressure, shearing forces, friction, and moisture lead to the death of tissue due to lack of blood supply. Also referred to as decubitus ulcer, pressure sore, or bedsore.

proprioception   Perception of movement and the body's position, mediated by sensory nerve endings in muscles and tendons.

psychoactive   Affecting the mind or behavior; there is a strong relationship between drugs of this type and the occurrence of falls.

psychological abuse   Infliction of anguish, emotional pain, or distress. Includes verbal assaults, threats, intimidation, harassment, and forced social isolation.

psychopathology of the abuser theory A theory that attempts to explain the cause of elder abuse; maintains that the abuser's problems (such as personality disorders or substance abuse) lead to the abuse or neglect.

psychotropic Capable of affecting the mental state; there is a strong relationship between drugs of this type and the occurrence of falls.

pulmonary edema A buildup of fluid in the lungs, usually as a result of congestive heart failure.

pulmonary embolism The lodging of a clot in the vessels of the lungs.

pulmonary embolus A blood clot that breaks off from a large vein and travels to the blood vessels of the lung, causing obstruction of blood flow.

pulsus paradoxicus A loss of more than 10 to 12 mm Hg of blood pressure during inspiration.

purulent sputum Sputum that contains pus; it is a physical finding in pneumonia.

Q

quadriplegia Paralysis of all four limbs, usually due to disease or injury of the spinal cord.

quality of life The interplay of four factors: physical and emotional health, social connections, economic security, and safety.

R

raccoon eyes Bruising around the eyes that indicates possible basal skull fracture.

reserve capacity The body's ability to respond to increased demands under stress, such as illness or exercise.

residual volume The amount of air left in the lungs after the maximum possible amount of air has been expired.

respite care Provides temporary relief for caregivers, ranging from hours to days.

retrograde amnesia The inability to remember events leading up to a head injury.

rhabdomyolysis Disintegration of muscle fibers that results in excretion of myoglobin (pigment of the muscle) in the urine.

rheumatoid arthritis (RA) A systemic inflammatory disease that affects the body's joints and whose symptoms include inflammation in and around the joints in the hands, wrists, ankles, and feet, and less often in the knees and spine.

rhonchi Coarse, low-pitched breath sounds heard in patients with chronic mucus in the airways.

rotator cuff A muscle supporting the shoulder joint, composed of four muscles that attach to the humerus to allow motion and provide stability to the arm and shoulder; highly susceptible to injury in older people due to progressive degeneration.

rule of double effect An ethical principle used to justify certain treatment decisions made by health care providers at the end of life, stating that it is morally acceptable to give a treatment that hastens death if the main intention is to provide relief of suffering.

Rule of Nines A system that assigns percentages to sections of the body, allowing calculation of the amount of skin surface involved in the burn area.

rule of symmetry The principle that physical findings found on both sides of the body are likely to be normal for that patient, and therefore, that findings found on only one side are not normal and a possible indication of a problem.

S

seatbelt-type fracture A fracture of the entire vertebral body and bony arch, caused by a distraction component (energy being dispersed in two opposite directions); typically results from an ejection or from wearing only a lap belt without a shoulder harness.

sedative A substance that decreases activity and excitement.

self-neglect Behaviors on the part of the older person that threaten his or her own health or safety. Generally manifests itself in refusal or failure to provide self with adequate food, shelter, or personal safety.

separation anxiety Anxiety that may be experienced by an older person when there is a threat of being taken away from family, friends, neighbors, or pets.

sepsis Disease state that results from the presence of microorganisms or their toxic products in the bloodstream.

sexual abuse Non-consensual sexual contact of any kind, including with a person incapable of giving consent. Includes but not limited to unwanted touching, sexual assault or battery such as rape, sodomy, coerced nudity, and sexually explicit photographing.

skin tenting A procedure for assessing dehydration in which a small section of skin is pinched upward (away from the body), forming a tent. In older people, skin that requires more than 2 to 5 seconds to return to a flat position is dehydrated.

social learning theory A theory that attempts to explain the cause of elder abuse; maintains that violence is learned—if a person was abused as a child, that person will abuse his or her parents. Also called the transgenerational theory.

spinal shock A temporary situation after transection of the spinal cord in which the volume of the intravascular space dramatically increases and leads to hypotension and a loss of reflexes below the point of injury.

stable spinal injury A spinal injury that has a low risk for leading to permanent neurological deficit or structural deformity.

status epilepticus The term used to describe a continuous seizure, or multiple seizures without a return to consciousness, for 30 minutes or more.

stressed caregiver theory   A theory that attempts to explain the cause of elder abuse; maintains that when the caretaker reaches a certain stress level, abuse and neglect will occur.

stridor   A harsh, high-pitched inspiratory sound that is often heard in acute laryngeal (upper airway) obstruction; may sound like crowing and be audible without a stethoscope.

stroke volume   The amount of blood pumped out of the heart in one beat.

subarachnoid hemorrhage   Bleeding between the arachnoid and the pia mater in the brain.

subdural hematoma   Bleeding into the area between the brain and the meningeal layer called the dura mater.

suicidal ideation   Thoughts about or plans of committing suicide.

synapse   The junction between two neurons.

T

tamponade   To close or block in order to stop bleeding.

tension pneumothorax   An accumulation of air or gas in the pleural cavity that progressively increases the pressure in the chest wall with potentially fatal results.

thermoreceptors   Temperature-sensing mechanisms throughout the body that send information to the hypothalamus.

thyroid storm   A rare, life-threatening condition of hyperthyroidism, usually triggered by a stressful event or increased volume of thyroid hormones in the circulation.

tolerance   The need for increasing amounts of a drug to obtain the same effect.

tracheostomy   A temporary or permanent surgical opening (stoma) through the third or fourth tracheal ring.

transgenerational theory   *See* Social learning theory.

transient ischemic attack (TIA)   A disorder of the brain in which brain cells temporarily stop working because of insufficient oxygen, causing stroke-like symptoms that resolve completely within 24 hours of onset.

type I diabetes   Insulin-dependent diabetes.

type II diabetes   Non-insulin-dependent diabetes.

U

ulcer   A hollowing out or disintegration of tissue; in older people, more commonly found in the gastrointestinal system and the skin.

unstable spinal injury   A spinal injury that has a high risk of permanent neurological deficit or structural deformity.

urine burn   Reddening of the skin that occurs around the inner thighs and buttocks when the older person is allowed repeatedly to lie for prolonged periods of time in his or her urine.

ureterostomy   A method of diverting urine in which the ureter is brought to the abdominal wall to form a stoma.

V

vasculitis   Inflammation or infection in a blood vessel.

venous ulceration   The presence of an ulcer, or disintegrated tissue, in a vein due to pressure in the lower extremities.

ventilation   Movement of air in and out of the lungs produced by chest wall motion.

verbal communication   The words a person uses to send a message.

vertigo   A sensation in which a person feels that he or she is spinning, the surroundings are spinning, or both the person and the environment are spinning; often caused by a problem in the inner ear, but can also be caused by low blood pressure, dehydration, or anemia.

vesicle   Tiny blister.

vital capacity   Volume of air moved during the deepest inspiration and expiration.

W

wheeze   A high-pitched, whistling breath sound caused by air traveling through narrowed air passages within the bronchioles, characteristically heard on expiration in patients with asthma or chronic obstructive pulmonary disease (COPD).

Index

Note: Page numbers followed by "f" refer to figures; page numbers followed by "t" refer to tables.

Photo Credits

Unless otherwise indicated, photographs have been supplied by the Maryland Institute of Emergency Medical Services System. Photographs have also been supplied by the American Academy of Orthopaedic Surgeons, and Jones and Bartlett Publishers. Illustrations were created by Imagineering and Rolin Graphics.

p. 3 © PhotoDisc; p. 7 © Steve Mason/PhotoDisc; p. 10 © Joel Gordon 1999; p. 13 (top) © Joel Gordon 1991; p. 16 © Steve Mason/PhotoDisc; p. 17 (left) © Steve Mason/PhotoDisc, (right) © PhotoDisc; p. 23 © PhotoDisc; p. 24 © PhotoDisc; p. 31 © Bill Aron/PhotoEdit; p. 54 © Joel Gordon 1991; p. 59 reprinted with permission from Partnership for Caring; p. 70 © PhotoDisc; p. 72 © Jeff Greenberg/PhotoEdit; p. 73 Marilyn Westlake; p. 77 (bottom) © Visuals Unlimited; p. 78 (bottom) © Susan Lerner/Design Conceptions/Joel Gordon 2000, (top) courtesy of Baltimore County Police Department, Baltimore, Maryland; p. 81 © Visuals Unlimited; p. 91 courtesy of Diagnostics Corporation; p. 97 (top) James Upchurch; p. 104 Marilyn Westlake; p. 105 © Visuals Unlimited; p. 109 parts A, B © Custom Medical Stock Photo; p. 110 (bottom) courtesy of e-pill, LLC (R); p. 111 March Networks' MainStreet Messenger personal emergency response system. courtesy Home Technology Systems, Dubuque, Iowa; p. 115 © Eddie Sperling/Scene 911 Pictures; p. 118 (left) © Visuals Unlimited, (right) © John A. Rizzo/PhotoDisc; p. 121 © Visuals Unlimited; p. 122 © Craig Jackson/In the Dark Photography; p. 123 (left) © Linda Gheen; p. 126 (bottom) © Dr. P. Marazzi/Science Photo Library/Custom Medical Stock Photo; p. 140 (top) © Steve Mason/PhotoDisc, (bottom) © Visuals Unlimited;

p. 146 Rhonda Beck; p. 158 © Dan Hatlestad/Tri-anim; p. 159 courtesy VIASYS Healthcare Critical Care Division © 2002; p. 175 © P. Stocklein/Custom Medical Stock Photo; p. 182 © Custom Medical Stock Photo; p. 186 (top) © Visuals Unlimited; p. 188 courtesy of Marian P. LaMonte, MD, MSN, and Peter Hu, MD, University of Maryland School of Medicine and National Library of Medicine; p. 204 Marilyn Westlake; p. 206 © Joel Gordon 1996; p. 208 © Linda Gheen; p. 223 © Spencer Grant/PhotoEdit; p. 235 © Visuals Unlimited; p. 236 (left) courtesy of Palco Labs, Inc.; p. 241 (parts A and C), Charles Stewart, MD, (parts B and D) courtesy of National Pressure Ulcer Advisory Board; p. 244 Charles Stewart, MD; p. 252 National Ski Patrol/Ingrid Tistaert; p. 261 © Visuals Unlimited; p. 283 © Mel Curtis/Getty Images; p. 285 © PhotoDisc; p. 291 courtesy of Baltimore County Police Department, Baltimore, Maryland; p. 295 parts A-C courtesy of Daniel J. Sheridan, PhD, RN, (bottom) © Visuals Unlimited; p. 305 © S. O'Brien/Custom Medical Stock Photo; p. 306 © PhotoDisc; p. 307 (right) © PhotoDisc; p. 319 James Upchurch; p. 331 James Upchurch; p. 333 James Upchurch; p. 335 (top) © SIU Bio Med/Custom Medical Stock Photo, (part A) © Visuals Unlimited, (part B) © M. English/Custom Medical Stock Photo; p. 338 James Upchurch.